# The Cardiology Intensive Board Review Question Book

2nd EDITION

# The Cardiology Intensive Board Review Question Book

**2nd EDITION**

*Editors*

## Leslie Cho, MD, FACC
Director, Women's Cardiovascular Center
Director, Preventive Cardiology and Rehabilitation
Department of Cardiovascular Medicine
Cleveland Clinic
Cleveland, Ohio, USA

## Brian P. Griffin, MD, FACC
Director, Cardiovascular Disease Training Program
The John and Rosemary Brown Endowed Chair in Cardiovascular Medicine
Cleveland Clinic
Cleveland, Ohio, USA

## Eric J. Topol, MD, FACC
Director, Scripps Translational Science Institute
Chief Academic Officer, Scripps Health
Professor of Translational Genomics, TSRI
Senior Consultant, Division of Cardiovascular Diseases
Scripps Clinic
La Jolla, California, USA

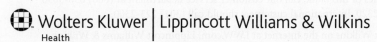

Wolters Kluwer | Lippincott Williams & Wilkins
Health
Philadelphia · Baltimore · New York · London
Buenos Aires · Hong Kong · Sydney · Tokyo

*Acquisitions Editor:* Frances R. DeStefano
*Managing Editor:* Julia Seto
*Project Manager:* Jennifer Harper
*Senior Manufacturing Manager:* Benjamin Rivera
*Marketing Manager:* Kimberly S. Schonberger
*Art Director:* Risa Clow
*Production Services:* International Typesetting and Composition

© 2009 by LIPPINCOTT WILLIAMS & WILKINS, a Wolters Kluwer business

**530 Walnut Street**
**Philadelphia, PA 19106 USA**
**LWW.com**

First edition, © 2003 by Lippincott Williams & Wilkins

Printed in China

**Library of Congress Cataloging-in-Publication Data**

The cardiology intensive board review question book / edited by Leslie Cho, Brian P. Griffin, Eric J. Topol.—2nd ed.
        p. ; cm.
    Includes bibliographical references and index.
    ISBN-13: 978-0-7817-7467-3
    ISBN-10: 0-7817-7467-5
    1. Cardiology—Examinations, questions, etc.   I. Cho, Leslie.   II. Griffin, Brian P., 1956-   III. Topol, Eric J., 1954-
    [DNLM: 1. Cardiovascular Diseases—Examination Questions.
2. Cardiovascular Diseases—drug therapy—Examination Questions.
3. Heart—physiology—Examination Questions.   WG 18.2 C2694 2009]
    RC669.2.C375 2009
    616.1'20076—dc22

                                     2008026595

Care has been taken to confirm the accuracy of the information presented and to describe generally accepted practices. However, the authors, editors, and publisher are not responsible for errors or omissions or for any consequences from application of the information in this book and make no warranty, expressed or implied, with respect to the currency, completeness, or accuracy of the contents of the publication. Application of the information in a particular situation remains the professional responsibility of the practitioner.

The authors, editors, and publisher have exerted every effort to ensure that drug selection and dosage set forth in this text are in accordance with current recommendations and practice at the time of publication. However, in view of ongoing research, changes in government regulations, and the constant flow of information relating to drug therapy and drug reactions, the reader is urged to check the package insert for each drug for any change in indications and dosage and for added warnings and precautions. This is particularly important when the recommended agent is a new or infrequently employed drug.

Some drugs and medical devices presented in the publication have Food and Drug Administration (FDA) clearance for limited use in restricted research settings. It is the responsibility of the health care providers to ascertain the FDA status of each drug or device planned for use in their clinical practice.

To purchase additional copies of this book, call our customer service department at (800) 638-3030 or fax orders to (301) 223-2320. International customers should call (301) 223-2300.

Visit Lippincott Williams & Wilkins on the Internet at LWW.com. Lippincott Williams & Wilkins customer service representatives are available from 8:30 am to 6 pm, EST.

10 9 8 7 6 5

*To the cardiovascular disease fellows at The Cleveland Clinic past, present, and future*

# *Preface*

The second edition of our book seeks to provide latest updates for topics addressed on the cardiovascular board examination. Like the first edition, we have included subjects, images and tracings that are important not only for examinations but are also very relevant to daily practice. We have revised all chapters and have included new chapters on peripheral vascular disease, cardiac imaging, and electrocardiograms. The questions are presented in formats that are commonly used on the boards.

We would like to thank all of those who have made this book possible, including the contributors, our colleagues, and our assistants. We hope you enjoy the book and find it useful.

Leslie Cho, M.D.
Brian P. Griffin, M.D.
Eric J. Topol, M.D.

# Preface

The second edition of our book seeks to provide latest updates for topics addressed on the cardiovascular board examination. Like the first edition, we have included subjects, images and tracings that are important not only for examinations but are also very relevant to daily practice. We have revised all chapters and have included new chapters on peripheral vascular disease, cardiac imaging, and electrocardiograms. The questions are presented in formats that are commonly used on the boards.

We would like to thank all of those who have made this book possible, including the contributors, our colleagues, and our assistants. We hope you enjoy the book and find it useful.

Leslie Cho, M.D.
Brian P. Griffin, M.D.
Eric J. Topol, M.D.

# Contributors

**Craig R. Asher, MD, FACC**
Cardiology Fellowship Director
Department of Cardiology
Cleveland Clinic
Weston, Florida

**Arman T. Askari, MD**
Staff Physician
Section of Clinical Cardiology
Associate Director, Cardiovascular Medicine Training
 Program
Cleveland Clinic
Cleveland, Ohio

**Deepak L. Bhatt, MD, FACC**
Chief of Cardiology
VA Boston Healthcare System
Director of the Integrated Cardiovascular Intervention
 Program
Brigham and Women's Hospital and the VA Boston
 Healthcare System
Boston, Massachusetts

**Leslie Cho, MD, FACC**
Director, Women's Cardiovascular Center
Medical Director, Preventive Cardiology and
 Rehabilitation
Department of Cardiovascular Medicine
Cleveland Clinic
Cleveland, Ohio

**Mary C. Downing, MD**
Department of Vascular Medicine
Cleveland Clinic Foundation
Cleveland, Ohio

**Jodie M. Fink, Pharm.D.**
Department of Pharmacy
Cleveland Clinic
Cleveland, Ohio

**Gary S. Francis, MD**
Professor of Medicine
Department of Cardiovascular Medicine
Cleveland Clinic
Cleveland, Ohio

**Sasan Ghaffari, MD**
Pacific Cardiovascular Associates
Laguna Hills, California

**Brian P. Griffin, MD**
Department of Cardiovascular Medicine
Cleveland Clinic
Cleveland, Ohio

**Christopher Ingelmo**
Department of Cardiovascular Medicine
Cleveland Clinic
Cleveland, Ohio

**Wael A. Jaber, MD, FACC**
Department of Cardiovascular Medicine
Section of Cardiovascular Imaging
Cleveland Clinic
Cleveland, Ohio

**Douglas E. Joseph, DO, RVT**
Associate Staff
Department of Cardiovascular Medicine
Cleveland Clinic
Cleveland, Ohio

**Richard A. Krasuski, MD**
Director of Adult Congenital Heart Disease Services
Department of Cardiovascular Medicine
Cleveland Clinic
Cleveland, Ohio

**Raymond Q. Migrino, MD**
Division of Cardiovascular Medicine
The Medical College of Wisconsin
Milwaukee, Wisconsin

**Michael A. Militello, Pharm.D.**
Cardiology Clinical Specialist
Department of Pharmacy
Cleveland Clinic
Cleveland, Ohio

**Debabrata Mukherjee, MD**
Gill Foundation Professor of Interventional Cardiology
University of Kentucky
Lexington, Kentucky

**Gian M. Novaro, MD, MS, FACC, FASE**
Director, Echocardiography Laboratory
Associate Director, Internal Medicine Residency Program
Department of Cardiology
Cleveland Clinic
Weston, Florida

**Olusegun Osinbowale, MD**
Department of Cardiovascular Medicine
Section of Vascular Medicine
Cleveland Clinic
Cleveland, Ohio

**Marc S. Penn, MD, PhD**
Department of Cardiovascular Medicine
Cleveland Clinic
Cleveland, Ohio

**Marco Roffi, MD**
Department of Cardiology
University of Geneva
Geneva, Switzerland

**Ellen Mayer Sabik, MD, FACC, FASE**
Department of Cardiovascular Medicine
Cleveland Clinic
Cleveland, Ohio

**Walid I. Saliba, MD**
Director, Electrophysiology Laboratories
Section of Cardiac Pacing and Electrophysiology
Department of Cardiovascular Medicine
Cleveland Clinic
Cleveland, Ohio

**Robert A. Schweikert, MD**
Section of Cardiac Pacing and Electrophysiology
Department of Cardiovascular Medicine
Cleveland Clinic
Cleveland, Ohio

**Monvadi B. Srichai, MD**
Department of Cardiovascular Medicine
Cleveland Clinic
Cleveland, Ohio

**Maran Thamilarasan, MD**
Department of Cardiovascular Medicine
Cleveland Clinic
Cleveland, Ohio

**Donald A. Underwood, MD**
Department of Cardiovascular Medicine
Cleveland Clinic
Cleveland, Ohio

# Abbreviations

| | | | | |
|---|---|---|---|---|
| **AAA** | abdominal aortic aneurysm | | **CPK** | creatine phosphokinase |
| **ABI** | ankle brachial index | | **CRP** | C-reactive protein |
| **ACC** | American College of Cardiology | | **CS** | coronary stenting |
| **ACE** | angiotensin-converting enzyme | | **CT** | computed tomography |
| **ACEI** | angiotensin-converting enzyme inhibitor | | **CTA** | computed tomography angiography |
| **ACS** | acute coronary syndrome | | **CTEPH** | chronic thromboembolic pulmonary hypertension |
| **ACTH** | adrenocorticotropic hormone | | **CXR** | chest x-ray |
| **AED** | automated external defibrillator | | **DC** | direct current |
| **AFib** | atrial fibrillation | | **DTI** | direct thrombin inhibitor |
| **AHA** | American Heart Association | | **DVT** | deep venous thrombosis |
| **AI** | aortic insufficiency | | **ECG** | electrocardiogram |
| **AMI** | acute myocardial infarction | | **EF** | ejection fraction |
| **AP** | action potential | | **EGD** | esophagogastroduodenoscopy |
| **aPTT** | activated partial thromboplastin time | | **EMD** | electromechanical dissociation |
| **AR** | aortic regurgitation | | **EMS** | emergency medical service |
| **ARBs** | angiotensin receptor blockers | | **EP** | electrophysiology |
| **AS** | aortic stenosis | | **ESR** | erythroctye sedimentation rate |
| **ASA** | atrial septal aneurysm | | **ET** | exercise training |
| **ASD** | atrial septal defect | | **FDA** | Food and Drug Administration |
| **AV** | atrioventricular | | **FEV$_1$** | forced expiratory volume in the first second of expiration |
| **AVNRT** | atrioventricular nodal reentrant tachycardia | | | |
| **AVR** | aortic valve replacement | | **GI** | gastrointestinal |
| **AVRT** | orthodromic atrioventricular reentrant tachycardia | | **GP** | glycoprotein |
| **β-AR** | beta-adrenoreceptor | | **GU** | genitourinary |
| **bFGF** | basic fibroblast growth factor | | **HBE** | His bundle electrogram |
| **BMI** | body mass index | | **HF** | heart failure |
| **BNP** | brain natriuretic peptide | | **HIT** | heparin-induced thrombocytopenia |
| **BP** | blood pressure | | **HR** | heart rate |
| **bpm** | beats per minute | | **HRA** | high right atrium |
| **BUN** | blood urea nitrogen | | **HRR** | hazard rate ratio |
| **CABG** | coronary artery bypass grafting | | **HTN** | hypertension |
| **CAD** | coronary artery disease | | **IABP** | intraaortic balloon pump |
| **cAMP** | cyclic adenosine monophosphate | | **ICD** | implantable cardioverter-defibrillator |
| **CBC** | complete blood count | | **IgE** | immunoglobulin E |
| **cDNA** | complementary DNA | | **IgG** | immunoglobulin G |
| **CHB** | complete heart block | | **INR** | international normalized ratio |
| **CHD** | coronary heart disease | | **IQR** | interquartile range |
| **CHF** | congestive heart failure | | **IRBBB** | incomplete right bundle branch block |
| **CI** | confidence interval | | **ISA** | intrinsic sympathomimetic activity |
| **CK-MB** | MB fraction of creatine kinase | | **ISR** | in-stent restenosis |

| | |
|---|---|
| **IV** | intravenous (-ly) |
| **IVC** | inferior vena cava |
| **JNC** | Joint National Committee |
| **JVP** | jugular venous pulse |
| **LA** | left atrium (-al) |
| **LAD** | left anterior descending artery |
| **LBBB** | left bundle branch block |
| **LCC** | left coronary cusp |
| **LCx** | left circumflex artery |
| **LDL** | low density lipoprotein |
| **LDH** | lactate dehydrogenase |
| **LMWH** | low-molecular-weight heparin |
| **LV** | left ventricle (-ular) |
| **LVEF** | left ventricle ejection fraction |
| **LVH** | left ventricular hypertrophy |
| **LVOT** | left ventricular outflow tract |
| **MAT** | multifocal atrial tachycardia |
| **METs** | metabolic equivalents |
| **MI** | myocardial infarction |
| **MR** | mitral regurgitation |
| **MRA** | magnetic resonance angiography |
| **MRI** | magnetic resonance image (-ing) |
| **MS** | mitral stenosis |
| **MTHFR** | methylenetetrahydrofolate reductase |
| **MV** | mitral valve |
| **MVP** | mitral valve prolapse |
| **NCC** | noncoronary cusp |
| **NSAIDs** | nonsteroidal anti-inflammatory drugs |
| **NSR** | normal sinus rhythm |
| **NTG** | nitroglycerin |
| **OR** | odds ratio |
| **P** | pulse |
| **PA** | pulmonary artery |
| **PAD** | peripheral arterial disease |
| **PCI** | percutaneous coronary intervention |
| **PCWP** | pulmonary capillary wedge pressure |
| **PDA** | patent ductus arteriosus |
| **PE** | pulmonary embolus |
| **PEA** | pulseless electrical activity |
| **PET** | positron emission tomography |
| **PFO** | patent foramen ovale |
| **PJRT** | permanent junctional reciprocating tachycardia |
| **PMI** | point of maximum impulse |
| **PO** | oral (-ly) |
| **PT** | prothrombin time |

| | |
|---|---|
| **PTCA** | percutaneous transluminal coronary angioplasty |
| **PVARP** | post-ventricular atrial refractory period |
| **PVC** | premature ventricular contraction |
| **QOL** | quality of life |
| **RA** | right atrium (-al) |
| **RAO** | right anterior oblique |
| **RAS** | renal artery stenosis |
| **RBBB** | right bundle branch block |
| **RCA** | right coronary artery |
| **RCC** | right coronary cusp |
| **RR** | risk ratio |
| **RT-PCR** | reverse transcriptase-polymerase chain reaction |
| **RUSB** | right upper sternal border |
| **RV** | right ventricle (-ular) |
| **RVH** | right ventricular hypertrophy |
| **RVSP** | right ventricular systolic pressure |
| **SAM** | systolic anterior motion |
| **SBE** | subacute bacterial endocarditis |
| **SC** | subcutaneous (-ly) |
| **SERCA2** | sarcoplasmic-endoplasmic reticulum calcium ATPase type 2 |
| **SL** | sublingual (-ly) |
| **SSS** | sick sinus syndrome |
| **STEMI** | ST-segment elevation myocardial infarction |
| **SVR** | systemic vascular resistance |
| **SVT** | supraventricular tachycardia |
| **TAO** | thromboangiitis obliterans |
| **TdP** | torsades de pointes |
| **TEE** | transesophageal echocardiography |
| **TIA** | transient ischemic attack |
| **TID** | transient ischemic dilation |
| **TIMI** | thrombolysis in myocardial infarction |
| **tPA** | tissue plasminogen activator |
| **TR** | tricuspid regurgitation |
| **TTE** | transthoracic echocardiogram |
| **TVR** | target vessel revascularization |
| **UA** | unstable angina |
| **UA/ NSTEMI** | unstable angina and non–ST-segment elevation myocardial infarction |
| **UFH** | unfractionated heparin |
| **VF** | ventricular fibrillation |
| **VSD** | ventricular septal defect |
| **VT** | ventricular tachycardia |
| **VTE** | venous thromboembolism |
| **VTI** | velocity time integral |

# Contents

# chapter 1

# *Arrhythmia*

ROBERT A. SCHWEIKERT · WALID I. SALIBA

## QUESTIONS

1. Which of the following antiarrhythmic medications would be the best choice for treatment of a patient with AFib and significant renal insufficiency?
   a. propafenone
   b. sotalol
   c. dofetilide
   d. flecainide

2. Which of the following antiarrhythmic drugs is not at least partially cleared by hemodialysis?
   a. disopyramide
   b. procainamide
   c. sotalol
   d. amiodarone

3. Which of the following antiarrhythmic medications has active metabolites?
   a. amiodarone
   b. sotalol
   c. dofetilide
   d. flecainide

4. A patient arrives at the emergency department with symptomatic narrow complex tachycardia. The patient is hemodynamically stable. The decision is made to administer IV adenosine. Under which of the following circumstances should the dosage of adenosine be reduced?
   a. The patient is taking theophylline.
   b. The patient is taking dipyridamole.
   c. The patient has significant valvular regurgitation.
   d. The patient has a significant left-to-right shunt.

5. Which of the following antiarrhythmic drugs increases serum digoxin levels?
   a. flecainide
   b. propafenone
   c. quinidine
   d. all of the above

6. Which of the following medications is contraindicated for use with dofetilide?
   a. digoxin
   b. diltiazem
   c. verapamil
   d. propranolol

7. Which of the following antiarrhythmic drugs is the least negative inotrope?

   **a.** dofetilide
   **b.** sotalol
   **c.** amiodarone
   **d.** flecainide

8. Which of the following antiarrhythmic drugs may be more likely to have proarrhythmia at increased heart rates?

   **a.** sotalol
   **b.** flecainide
   **c.** quinidine
   **d.** dofetilide

9. Which of the following statements is *true* regarding antiarrhythmic drugs with reverse-use dependence?

   **a.** Antiarrhythmic drugs with reverse-use dependence have greater efficacy for arrhythmia prevention than termination and have less risk for ventricular proarrhythmia after AFib termination (at slower sinus rates) than during AFib.
   **b.** Antiarrhythmic drugs with reverse-use dependence have less efficacy for arrhythmia prevention than termination and have greater risk for ventricular proarrhythmia after AFib termination (at slower sinus rates) than during AFib.
   **c.** Antiarrhythmic drugs with reverse-use dependence have greater efficacy for arrhythmia prevention than termination and have greater risk for ventricular proarrhythmia after AFib termination (at slower sinus rates) than during AFib.
   **d.** Antiarrhythmic drugs with reverse-use dependence have less efficacy for arrhythmia prevention than termination and have less risk for ventricular proarrhythmia after AFib termination (at slower sinus rates) than during AFib.

10. Which of the following is *true* regarding the Cardiac Arrhythmia Suppression trials (CAST I and II)?

    **a.** The treatment drugs increased mortality for patients without heart disease.
    **b.** All class IC antiarrhythmic drugs were found to increase mortality.
    **c.** The treatment drugs effectively suppressed PVCs.
    **d.** The antiarrhythmic drugs studied were flecainide, propafenone, and moricizine.

11. Which of the following antiarrhythmic drugs is the most potent sodium channel blocker?

    **a.** flecainide
    **b.** lidocaine
    **c.** disopyramide
    **d.** procainamide

12. The serum concentration or drug effect of which of the following medications is *not* increased in the presence of amiodarone?

    **a.** digoxin
    **b.** cyclosporine
    **c.** warfarin
    **d.** none of the above

13. Which of the following antiarrhythmic drugs is *not* a Vaughan Williams class III drug?

    **a.** sotalol
    **b.** ibutilide
    **c.** mexiletine
    **d.** dofetilide

14. Which of the following antiarrhythmic drugs is approved by the FDA for acute pharmacologic conversion of AFib to sinus rhythm?

    **a.** procainamide
    **b.** amiodarone

    **c.** ibutilide

    **d.** all of the above

**15.** Which of the following effects is expected when administering adenosine to a patient with recent cardiac transplantation (denervated heart)?

    **a.** no effect

    **b.** diminished effect

    **c.** enhanced effect

    **d.** delayed effect

**16.** For which of the following antiarrhythmic drugs is proarrhythmia *not* dose related?

    **a.** dofetilide

    **b.** quinidine

    **c.** sotalol

    **d.** ibutilide

**17.** Which of the following is not typically a "short RP" regular narrow QRS tachycardia?

    **a.** orthodromic atrioventricular reentrant tachycardia (AVRT)

    **b.** atrioventricular nodal reentrant tachycardia (AVNRT)

    **c.** permanent junctional reciprocating tachycardia (PJRT)

    **d.** nonparoxysmal junctional tachycardia

**18.** A patient presents with regular narrow QRS tachycardia. An esophageal electrode shows a 1:1 atrial-to-ventricular relationship during tachycardia. The VA interval is measured as 55 milliseconds. Which of the following is the most likely diagnosis?

    **a.** orthodromic AVRT

    **b.** atrial tachycardia

    **c.** AVNRT

    **d.** PJRT

**19.** A 17-year-old patient who is known to have Wolff-Parkinson-White syndrome presents with a regular narrow complex tachycardia with a cycle length of 375 milliseconds (160 bpm) that occurred with a sudden onset. You note that there is a 1:1 atrial-to-ventricular relationship and that the RP interval is 100 milliseconds. The best initial treatment is

    **a.** IV procainamide

    **b.** atropine

    **c.** IV verapamil

    **d.** catheter ablation

**20.** A 25-year-old patient presents with the sudden onset of tachycardia and is found to have a regular narrow QRS tachycardia with a cycle length of 340 milliseconds (176 bpm). An ECG appears to show P waves visible just after each QRS complex. You place an esophageal electrode and confirm a 1:1 atrial-to-ventricular relationship with a VA interval of 110 milliseconds. During the tachycardia, there is spontaneous development of LBBB, and a slower tachycardia with a VA interval of 150 milliseconds is now seen. What is the most likely diagnosis for the second tachycardia?

    **a.** AVNRT

    **b.** orthodromic AVRT using a right-sided accessory pathway

    **c.** orthodromic AVRT using a left-sided accessory pathway

    **d.** VT with 1:1 VA conduction

**21.** A 65-year-old man presents after an arrest while eating at a local restaurant. On arrival, paramedics documented VF, and he was successfully resuscitated. He has a history of MI and CHF. Serum electrolytes are remarkable only for mild hypokalemia. MI is ruled out by ECG and serial blood tests of myocardial enzymes. Subsequent evaluation includes cardiac catheterization, which shows severe three-vessel CAD and severe LV systolic dysfunction. A nuclear myocardial perfusion scan shows a large area of myocardial scar without significant viability in the territory of the left anterior descending coronary artery. The decision is made to treat the CAD medically. Which of the following is the best management strategy for his arrhythmia?

a. PO amiodarone
b. ICD implantation if an EP study shows inducible VT or VF
c. ICD implantation
d. beta-blocker medication

22. A 55-year-old woman has CAD and moderately severe LV systolic dysfunction (LVEF, 34%). Routine ambulatory Holter monitoring shows asymptomatic frequent ventricular ectopy with PVCs and occasional runs of nonsustained VT. Which of the following statements about the management of this patient is *true*?

a. Implantation of an ICD is indicated.
b. Implantation of an ICD is indicated if an EP study shows inducible VT.
c. Treatment with amiodarone is indicated, and if the arrhythmia recurs, then an EP study is indicated.
d. No treatment is indicated unless the arrhythmia becomes symptomatic.

23. Which of the following is *false* regarding ICDs?

a. ICDs are programmable devices with antibradycardia and antitachycardia capabilities.
b. Biphasic shocks require more energy for cardioversion and defibrillation than monophasic shocks.
c. ICDs may terminate VT with cardioversion shocks or antitachycardia pacing.
d. The use of MRI is contraindicated for the patient with an ICD.

24. All of the following are *true* statements about the ICD implantation procedure *except*

a. The right-chest site is preferred over the left-chest site for ICD systems with an "active can," in which the ICD pulse generator acts as one component of the shocking electrode system.
b. Implantation of an ICD system is similar to implantation of a pacemaker system.
c. The incidence of postoperative infection is generally 1% to 4%.
d. The incidence of operative mortality is <1%.

25. A patient arrives at the emergency department after experiencing multiple shocks from his ICD. The shocks were not preceded by any symptoms. He is noted to be in sinus rhythm on presentation, and, while on the monitor, he receives several more shocks from the ICD without any arrhythmias noted. Which of the following is the most appropriate initial step in the management of this patient?

a. Immediately arrange for a programmer for interrogation and reprogramming of the ICD.
b. Arrange for urgent surgery in the EP lab.
c. Initiate antiarrhythmic drug therapy.
d. Place a "donut" magnet over the ICD site.

26. All of the following patients have indications for ICD implantation *except*

a. a 35-year-old man with hypertrophic cardiomyopathy with clinical features indicating high risk for sudden cardiac death
b. a 17-year-old girl with congenital long-QT syndrome and recurrent syncope despite optimal medical therapy
c. a 60-year-old man with CAD, prior MI, LV dysfunction, and incessant sustained VT
d. an 80-year-old man with leukemia in remission and CAD who survived an episode of cardiac arrest with documented VF

**27.** Which of the following is most important for successful resuscitation of an adult patient with out-of-hospital cardiac arrest?

    **a.** IV epinephrine
    **b.** early DC-shock defibrillation
    **c.** IV antiarrhythmic drugs
    **d.** early intubation

**28.** Which of the following rhythms documented at the time of resuscitation from cardiac arrest carries the poorest prognosis for long-term survival?

    **a.** asystole
    **b.** electromechanical dissociation (EMD) or pulseless electrical activity (PEA)
    **c.** VF
    **d.** VT

**29.** Which of the following rhythm disturbances is most commonly documented for an adult with out-of-hospital sudden cardiac death resuscitated within the first 4 minutes after arrest?

    **a.** asystole
    **b.** EMD or PEA
    **c.** monomorphic VT
    **d.** VF

**30.** Which of the following may be responsible for multiple ("cluster") shocks from an ICD?

    **a.** recurrent VT
    **b.** AFib with rapid ventricular response
    **c.** lead malfunction
    **d.** all of the above

**31.** Which of the following treatments is *not* useful for a patient with frequent episodes of vasovagal syncope?

    **a.** dual-chamber pacemaker implantation
    **b.** midodrine
    **c.** beta-blocker medications
    **d.** diuretics

**32.** Which of the following statements about syncope are *true*?

    **a.** A carefully performed initial evaluation (history, physical examination, basic hematologic or biochemical studies, and an ECG) may provide an etiology for syncope in 50% to 60% of cases.
    **b.** The majority of syncopal episodes occurs in patients without cardiac or neurologic disease.
    **c.** Neurally mediated syncope is the most common cause of syncope.
    **d.** All of the above are true.

**33.** Which of the following treatment options has been most consistently shown to be effective for the primary prevention of sudden cardiac death in patients with CAD and recent MI?

    **a.** D-sotalol
    **b.** beta-blocker medications
    **c.** amiodarone
    **d.** dofetilide

**34.** Which of the following is the most common condition associated with sudden cardiac death in the United States?

    **a.** hypertrophic cardiomyopathy
    **b.** CAD
    **c.** valvular heart disease
    **d.** dilated cardiomyopathy

**35.** A 55-year-old man is referred for recurrent syncope. The episodes consist of a prodrome of weakness and nausea followed by loss of consciousness. Physical examination is unremarkable. ECG and exercise treadmill stress test were normal. Which of the following is the most appropriate next step?

  **a.** EP study
  **b.** signal-averaged ECG
  **c.** head-upright tilt table testing
  **d.** ambulatory Holter monitoring

**36.** Which of the following is the most common type of response during vasovagal syncope?

  **a.** predominantly cardioinhibitory (decreased heart rate)
  **b.** predominantly vasodepressor (decreased BP)
  **c.** combination of cardioinhibitory and vasodepressor
  **d.** none of the above

**37.** A 25-year-old man is referred for evaluation of an abnormal ECG that was found at the time of a routine examination. The ECG shows a short PR interval with ventricular pre-excitation consistent with the Wolff-Parkinson-White pattern. He has not had any symptoms such as palpitations, lightheadedness, near syncope, or syncope. You order an ambulatory Holter monitor, which shows intermittent ventricular pre-excitation. What is the most appropriate next step in the evaluation of this patient?

  **a.** exercise test
  **b.** catheter ablation
  **c.** EP study
  **d.** none of the above

**38.** A 40-year-old woman presents to the emergency department with tachycardia. An ECG shows regular narrow complex tachycardia at 160 bpm. Atrial activity is difficult to discern in the tracing, but during tachycardia, there appears to be an "r prime" in lead V$_1$ that is not present on an ECG during sinus rhythm recorded a few months earlier. Which of the following is the most likely diagnosis?

  **a.** AVNRT
  **b.** AVRT
  **c.** atrial tachycardia
  **d.** atrial flutter

**39.** Which of the following statements is *false* regarding multifocal atrial tachycardia (MAT)?

  **a.** MAT is defined as an atrial arrhythmia with at least three distinct P-wave morphologies, an irregular PR interval, and an irregular ventricular response.
  **b.** MAT can be confused with AFib.
  **c.** DC cardioversion is effective in the treatment of MAT.
  **d.** The initial treatment for MAT is correction of the underlying condition.

**40.** Which of the following statements about head-upright tilt table testing is *true*?

  **a.** The specificity of the test is approximately 80%.
  **b.** The sensitivity of the test is approximately 80%.
  **c.** The reproducibility of the test is approximately 80%.
  **d.** All of the above are true.

**41.** Patients with an implanted pacemaker may safely use all of the following equipment *except*

  **a.** cellular phones
  **b.** weapon detectors
  **c.** arc welding equipment
  **d.** microwave ovens
  **e.** electric power tools

**42.** An 80-year-old man with chronic AFib of 15 years' duration is admitted with recurrent episodes of dizziness and a recent episode of syncope. He has normal LV function and no evidence of CAD. In-hospital telemetry confirms the presence of slow ventricular rate and frequent pauses (4 seconds) that correlate with his lightheadedness. His medications consist of warfarin sodium (Coumadin). The most appropriate course of action includes which of the following?

  **a.** reassuring the patient and instructing him to come back if he has recurrence of syncope
  **b.** prolonged monitoring with a loop recorder
  **c.** EP testing to evaluate for ventricular arrhythmia
  **d.** permanent pacemaker implant
  **e.** ICD implant

**43.** A decision was made in the previous case to proceed with a permanent pacemaker. Which would be the most suitable pacing modality?

  **a.** dual-chamber system programmed to DDDR
  **b.** dual-chamber system programmed to DDDR with mode switching
  **c.** dual-chamber system programmed to DDIR
  **d.** single-chamber system in the ventricle programmed to VVIR
  **e.** single-chamber system in the atrium programmed to AAIR

**44.** Which one of the following is *true* about "pacemaker syndrome"?

  **a.** Symptoms usually include fatigue, dizziness, and hypotension.
  **b.** It occurs equally in atrial-based and ventricular-based pacing systems.
  **c.** It does not occur in patients who have 1:1 ventriculoatrial conduction.
  **d.** It can be treated with fludrocortisone.
  **e.** It is treated by increasing the VVI baseline pacing rate.

**45.** In hypertrophic cardiomyopathy, dual-chamber pacing has been associated with all of the following *except*

  **a.** increased LV systolic dimension
  **b.** increased LV diastolic dimension
  **c.** reduced MR
  **d.** changed activation of the septum activation
  **e.** reduced LV outflow gradient

**46.** Of the following patients, who is the most likely to carry the diagnosis of sick sinus syndrome (SSS)?

  **a.** a 65-year-old woman with a resting sinus arrhythmia varying from 70 to 85 bpm
  **b.** a 30 year old with sinus pauses 1.5 seconds in duration
  **c.** a 20-year-old athletic man with sinus bradycardia at 25 bpm while sleeping
  **d.** a 73-year-old man with chronic AFib and a ventricular rate of 40 bpm during peak treadmill test
  **e.** a 70 year old with sinus bradycardia and AV block secondary to a beta-blocker overdose

**47.** A 76-year-old patient with dilated cardiomyopathy and LBBB on baseline TTE is undergoing evaluation for syncope. Placement of a catheter near his bundle during EP testing is most likely to

  **a.** induce AFib
  **b.** induce VT
  **c.** perforate the atrium
  **d.** perforate the ventricle
  **e.** induce CHB

**48.** A 25-year-old patient with a history of depression is brought to the emergency room after ingesting some of her mother's prescription medications, including diltiazem and metoprolol. Her pulse rate is 25 bpm, and her BP is 90/50. Her ECG shows sinus bradycardia and high-grade AV block. In preparation for temporary pacemaker placement, which of the following is most likely to be effective?

**a.** IV calcium gluconate
**b.** isoproterenol infusion
**c.** IV atropine
**d.** IV magnesium sulfate
**e.** IV glucagon

**49.** To which of the following is the EP mechanism of typical atrial flutter most likely related?

**a.** intra-atrial reentry
**b.** ectopic automatic atrial focus
**c.** triggered activity secondary to delayed afterdepolarization
**d.** triggered activity secondary to early afterdepolarization
**e.** none of the above

**50.** A young patient is admitted to the intensive care unit with amitriptyline overdose. Three hours after gastric lavage, he develops hypotension and wide complex tachycardia that is recurrent despite cardioversion. Appropriate management includes which of the following?

**a.** IV bretylium
**b.** temporary pacemaker with overdrive pacing
**c.** IV calcium gluconate
**d.** administration of sodium-containing solution
**e.** IV magnesium sulfate

**51.** Which of the following mechanisms is believed to cause sudden death related to the use of terfenadine?

**a.** $Na^+$ channel blockade with increase in QRS duration
**b.** $K^+$ channel blockade with increase in the QT interval
**c.** $Ca^{2+}$ channel blockade with no change in the QRS or QT intervals
**d.** myocardial ischemia secondary to coronary spasm
**e.** none of the above

**52.** An 80 year old undergoes dual-chamber pacemaker placement for CHB. Excellent ventricular and atrial capture thresholds were obtained at the time of the implant. The pacemaker programmed parameters are as follows: mode DDD; lower rate, 70 bpm; upper rate, 130 bpm; atrial sensitivity, 0.25 mV (most sensitive setting); ventricular sensitivity, 1.00 mV; AV delay, 175 milliseconds; pace/sense configuration, bipolar. The next day, the following rhythm strip was recorded (Fig. 1–1): This rhythm strip shows

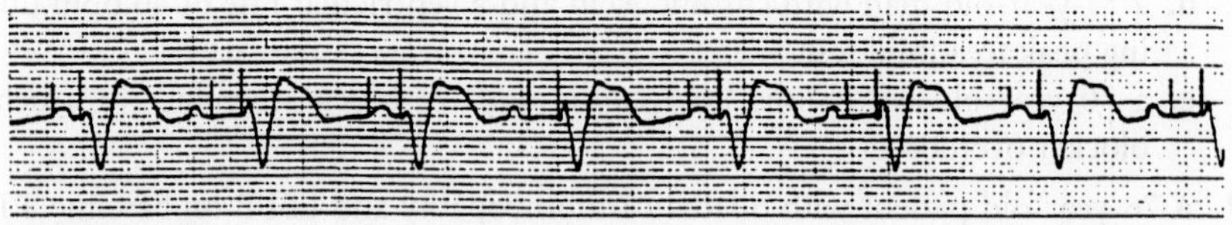

**FIGURE 1–1**

**a.** normal pacemaker function for the programmed parameters
**b.** atrial noncapture
**c.** ventricular noncapture
**d.** atrial undersensing
**e.** ventricular undersensing

**53.** A 50-year-old man with chronic obstructive pulmonary disease related to chronic smoking presents to the emergency room with palpitations. ECG shows narrow

QRS tachycardia at 165 bpm. His BP is 125/60. Expiratory wheezes are heard on lung examination. His medications include albuterol inhaler and theophylline. The most appropriate initial treatment includes which of the following?

a. adenosine IV bolus
b. digoxin loading over 6 hours
c. verapamil IV bolus
d. propafenone IV bolus
e. immediate cardioversion

54. A 55-year-old woman returns to the clinic after a recent dual-chamber pacemaker placement. She reports frequent palpitations and fatigue. These episodes last for several minutes before stopping. A Holter monitor recorded the following rhythm (Fig. 1–2): The pacemaker is programmed to mode DDD; lower rate, 80 bpm; upper rate, 150 bpm; AV delay, 200 milliseconds; postventricular atrial RP, 150 milliseconds. The latter part of this rhythm strip shows

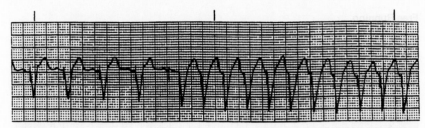

**FIGURE 1–2**

a. VT induced by the pacemaker
b. initiation of atrial tachycardia with atrial tracking
c. pacemaker-mediated tachycardia
d. pacemaker function failure with inappropriate rapid ventricular pacing
e. artifact

55. A 60-year-old man is having a transtelephonic pacemaker check. He has recently undergone a pacemaker upgrade from a single-chamber–ventricular to a dual-chamber system. He is reporting the same "old" symptoms he had with the VVI system. The following rhythm was recorded (Fig. 1–3). Which of the following is *true*?

**Free Running**

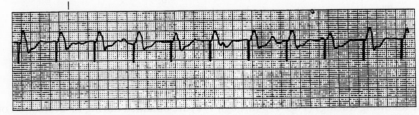

**Magnet**

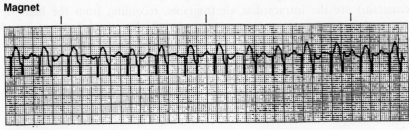

**FIGURE 1–3**

   **a.** A CXR should be obtained to check atrial-lead position.
   **b.** The rhythm strip shows normal dual-chamber pacemaker function.
   **c.** The pacemaker is programmed to VVI mode.
   **d.** Underlying rhythm is AFib with expected auto mode switch response to VVI.
   **e.** None of the above is true.

56. As related to the previous case, the most appropriate corrective action is to

   **a.** reassure the patient and schedule a follow-up in 6 months for re-evaluation
   **b.** increase the energy output on the atrial channel to assure atrial capture
   **c.** change the atrial sensitivity setting
   **d.** suspect a pulse generator defect and replace it with a new one
   **e.** obtain a CXR to document atrial-lead dislodgment and reposition the lead

57. An 82-year-old man receives a dual-chamber pacemaker for SSS. Routine transtelephonic check (without and with magnet) shows the following strips (Fig. 1–4). Which of the following is *true*?

**Free Running**

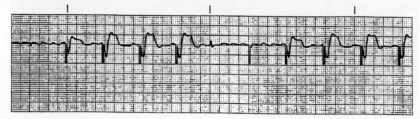

**Magnet**

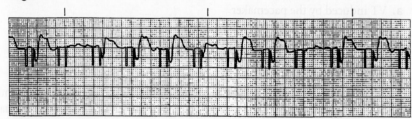

**FIGURE 1–4**

   **a.** The pacing mode is VVI secondary to automatic mode switch.
   **b.** There is consistent atrial capture on the magnet strip.
   **c.** There is consistent ventricular capture.
   **d.** Ventricular sensing cannot be determined by the available strips.
   **e.** Atrial sensing cannot be determined by the available strips.

## Questions 58–61

The following tracings (Figs. 1–5 through 1–8) are obtained during EP evaluation of AV conduction in different patients. HRA (*high right atrium*) and HBE (*His bundle electrogram*) are the intracardiac electrograms, recording from the high right atrium and the His bundle regions, respectively. Which of the following is *true* for these tracings?

58.

59.

60.

61.

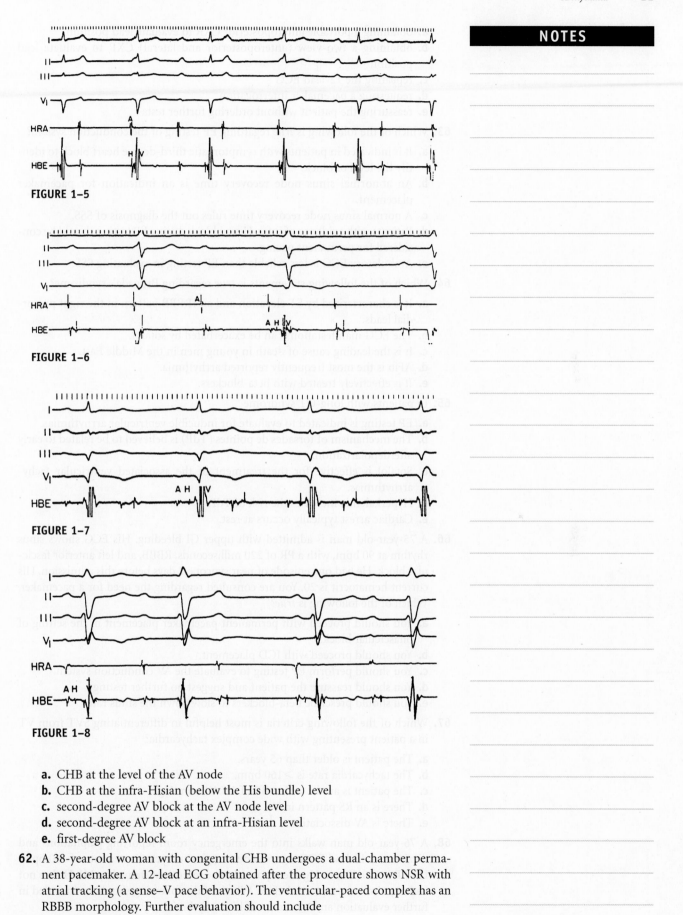

FIGURE 1–5

FIGURE 1–6

FIGURE 1–7

FIGURE 1–8

    **a.** CHB at the level of the AV node

    **b.** CHB at the infra-Hisian (below the His bundle) level

    **c.** second-degree AV block at the AV node level

    **d.** second-degree AV block at an infra-Hisian level

    **e.** first-degree AV block

**62.** A 38-year-old woman with congenital CHB undergoes a dual-chamber permanent pacemaker. A 12-lead ECG obtained after the procedure shows NSR with
atrial tracking (a sense–V pace behavior). The ventricular-paced complex has an
RBBB morphology. Further evaluation should include

a. obtaining a portable anteroposterior CXR to evaluate lead position
b. obtaining a two-view (anteroposterior and lateral) CXR to evaluate lead position
c. repeating the 12-lead ECG
d. requesting a pacemaker interrogation
e. reassuring the patient without ordering further tests

63. Which of the following is *true* regarding EP testing of the conduction system?

a. It is indicated in patients with symptomatic third-degree heart block to identify the level of block.
b. An abnormal sinus node recovery time is an indication for pacemaker placement.
c. A normal sinus node recovery time rules out the diagnosis of SSS.
d. Patients with evidence of infra-Hisian block during EP testing should be considered for permanent pacing.
e. Ambulatory ECG is less reliable than EP testing in evaluating SSS.

64. Which of the following statements is *true* regarding Brugada's syndrome?

a. It is characterized by ST elevation and an IRBBB pattern in the right precordial leads.
b. The ECG manifestations can be exacerbated by sotalol.
c. It is the leading cause of death in young men in the Middle East.
d. AFib is the most frequently reported arrhythmia.
e. It is effectively treated with beta-blockers.

65. In patients with long-QT syndrome

a. EP testing is indicated to evaluate for inducible ventricular arrhythmias.
b. The mechanism of torsades de pointes (TdP) is believed to be related to early afterdepolarization.
c. Sotalol is effective for the treatment of the associated ventricular tachyarrhythmias.
d. Hyperkalemia increases the risk of TdP.
e. Cardiac arrest typically occurs at rest.

66. A 75-year-old man is admitted with upper GI bleeding. His ECG shows sinus rhythm at 90 bpm, with a PR of 220 milliseconds, RBBB, and left anterior fascicular block. He had one episode of near syncope 2 days before this admission. His current hematocrit is 20. You are consulted regarding the need for a pacemaker. Which of the following is *true*?

a. You should proceed with permanent pacemaker placement in the setting of bifascicular block.
b. You should proceed with ICD placement.
c. You should perform EP testing to evaluate the AV conduction system.
d. You should reassure the patient and suggest no further testing.
e. You should prescribe beta-blockers to slow down the sinus rate.

67. Which of the following criteria is most helpful in differentiating SVT from VT in a patient presenting with wide complex tachycardia?

a. The patient is older than 65 years.
b. The tachycardia rate is >160 bpm.
c. The patient is awake with a BP of 110/65 mm Hg.
d. There is an RS pattern in $V_2$.
e. There is AV dissociation.

68. A 76-year-old man walks into the emergency room reporting palpitations and dizziness. A 12-lead ECG shows wide complex tachycardia at a rate of 160 bpm. His BP is 110/50 mm Hg. He reports that he recently sustained an MI. He has not had any similar symptoms before. Which of the following should be included in further evaluation and treatment of his arrhythmia?

**a.** verapamil, 10-mg IV bolus, to treat SVT with aberrancy, as the patient is hemodynamically stable

**b.** immediate DC cardioversion

**c.** procainamide, 15 mg/kg IV over 30 to 60 minutes

**d.** immediate cardiac catheterization and angioplasty, as needed

**e.** digoxin, 1 mg IV over 6 hours in four divided doses

**69.** A 55-year-old man had a pacemaker initially implanted 8 years ago over the left prepectoral area. Two months earlier, his old pacemaker reached end-of-life, and he underwent replacement of the pacemaker using the existing leads. He is presenting now with dull pain, swelling, and mild erythema over the pacemaker pocket site that started 1 week earlier, together with low-grade fever. He reports some purulent drainage from the incision site. Blood cultures were drawn. The best course of action is

**a.** to prescribe PO antibiotics for 2 weeks

**b.** to admit the patient for IV antibiotics and pacemaker-system extraction

**c.** to prescribe long-term suppressive PO antibiotics, as the pacemaker and leads system are too old to be extracted

**d.** to remove the recently implanted pulse generator on the left, leaving the old leads in place, and implant a new pacemaker system on the right prepectoral area

**e.** to incise and drain the pacemaker pocket and allow it to heal with secondary intention with daily change of dressing

**70.** Which of the following is a *correct* statement concerning external cardioversion of AFib?

**a.** Acute MI is a contraindication to cardioversion, as it results in further myocardial damage.

**b.** A nonsynchronized shock should be delivered because the rhythm is irregular.

**c.** Inadequate synchronization may occur with peaked T waves, low-amplitude signal, and malfunctioning pacemakers.

**d.** Digoxin therapy should be discontinued for 48 hours before elective cardioversion.

**e.** Patients with pacemakers should not undergo cardioversion because of the risk of pacemaker damage.

**71.** In patients with Wolff-Parkinson-White syndrome, with which of the following is acute pharmacologic treatment of AFib best achieved?

**a.** diltiazem

**b.** lidocaine

**c.** verapamil

**d.** procainamide

**e.** adenosine

**72.** A 75-year-old patient with a history of ischemic cardiomyopathy develops worsening heart failure symptoms during episodes of AFib despite a controlled ventricular rate. Which of the following is included in a reasonable trial of pharmacologic therapy?

**a.** flecainide

**b.** sotalol

**c.** verapamil

**d.** disopyramide

**e.** amiodarone

**73.** Which of the following is *true* regarding the use of digoxin in AFib?

**a.** It is superior to placebo for the acute conversion of AFib.

**b.** It controls ventricular rate during exercise in most patients.

**c.** It can control ventricular rate at rest in many patients.

**NOTES**

**d.** It effectively maintains sinus rhythm after cardioversion.

**e.** Because of its hepatic clearance, it is safe to use in patients with renal insufficiency.

**74.** Which of the following patients does *not* need anticoagulation with warfarin?

**a.** a 71-year-old man with dilated cardiomyopathy and paroxysmal AFib

**b.** a 74-year-old woman with chronic AFib who had ablation of the AV junction and a single-chamber permanent pacemaker

**c.** a 40-year-old woman with paroxysmal AFib and hypertrophic cardiomyopathy

**d.** a 35-year-old woman with mitral stenosis who underwent elective cardioversion 1 week ago

**e.** a 45-year-old man with paroxysmal AFib and no structural heart disease

**75.** Which of the following statements regarding flecainide as a treatment of AFib is *true*?

**a.** It may contribute to an increase in the digoxin level.

**b.** It may be used without an AV nodal blocking agent because of its potent effect on the AV conduction system.

**c.** It has been shown to be effective and safe for use in patients with hypertrophic cardiomyopathy.

**d.** It has no effect on the acute conversion of AFib but only on maintenance of sinus rhythm postcardioversion.

**e.** It is used for the treatment of AFib but not atrial flutter.

**76.** Which of the following mechanisms is responsible for AFib occurring in the immediate postoperative period after a maze procedure?

**a.** change in the atrial refractory period as a result of the surgical manipulation

**b.** autonomic imbalance as a result of the surgical intervention

**c.** misplacement of a suture line

**d.** an incomplete or omitted suture line

**e.** inhibition of atrial natriuretic peptide secretion as a result of the surgical manipulation

**77.** Characteristics of arrhythmogenic RV dysplasia include all the following *except*

**a.** fatty infiltration of the RV

**b.** fatty infiltration of the right atrium

**c.** monomorphic VT

**d.** abnormal signal-averaged ECG

**e.** possible detection by cardiac MRI

**78.** Concerning the cardiac AP, all of the following are true *except*

**a.** The AP duration in the atrium is shorter than that in the ventricle.

**b.** Myocytes located within the ventricular myocardium (so-called M cells) have longer AP duration than those located in the endocardial region.

**c.** Phase 3 (repolarization) is predominantly mediated by the $Na^+$ outward current.

**d.** The transient outward current that mediated phase I of the AP is more prominent in atrial than ventricular myocytes.

**e.** In atrial and ventricular myocytes, phase 0 of the AP (depolarization) is mediated by the $Na^+$ inward current.

**79.** Which of the following statements is *not* true concerning anticoagulation and AFib?

**a.** In patients with chronic AFib, anticoagulation for 3 weeks is indicated before cardioversion.

**b.** If AFib has been present for less than 2 days, anticoagulation for 3 weeks is not considered necessary before cardioversion.

**c.** In patients with chronic AFib, if no atrial thrombi are detected by TEE, cardioversion may be performed while maintaining anticoagulation during and for at least 4 weeks after the procedure.

**d.** Patients with chronic AFib in whom pharmacologic conversion with ibutilide is planned need not be anticoagulated.

**e.** An international normalized ratio of 2:3 is considered an adequate anticoagulation level.

**80.** The following tachycardia was induced during EP testing of a 36-year-old woman with recurrent palpitations (Fig. 1–9). Which of the following is the most likely diagnosis?

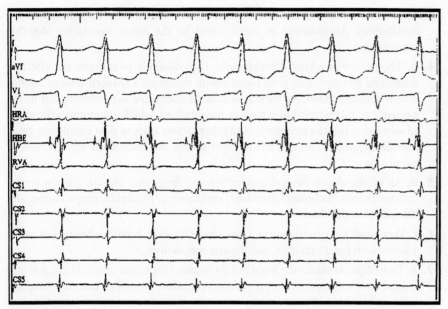

**FIGURE 1–9**

**a.** AVNRT
**b.** orthodromic reentrant tachycardia
**c.** antidromic reentrant tachycardia
**d.** VT
**e.** idiopathic left VT

## ANSWERS

1. **a.** Propafenone. Sotalol and dofetilide are primarily excreted by the renal route and should be used cautiously, if at all, in patients with significant renal insufficiency. Flecainide primarily undergoes hepatic elimination (approximately 70%) but has 25% renal elimination. The route of elimination for propafenone is 99% hepatic.

2. **d.** Amiodarone.

3. **a.** Amiodarone. Sotalol, dofetilide, and flecainide do not have significant active metabolites. Amiodarone is metabolized to the active metabolite desethyl amiodarone.

4. **b.** The patient is taking dipyridamole. Dipyridamole potentiates the effect of adenosine by interfering with metabolism; therefore, a reduced dose of adenosine is recommended. An increased dose of adenosine is recommended in the presence of methylxanthines such as theophylline, which antagonizes the effect of adenosine (blocks receptors), and other factors such as slow circulation time, valvular regurgitation, and left-to-right shunts that reduce the effectiveness of adenosine.

5. **d.** All of the above. Several antiarrhythmic drugs may elevate digoxin serum concentrations, including quinidine, amiodarone, flecainide, propafenone, and calcium channel blockers.

6. **c.** Verapamil. Verapamil may increase serum levels of dofetilide because of interference with renal excretion and hepatic metabolism.

7. **a.** Dofetilide. Amiodarone has a mildly negative inotropic effect. Flecainide and sotalol have a moderately negative inotropic effect. Dofetilide does not have significant inotropic effects.

8. **b.** Flecainide. Flecainide is a class IC antiarrhythmic drug, and these agents exhibit "use dependence." This refers to the property of increased drug effect at increased heart rates. Sotalol and dofetilide are class III antiarrhythmic drugs that exhibit "reverse use dependence"—that is, greater drug effect at slower heart rates.

9. **c.** Antiarrhythmic drugs with reverse-use dependence have greater efficacy for arrhythmia prevention than termination and have greater risk for ventricular proarrhythmia after AFib termination (at slower sinus rates) than during AFib. Antiarrhythmic drugs with use dependence, such as sotalol and dofetilide, have greater antiarrhythmic effect at slower heart rates. Consequently, drug efficacy is enhanced at the relatively slower rates in sinus rhythm, making these drugs more effective for prevention of AFib than those drugs with use dependence. Likewise, for proarrhythmia, the antiarrhythmic drugs with reverse-use dependence are more likely to produce ventricular proarrhythmia after conversion to sinus rhythm at the relatively slower sinus rate or with a postconversion pause.

10. **c.** The treatment drugs effectively suppressed PVCs. CAST studied the concept that PVC suppression in the postinfarction period would reduce the incidence of sudden cardiac death. Patients without heart disease were, therefore, excluded from these studies. CAST I studied flecainide, encainide, and moricizine versus placebo. Demonstration of effective suppression of PVCs by one of the drugs was necessary before a patient could be randomized to drug or placebo treatment. Propafenone, another class IC antiarrhythmic drug, was not studied. CAST I was prematurely terminated by the safety committee after only a 10-month average follow-up because of significantly increased incidence of arrhythmic death and nonfatal cardiac arrests in the flecainide and encainide treatment groups. CAST II was a continuation of the study with only moricizine versus placebo, but this study was also terminated early because of an increased incidence of cardiac arrest in the moricizine treatment group.

11. **a.** Flecainide. All of these drugs are class I antiarrhythmic medications and have sodium channel–blocking properties to various degrees. The class IC agents, such as flecainide, have the most potent sodium channel–blocking effects, and the class IB agents, such as lidocaine, have the least potent sodium channel–blocking effects.

12. **d.** None of the above. Amiodarone increases serum digoxin and cyclosporine concentrations and enhances warfarin effect.

13. **c.** Mexiletine is not a Vaughn Williams class III drug. Mexiletine is a class IB antiarrhythmic drug.

14. **c.** Ibutilide. Ibutilide is the only antiarrhythmic drug approved by the FDA for acute pharmacologic conversion of AFib to sinus rhythm.

15. **c.** Enhanced effect. Patients with denervated hearts are supersensitive to the effects of adenosine.

16. **b.** Quinidine. Proarrhythmia with quinidine is idiosyncratic and not dose related. The other drugs listed have dose-related proarrhythmia.

17. **c.** PJRT. Regular narrow QRS tachycardias can be grouped into two categories based on the timing of the atrial and ventricular relationship during the arrhythmia— that is, the position of the P wave relative to the QRS or R wave. Tachycardias that have a shorter RP than PR interval are termed *short RP tachycardias,* and tachycardias that have a longer RP than PR interval are termed *long RP tachycardias.* Orthodromic AVRT is an accessory pathway–mediated reentrant tachycardia that uses the AV node as the antegrade limb and the accessory pathway as the retrograde limb of the arrhythmia circuit. The P wave, representing the retrograde activation of the atria, is generally seen just after the QRS complex within the ST segment and is, therefore, a short RP tachycardia. AVNRT in its typical form uses the AV-nodal slow pathway for the antegrade limb and the AV-nodal fast pathway for the retrograde limb of the arrhythmia circuit. The P wave, representing the retrograde activation of the atria, is, therefore, within or shortly after the QRS complex and is, therefore, a short RP tachycardia. Nonparoxysmal junctional tachycardia is an automatic or triggered arrhythmia that originates in the AV junction. The P wave may be just before, within, or just after the QRS complex. The permanent form of junctional reciprocating tachycardia is a special type of orthodromic AVRT that involves a posteroseptal accessory pathway with decremental (AV nodal-like) conduction properties. This decremental retrograde conduction property results in delay in the retrograde activation of the atria during the tachycardia, and, consequently, the P wave is seen well beyond the QRS/ST segment and closer to the next QRS complex (a long RP interval).

18. **c.** AVNRT. Atrial tachycardia and PJRT are long RP tachycardias and, therefore, would not have such a short VA interval. PJRT is a special type of orthodromic AVRT that involves a posteroseptal accessory pathway with decremental (AV nodal-like) conduction properties and, hence, has a long RP (long VA) interval. Because of the time required to reach the accessory pathway for the retrograde portion of the arrhythmia circuit, orthodromic AVRT generally has a VA interval longer than 70 milliseconds. Therefore, a VA interval shorter than 70 milliseconds excludes orthodromic AVRT and makes AVNRT the most likely diagnosis.

19. **c.** IV verapamil. A sudden onset of a regular narrow complex tachycardia with a cycle length of 375 milliseconds and an RP interval of 100 milliseconds is a short RP tachycardia (the PR interval would be 375 milliseconds − 100 milliseconds = 275 milliseconds, so the RP is shorter than the PR). This patient most likely presents with orthodromic AV reentrant tachycardia, a reciprocating tachycardia circuit that involves antegrade conduction through the AV node and retrograde conduction through the accessory pathway (however, AV node reentrant tachycardia is also possible). As the AV node is a necessary component of the arrhythmia circuit, AV nodal blockade effectively terminates this type of tachycardia. Although not

listed as an option in this exercise, vagal maneuvers, such as Valsalva, coughing, or carotid sinus massage, may be quite effective and avoid the potential risks associated with administration of medications. Verapamil and other drugs that block AV conduction, such as beta-blockers and adenosine, may be quite useful for termination of AV reentrant tachycardia. This should not be confused with the management of AFib in the setting of Wolff-Parkinson-White syndrome, in which administration of AV nodal blocking drugs, such as verapamil, is contraindicated. In that situation, IV procainamide or DC cardioversion is the correct management. A precautionary note regarding the use of adenosine for regular narrow QRS tachycardia in patients with Wolff-Parkinson-White syndrome: Adenosine may precipitate AFib and result in a very rapid ventricular response (pre-excited tachycardia). Atropine has no role in the treatment of these types of arrhythmia. Catheter ablation is not generally an acute treatment option for this arrhythmia, although this approach may be an excellent option for chronic treatment (cure).

20. **c.** Orthodromic AVRT using a left-sided accessory pathway. A regular narrow QRS tachycardia that has VA interval prolongation with the development of bundle branch block is most consistent with an orthodromic AVRT using an accessory pathway ipsilateral to the bundle branch. During AVRT, the antegrade limb of the circuit is the AV node and His Purkinje/bundle branch system, and the retrograde limb is the accessory pathway. Block in a bundle branch ipsilateral to an accessory pathway creates a larger circuit, as the antegrade limb must now use the contralateral bundle branch, and, therefore, the VA interval increases. This results in an increase in the tachycardia cycle length (a slower tachycardia). Of note, a slower tachycardia with bundle branch block itself does not necessarily have the same significance. Other types of tachycardia may slow because of a change in conduction of other components of the tachycardia circuit, such as the conduction through the AV node (A-H interval). Thus, it is important to demonstrate VA interval prolongation during bundle branch block to implicate an ipsilateral accessory pathway participating in AV reentrant tachycardia.

21. **c.** ICD implantation. Cardiac arrest with VT or VF in the absence of reversible causes (e.g., MI, severe electrolyte or metabolic disorders) is a class I indication for ICD implantation. ICD implantation for such patients is superior to amiodarone drug therapy, as demonstrated in the Antiarrhythmics Versus Implantable Defibrillator (AVID) trial. The Canadian Implantable Defibrillator Study examined a similar population of patients and, although not statistically significant, showed a strong trend for the superiority of ICDs. Demonstration of inducible VT or VF in these types of patients is not necessary.

22. **b.** Implantation of an ICD is indicated if an EP study shows inducible VT. The Multicenter Automatic Defibrillator Implantation Trial (MADIT) evaluated patients with CAD, ischemic cardiomyopathy with an LV EF of <35%, and non-sustained VT. This study showed that for patients with inducible VT at baseline EP study and after administration of IV procainamide, treatment with an ICD was superior to treatment with antiarrhythmic drugs. This is a class I indication for ICD implantation.

23. **b.** Biphasic shocks require less energy for cardioversion and defibrillation than monophasic shocks. All of the modern ICDs use biphasic-shock waveforms for cardioversion and defibrillation. All of the other statements about ICDs are true.

24. **a.** Modern ICD systems employ the pulse generator as a component of the shocking electrode configuration ("active can"). In general, the left-chest site for the pulse generator results in lower energy requirements for cardioversion and defibrillation.

25. **d.** Place a "donut" magnet over the ICD site. The patient is having inappropriate or spurious shocks from the ICD, most likely caused by detection of electrical

noise from a malfunction of the ICD lead. It is imperative that further shocks be prevented immediately, not only for patient comfort, but also to prevent induction of life-threatening ventricular arrhythmias (including ventricular arrhythmia storm) caused by the ICD shocks. The most effective action at this point is placement of a magnet over the ICD site. This prevents the ICD from delivering any therapies. It would not be optimal to delay the prevention of further shocks while waiting for an ICD programmer. Of note, unlike pacemakers, ICDs do not have an asynchronous pacing response to application of a magnet.

26. **c.** A 60-year-old man with CAD, prior MI, LV dysfunction, and incessant sustained VT would not be a candidate for ICD implantation. Incessant VT is a contraindication to ICD implantation. An ICD in this situation would lead to an excessive number of shocks. Better control of the arrhythmia would be necessary before ICD implantation could be considered. An ICD may be indicated for some patients with certain familial or inherited conditions with a high risk for life-threatening ventricular tachyarrhythmias, such as congenital long-QT syndrome or hypertrophic cardiomyopathy. Patients who survive a cardiac arrest caused by VF without reversible causes are candidates for ICD implantation, even with comorbid conditions such as cancer, unless the life expectancy is 6 months or shorter.

27. **b.** Early DC-shock defibrillation. The two most crucial factors that determine the value of out-of-hospital resuscitation for patients who experience sudden cardiac death are citizen-bystander cardiopulmonary resuscitation and early DC-shock defibrillation.

28. **a.** Asystole. EMD or PEA and, in particular, asystole tend to be found in increasing proportions as the time since arrest increases. This is likely caused by degeneration of prolonged VF. When VF is the documented rhythm at the time of resuscitation, the long-term survival is approximately 25%. When EMD or PEA is the documented rhythm, the long-term survival rate drops to approximately 6%, and it drops even further, to approximately 1%, when asystole is documented.

29. **d.** VF. The initial rhythm documented in a patient who undergoes sudden cardiac death is dependent on the time elapsed since the arrest. Most episodes of sudden cardiac death (approximately 65% to 85%) that are documented electrocardiographically are caused by malignant ventricular arrhythmias such as VF. Monomorphic VT is uncommonly documented as a cause of out-of-hospital sudden cardiac death, perhaps caused by degeneration of unstable VT to VF. Asystole and EMD or PEA are found in greater proportions as the time since arrest increases, as these rhythms are likely the result of prolonged VF.

30. **d.** All of the above. Multiple ICD shocks in a short period ("cluster shocks") may occur from all of the conditions listed. The absence of symptoms is not a reliable method of discriminating between these causes.

31. **d.** Diuretics. The treatment of vasovagal syncope is generally focused on volume maintenance and expansion (fluids, salt supplementation, mineralocorticoids) and vasoconstriction (midodrine). Diuretics are, therefore, to be avoided, as the relative hypovolemia produced by these drugs may exacerbate episodes of vasovagal syncope. Beta-blocker medications may be useful for suppressing the triggering events of the vasovagal episodes. Cardiac pacing for patients with frequent vasovagal syncopal episodes has recently been shown to be effective for suppression of these episodes in a randomized clinical trial, the North American Vasovagal Pacemaker Study.

32. **d.** All of the above are true. A carefully performed initial evaluation has been reported to provide an etiology for syncope in 50% to 60% of cases. This evaluation includes a detailed medical history (including history from witnesses to the event), physical examination, basic hematologic and biochemical studies, and an ECG. Neurally mediated syncope is the most common cause of syncope, particularly in the absence of structural heart disease.

**33. b.** Beta-blocker medications. Several randomized trials of the use of beta-blocker medications for patients after MI have shown efficacy for the prevention of sudden cardiac death (including propranolol, timolol, metoprolol, and acebutolol). Trials of amiodarone in this setting have provided mixed results. Two large randomized trials, the European Myocardial Infarct Amiodarone Trial (EMIAT) and the Canadian Amiodarone Myocardial Infarction Arrhythmia Trial (CAMIAT), examined the use of amiodarone in patients after MI and did not show a reduction in overall mortality with the use of amiodarone. The Polish Amiodarone trial showed that amiodarone improved survival only in patients with preserved LV function after MI. The Survival with Oral D-sotalol (SWORD) trial studied the use of the D-isomer of sotalol (D-sotalol) in patients with recent MI and LV dysfunction. This study found worse survival in the group treated with D-sotalol than in the group treated with placebo. The Danish Investigations of Arrhythmias and Mortality on Dofetilide (DIAMOND) studies showed that dofetilide had a neutral effect on total mortality compared with placebo in the treatment of post-MI patients with LV dysfunction.

**34. b.** CAD. CAD is the predominant disease process associated with sudden cardiac death in the United States, accounting for 64% to 90% of cases. The other cardiomyopathies, such as dilated and hypertrophic cardiomyopathies, together account for approximately 10% to 15% of cases of sudden cardiac death.

**35. c.** Head-upright tilt table testing. Syncope in the absence of structural heart disease is most likely neurally mediated (vasovagal). The head-upright tilt table test is the most appropriate test to evaluate for this condition. This test initiates the vasovagal episode by maximizing venous pooling, sympathetic activation, and circulating catecholamines. In general, the test involves at least 30 minutes of 70-degree head-up tilt angle without a saddle support. An addition of a catecholamine challenge with isoproterenol is sometimes used. Among symptomatic patients, the sensitivity of the head-upright tilt table test is approximately 85%. The specificity of the head-upright tilt table test is good, with the frequency of an abnormal tilt table test in control subjects being 0% to 15%. In the absence of structural heart disease, EP study, ambulatory Holter monitoring, and the signal-averaged ECG are low yield.

**36. c.** Combination of cardioinhibitory and vasodepressor. Vasovagal syncopal episodes may be classified according to the response of the BP and heart rate during an episode. Predominant cardioinhibition involves an episode in which the drop in heart rate is the prevailing event, whereas a vasodepressor response involves an episode in which the drop in BP is the prevailing event. Most vasovagal syncopal episodes are of the mixed variety. Note that the same patient may have any of these types of vasovagal responses with each episode.

**37. d.** None of the above. No further evaluation or treatment is indicated for an asymptomatic patient with intermittent ventricular pre-excitation. In an asymptomatic patient with a manifest accessory pathway (i.e., Wolff-Parkinson-White pattern by ECG), the main concern is risk stratification. With such patients, there may be an increased risk of sudden cardiac death caused by very rapid ventricular response across the accessory pathway during AFib. Demonstration of intermittent pre-excitation by ambulatory Holter monitoring or by exercise treadmill testing indicates that the accessory pathway does not support very rapid 1:1 AV conduction, and, hence, the likelihood of sudden cardiac death from AFib would be low.

**38. a.** AVNRT. An "r prime" in lead $V_1$ during regular narrow complex tachycardia that is not present during sinus rhythm indicates the inscription of the P wave in the terminal QRS, and this is very specific for AVNRT.

**39. c.** DC cardioversion is not an effective treatment for MAT. The other statements about MAT are true. If correction of the underlying condition is not effective or not possible, then treatment with calcium channel blockers and supplementation with potassium or magnesium may be effective. Treatment with beta-blocker medications may be problematic for patients with chronic pulmonary disease.

40. **d.** All of the above are true. All of the statements about head-upright tilt table testing are true.

41. **c.** Arc welding equipment may not be safely used. Normally functioning electrical power tools and home appliances usually have no effect on modern pacemakers. However, arc welding produces a strong electromagnetic field, that may result in pacemaker inhibition or noise reversion, and should be avoided in pacemaker-dependent patients. Other potential sources of interference include MRI imaging, lithotripsy, and betatron radiation.

42. **d.** Permanent pacemaker implant. This patient has evidence of symptomatic bradycardia on Holter monitoring, which constitutes a class I indication for permanent pacemaker placement. He has AV conduction system disease with no obvious reversible causes, which is most probably caused by idiopathic fibrosis (Lev's disease). Prolonged monitoring will probably show more episodes of bradycardia, which was already seen during telemetry, and which places this elderly patient at risk for syncope and injury. EP testing for ventricular arrhythmia is not indicated in view of the absence of structural heart disease. Likewise, ICD is not indicated.

43. **d.** Single-chamber system in the ventricle programmed to VVIR. This patient is in chronic AFib, and, therefore, physiologic pacing in the atrium cannot be achieved. Furthermore, conversion and long-term maintenance of sinus rhythm in this situation are very unlikely. Therefore, there is no indication for placement of an atrial lead. DDDR with mode switching and DDIR will behave like a VVIR system in this patient, at the expense, however, of an additional lead (atrial) and a more expensive dual-chamber pacemaker.

44. **a.** Pacemaker syndrome is caused by pacing the ventricle asynchronously, which results in AV dissociation or VA conduction. Symptoms consist of fatigue, dizziness, dyspnea, and weakness, with or without hypotension. The mechanism is believed to be related in part to atrial contraction against a closed AV valve and release of atrial natriuretic peptide. It occurs with ventricular pacing and therefore is worsened by increasing pacing rate and relieved by allowing intrinsic conduction (if present) by lowering the pacing rate, programming rate hysteresis, or upgrading to a dual-chamber system. Therapy with fludrocortisone and other volume-expansion modalities is not helpful.

45. **b.** Dual-chamber pacing in hypertrophic cardiomyopathy alters activation of the septum and has been shown echocardiographically to increase the LV end-systolic dimension without changing the LV end-diastolic dimension. It also reduces the LV outflow gradient; this can persist for up to 2 months after discontinuation of pacing. MR was also shown to decrease, a finding that is also related to change in septal activation.

46. **d.** A 73-year-old man with chronic AFib and a ventricular rate of 40 bpm during peak treadmill test. The 73-year-old man with AFib and slow ventricular rate during exercise is the classic example of SSS. This usually indicates degenerative disease of the cardiac conduction system involving the AV node as well as the sinus node. The finding of sinus arrhythmia varying by 15 bpm in an older patient, the profound nocturnal bradycardia in young athletes, and the sinus pauses in young patients are related mostly to a high vagal tone and do not indicate sinus node disease.

47. **e.** Induce CHB. Patients with true complete LBBB are at risk for developing transient CHB during catheter manipulation in the septal region of the tricuspid valve. This is caused by transient traumatic block of the right bundle branch.

**48. e.** IV glucagon. This patient has an overdose of diltiazem and metoprolol. These drugs slow sinoatrial and AV conduction. Calcium and magnesium have no effect in reversing these bradycardic effects. Isuprel and atropine are not likely to overcome the beta-blockade of metoprolol. IV glucagon acts on a specific receptor. This results in an increase in intracellular cyclic adenosine monophosphate, which enhances both sinoatrial and AV node conduction despite the presence of beta-blockade.

**49. a.** Intra-atrial reentry. The mechanism of typical atrial flutter has been shown to be related to a reentrant circus movement, most commonly in the right atrium along the tricuspid valve, involving the posterior cavotricuspid isthmus. Radiofrequency ablation of this isthmus is an effective treatment. Early afterdepolarizations are related to conditions that prolong repolarization, such as arrhythmia in the long-QT syndrome. Delayed afterdepolarizations are usually related to digoxin toxicity.

**50. d.** Administration of sodium-containing solution. Amitriptyline has sodium channel–blocking properties and induced QRS widening and VT. Increasing the extracellular sodium concentration by the administration of sodium-containing solution decreases the association of this drug with the sodium channel.

**51. b.** $K^+$ channel blockade with increase in QRS duration. Like other QT-prolonging drugs, terfenadine (a nonsedating $H_1$-receptor blocker) has $K^+$ channel–blocking properties, which delay myocardial repolarization and predispose to a specific form of polymorphic VT: TdP. Exacerbating factors include, among others, baseline QT prolongation, concomitant ingestion of other QT-prolonging drugs, and hypokalemia.

**52. d.** Atrial undersensing. This rhythm shows evidence of atrial undersensing. The pacemaker is programmed to DDD. In this mode, an appropriately sensed P wave should cause inhibition of the atrial spike; a ventricular spike is then delivered after the programmed AV interval or inhibited by an intrinsic R wave. In this strip, the P wave is present in each complex. However, in complexes 2, 4, 6, and 8, an atrial spike follows the intrinsic P wave because the intrinsic P wave was not appropriately sensed by the pacemaker.

**53. c.** Verapamil IV bolus. Adenosine is commonly used to terminate SVT. However, this patient is on theophylline, which is an effective blocker of adenosine receptor. Propafenone might be poorly tolerated by this patient because of its associated beta-blocking activity, which might increase airway resistance. Digoxin shortens the refractory period of the atrium and might potentially accelerate an atrial tachycardia. Immediate cardioversion is not needed, as the patient appears hemodynamically stable, and it would be reasonable to attempt pharmacologic therapy initially with verapamil.

**54. c.** Pacemaker-mediated tachycardia. In this strip, there is evidence of atrial undersensing (fifth complex) with loss of AV synchrony. This causes retrograde P-wave conduction, which is sensed by the pacer (because of short programmed PVARP), and results in ventricular pacing, causing a pacemaker-mediated tachycardia or endless-loop tachycardia. Acute treatment of this condition includes the application of a magnet to inhibit atrial sensing, thereby breaking the tachycardia loop. The spontaneous termination of these episodes in this patient is most probably related to intermittent atrial undersensing, which interrupts the tachycardia loop. Further prevention of these episodes includes reprogramming the PVARP, AV delay, or atrial sensitivity. Pacemaker-mediated tachycardia is an abnormal consequence of normal pacemaker function.

**55. a.** A CXR should be obtained to check atrial-lead position. On the magnet mode, there are AV sequential spikes, with capture of the ventricle by the atrial stimulus. So, the programmed mode is DDD. In the nonmagnet mode, there is no atrial sensing, with only ventricular pacing. This strongly suggests that the recently placed atrial lead has dislodged into the ventricle. A CXR will be diagnostic. The other possibility is swapping of the atrial and ventricular leads, but one might expect atrial capture with the second stimulus in the magnet mode, which is not the case.

**56. e.** Obtain a CXR to document atrial-lead dislodgment and reposition the lead. Atrial undersensing occurring early after implantation commonly results from lead dislodgment. Other possibilities include inappropriate programmed sensitivity and lead maturation process, which usually occurs at 2 to 4 weeks postimplant. This event occurred very early postimplant, making lead maturation an unlikely possibility. Atrial sensitivity is already programmed to the most sensitive setting available on most pacemakers. In this case, CXR confirmed lead dislodgment and the lead was repositioned, with adequate pacing and capture thresholds confirmed on follow-up.

**57. a.** The initial rhythm strip shows background AFib with VVI pacing, most probably related to automatic mode switch. The absence of atrial pacing suggests adequate atrial sensing (of the fibrillation), which resulted in the mode switch behavior. Atrial pacing cannot be determined in the presence of AFib. There is adequate ventricular sensing, as determined on the nonmagnet strip (th complex); however, there is intermittent ventricular capture noted.

**58. a.** CHB at the level of the AV node. In this tracing, there are background NSR with CHB and a narrow escape rhythm that is junctional in origin. This is apparent in the HBE tracing, in which the atrial deflections are completely dissociated from the H-V deflections. Therefore, the atrial impulse entering the AV node is not conducting down to the His bundle (A is not followed by His potential), indicating that the level of block is at the level of the AV node.

**59. b.** CHB at the infra-Hisian (below the His bundle) level. In this tracing, there is background NSR with CHB and a relatively wide escape rhythm. In the HBE tracing, each atrial deflection is followed by an initial His deflection and a third, smaller deflection, H′, indicating that there is conduction delay within the His bundle itself. This is suggestive of significant His-Purkinje conduction disease. Therefore, the atrial impulse enters the AV node, conducts down to the His bundle (normal AH interval), where it encounters conduction delay (HH′), and then fails to propagate to the ventricle, indicating that the level of block is at or below the level of the bundle of His. There is obvious AV dissociation with a ventricular escape rhythm.

**60. d.** Second-degree AV block at an infra-Hisian level. In this tracing, the surface ECG shows NSR with 2:1 AV block. The HBE tracing shows constant AH with 2:1 block below the level of the His bundle.

**61. d.** Second-degree AV block at an infra-Hisian level. In this tracing, the surface ECG shows NSR with second-degree type I AV block (Wenckebach). Because the QRS is wide, this type of block is usually localized either to the AV node or within or below the His bundle. In this situation, the HBE tracing shows progressive prolongation in the HV interval before it blocks in a 3:2 conduction pattern. Therefore, the conduction delay is not at the level of the AV node but at or below the His bundle. As opposed to Wenckebach in the AV node, which is usually benign in nature, this type of infra-Hisian block indicates His-Purkinje conduction system disease and is an indication for pacemaker placement, as it may progress to CHB.

**62. b.** Obtaining a two-view (anteroposterior and lateral) CXR to evaluate lead position. The presence of an RBBB-paced QRS complex pattern suggests that the ventricular lead is in the LV. The lead may enter the LV through an atrial or VSD or via perforation of the interventricular septum. It may also be inadvertently introduced into an artery and passed retrogradely through the aortic valve. Another possibility is placement into one of the LV branches of the coronary sinus. Although sometimes an apical position in the RV in a rotated heart can potentially give an RBBB paced pattern, a two-view CXR should be obtained to rule out LV positioning. A single-view portable AP will not distinguish an LV from an apical RV placement. If LV placement is confirmed on the lateral radiograph, repositioning of the lead is indicated.

63. **d.** Patients with evidence of infra-Hisian block during EP testing should be considered for permanent pacing. Patients with symptomatic CHB do not need EP testing because the decision for a permanent pacemaker is already made. The sensitivity and specificity of sinus node recovery time is approximately 70%, making this test less than ideal; in most cases, the decision as to whether to implant a pacemaker in cases of suspected sinus node dysfunction depends on symptoms and correlation with ambulatory monitoring rather than results of EP testing. Patients with infra-Hisian block tend to have an unpredictable course and should be considered for permanent pacing.

64. **a.** Brugada's syndrome has been described worldwide but is most common in Asian countries and is the leading cause of death in young men in part of Thailand. It is characterized by ST-segment elevation and an IRBBB pattern in the right precordial leads. These features can be induced with sodium channel blockers such as flecainide or ajmaline. (Sotalol is a potassium channel blocker.) It is believed to be related to a mutation in the sodium channel gene. It is associated with a high incidence of sudden cardiac death resulting from VF. Risk assessment and therapy appear to be poorly defined at this time, but the implantation of an ICD has been advocated.

65. **b.** The pathognomic arrhythmia associated with long-QT syndrome is TdP. The mechanism is believed to be related to early afterdepolarization and triggered activity. Sotalol causes QT prolongation and is contraindicated in patients with long QT. Hypokalemia, not hyperkalemia, is associated with an increase of TdP in this situation. EP testing is of no value and is not indicated for the risk stratification of patients with long-QT syndrome. Cardiac arrest occurs typically with vigorous activity and infrequently during sleep.

66. **c.** You should perform EP testing to evaluate the AV conduction system. The patient had an episode of near syncope, which could be related to his GI bleeding, but the possibility of intermittent heart block in the setting of bifascicular block cannot be ruled out. This is a class I indication for EP testing to evaluate AV conduction. If there is evidence of abnormally prolonged HV interval, then a permanent pacemaker should be considered. There is no indication for ICD placement in this setting. Beta-blockers would blunt a reactive tachycardia resulting from the patient's anemia.

67. **e.** There is AV dissociation. In patients presenting with wide complex tachycardia, the presence of AV dissociation is highly specific for VT. All the other listed parameters suffer from significant overlap between SVT and VT.

68. **c.** Procainamide, 15 mg/kg IV over 30 to 60 minutes. Wide complex tachycardia occurring after MI is most likely to be VT. Verapamil is contraindicated in this setting, as it might lead to hypotension and VF. DC cardioversion can be used if the patient does not respond to antiarrhythmic therapy or if he becomes hemodynamically unstable. Procainamide is the drug of choice because it treats ventricular as well as supraventricular arrhythmia. There is no role for digoxin and no need for urgent cardiac catheterization in this situation.

69. **b.** To admit the patient for IV antibiotics and pacemaker-system extraction. This presentation is consistent with pacemaker-system infection, which occurred following the recent pulse generator replacement. Antibiotics PO or IV without extraction of the pacemaker system have limited efficacy in eradicating the infection. The patient should undergo pacemaker-system extraction, followed by IV antibiotics, until negative blood cultures are obtained. A new pacemaker system can then be implanted on the right side.

**70. c.** Inadequate synchronization may occur with peaked T waves, low-amplitude signal, and malfunctioning pacemakers. Cardioversion is the delivery of electric energy synchronized on the R wave. A synchronized shock should be used in AFib. A nonsynchronized shock may result in VF. Improper synchronization may occur in a situation in which more than one peaked signal exists, such as with pacemakers and peaked T waves. On the other hand, a low QRS signal may not synchronize at all. In patients with pacemakers, the pads are positioned at least 3 inches away from the pulse generator to minimize damage. MI and digoxin intake are not contraindications for DC cardioversion as long as digoxin toxicity is not suspected.

**71. d.** Procainamide. Procainamide can slow down conduction across the accessory pathway and potentially converts AFib. Diltiazem (Cardizem) and verapamil cause hypotension and reflex increase in sympathetic activation and may result in increased ventricular response. Adenosine is of no use in this setting. Lidocaine has little effect on the refractory period of the accessory pathway.

**72. e.** Amiodarone. Amiodarone may allow maintenance of sinus rhythm in patients with AFib and cardiomyopathy. In low doses, the side effects are minimized. Flecainide and disopyramide are not used in patients with cardiomyopathy because of their potential for proarrhythmia and their negative inotropic effects. Verapamil is not effective for maintenance of sinus rhythm. Sotalol might not be tolerated in patients with heart failure and has the potential for proarrhythmia in patients on diuretics prone to hypokalemia.

**73. c.** Digoxin can control the ventricular rate at rest in patients with AFib, but not with exercise. It is as effective as placebo for the acute conversion of AFib and does not help in maintaining NSR.

**74. e.** A 45-year-old man with paroxysmal AFib and no structural heart disease. The risk of stroke in patients younger than 60 years of age and with a normal heart is low and does not warrant anticoagulation. Patients with structural heart disease, such as ischemic, dilated, or hypertrophic cardiomyopathy, have a significant risk of stroke and should be anticoagulated if there are no contraindications otherwise. After AV junction ablation, AFib persists, and anticoagulation should be continued. Anticoagulation should be continued for at least 4 weeks postcardioversion, as atrial function does not normalize immediately after restoration of normal rhythm.

**75. a.** It may contribute to an increase in the digoxin level. Flecainide (amiodarone, propafenone [Rythmol], and verapamil) can increase digoxin level. Flecainide can regularize and slow the atrial rhythm in patients with AFib and can, therefore, lead to increased ventricular response because of improved conduction of the atrial impulses through the AV node. It is, therefore, important to use an AV nodal blocking agent in patients with AFib treated with flecainide. It is used for AFib as well as flutter. There are no definite data on its safety in patients with hypertrophic cardiomyopathy. It is effective for acute conversion as well as maintenance of NSR postconversion.

**76. a.** Change in the atrial refractory period as a result of the surgical manipulation. The occurrence of AFib post–cardiac surgery is believed to be related to shortening of the refractory period of atrial tissue as it recovers from surgical manipulation, cardioplegia, and, potentially, ischemia. This nonuniformity of recovery results in reentry as the mechanism of AFib.

**77. b.** Fatty infiltration of the right atrium is not a characteristic of arrhythmogenic RV dysplasia. Arrhythmogenic RV dysplasia refers to fatty infiltration or deposition of the myocardium. It involves predominantly the RV and may extend to involve the LV. The atrial myocardium is not involved. MRI scanning has been used for diagnosis and follow-up of this condition. Late potentials and VT arising predominantly from the RV are typical findings. Treatment with sotalol, radiofrequency ablation, or ICD placement depends on the degree of ventricular involvement and the presenting spectrum of arrhythmia.

**78. c.** All the other statements are true concerning the AP.

**79. d.** In patients with AFib of longer than 3 days' duration, anticoagulation should be used for 3 weeks before electrical or pharmacologic cardioversion and continued for at least 4 weeks after conversion, keeping a therapeutic international normalized ratio level of 2:3. TEE-guided cardioversion has recently been shown to be safe, provided anticoagulation is maintained during and for 4 weeks after cardioversion. Anticoagulation is not required before cardioversion if AFib is known to be of shorter than 48 hours' duration.

**80. a.** AVNRT. This tracing shows AVNRT. It is a narrow complex tachycardia using the slow pathway of the AV node in the antegrade direction (long AH) and the fast pathway of the AV node in the retrograde direction (short HA). It is unlikely to be orthodromic reentrant tachycardia in which the retrograde limb of the circuit is an accessory pathway, because the QRS-A time is very short, not long enough to involve ventricular activation as part of the circuit. Because the QRS is narrow, VT is not a likely diagnosis. Idiopathic LV-VT can sometimes be narrow but has an RBBB morphology on the surface ECG.

## Suggested Reading

The Antiarrhythmics Versus Implantable Defibrillators (AVID) Investigators. A comparison of antiarrhythmic-drug therapy with implantable defibrillators in patients resuscitated from near-fatal ventricular arrhythmias. *N Engl J Med.* 1997;337:1576–1583.

Budaj A, Kokowicz P, Smielak-Korombel W, et al. Lack of effect of amiodarone on survival after extensive infarction. Polish Amiodarone Trial. *Coron Artery Dis.* 1996;7:315–319.

Cairns JA, Connolly SJ, Roberts R, et al. Randomised trial of outcome after myocardial infarction in patients with frequent or repetitive ventricular premature depolarisations: CAMIAT. Canadian Amiodarone Myocardial Infarction Arrhythmia Trial Investigators [published erratum appears in *Lancet.* 1997;349(9067):1776]. *Lancet.* 1997;349:675–682.

The Cardiac Arrhythmia Suppression Trial (CAST) Investigators. Preliminary report: effect of encainide and flecainide on mortality in a randomized trial of arrhythmia suppression after myocardial infarction. *N Engl J Med.* 1989;321:406–412.

The Cardiac Arrhythmia Suppression Trial II Investigators. Effect of the antiarrhythmic agent moricizine on survival after myocardial infarction. *N Engl J Med.* 1992;327:227–233.

Connolly SJ, Gent M, Roberts RS, et al. Canadian Implantable Defibrillator Study (CIDS): study design and organization. CIDS Co-Investigators. *Am J Cardiol.* 1993;72:103F–108F.

Connolly SJ, Sheldon R, Roberts RS, et al. The North American Vasovagal Pacemaker Study (VPS). A randomized trial of permanent cardiac pacing for the prevention of vasovagal syncope. *J Am Coll Cardiol.* 1999;33:16–20.

Julian DG, Camm AJ, Frangin G, et al. Randomised trial of effect of amiodarone on mortality in patients with left-ventricular dysfunction after recent myocardial infarction: EMIAT. European Myocardial Infarct Amiodarone Trial Investigators [published erratum appears in *Lancet.* 1997;349(9059):1180 and 1997;349(9067):1776]. *Lancet.* 1997; 349:667–674.

Moller M. DIAMOND antiarrhythmic trials. Danish Investigations of Arrhythmia and Mortality on Dofetilide. *Lancet.* 1996;348:1597–1598.

Moss AJ, Hall WJ, Cannom DS, et al. Improved survival with an implanted defibrillator in patients with coronary disease at high risk for ventricular arrhythmia. Multicenter Automatic Defibrillator Implantation Trial Investigators. *N Engl J Med.* 1996;335:1933–1940.

Waldo AL, Camm AJ, de Ruyter H, et al. Survival with oral D-sotalol in patients with left-ventricular dysfunction after myocardial infarction: rationale, design, and methods (the SWORD trial). *Am J Cardiol.* 1995;75:1023–1027.

# chapter 2

# Valvular Heart Disease

MARAN THAMILARASAN

## QUESTIONS

### Case 1

A 35-year-old woman is referred to your office for a murmur heard during a routine physical examination. She is asymptomatic. She jogs 2 to 3 miles a day without problems. She had frequent febrile illnesses as a child, but her past medical history is otherwise unremarkable.

#### Physical Examination

Blood pressure 120/70 mm Hg, pulse 73.
She is in no acute distress.
JVP is not elevated.
Chest is clear.
Cardiac—PMI not displaced. Regular rate and rhythm. $S_1$ is increased in intensity. $S_2$ is normal. A high-pitched diastolic sound is heard and is heard best between the apex and left sternal border, 0.12 seconds after $S_2$. No murmur is heard.
Abdomen—No organomegaly.
Extremities—No edema. Normal distal pulses. Good capillary refill.

1. Which of the following maneuvers would be most useful in helping to confirm your diagnosis?
   a. Valsalva
   b. exercise
   c. squatting
   d. handgrip

2. After exercise, a short decrescendo, low-pitched diastolic murmur is heard over the apex, ending by mid diastole. An echocardiogram is obtained. Which of the following would you *not* expect to find?
   a. a mitral pressure half-time of 230 milliseconds
   b. a planimetered mitral valve area of 1.7 cm$^2$
   c. a maximum velocity of the tricuspid insufficiency jet of 2.1 m/s
   d. a mean mitral gradient of 4 mm Hg

3. The echocardiogram reveals classic rheumatic changes of the mitral valve. Mitral valve area is 1.8 cm$^2$ by planimetry, pressure half-time is 110 milliseconds, mean gradient is 3 mm Hg. Left atrial dimension is 3.7 cm (planimetered area in apical four-chamber view is 15 cm$^2$). Left and right ventricular function is normal. Which of the following is appropriate?
   a. Endocarditis prophylaxis alone
   b. Endocarditis prophylaxis alone plus warfarin

c. Stress echocardiography to assess PA pressures post stress
d. Digoxin
e. None of the above

## Case 2

The above patient is referred back to your office 5 years later for a follow-up evaluation. She denies any symptoms, but is no longer exercising. She remains in sinus rhythm. $S_1$ remains loud, the opening snap is still quite audible (0.10 seconds after $S_2$). The murmur is now heard at rest and is longer. A repeat echocardiogram reveals a mitral valve area of 1.3 cm$^2$ with an estimated resting PA pressure of 35 mm Hg. Splittability score is given a six. LV size and function are normal.

4. Which of the following would be the most reasonable next step in management?

   a. immediate referral for surgery
   b. immediate referral for percutaneous valvuloplasty
   c. stress echocardiogram, to assess for mitral and pulmonary pressures post stress
   d. follow-up in 5 years

5. A stress echocardiogram is performed. Patient exercises for 6 METs. RVSP post stress is estimated at 70 mm Hg. Which of the following would be an appropriate next step?

   a. consideration for percutaneous valvuloplasty
   b. mitral valve replacement
   c. start beta blocker and return for follow-up in another 2 years
   d. start digoxin

## Case 3

A 50-year-old woman presents to you for evaluation. She complains of easy fatigability, as well as abdominal fullness and right upper quadrant pain. She also notes marked swelling in her legs. She has recently been diagnosed with asthma, and is also undergoing evaluation for recurrent diarrhea. On examination, she has a blood pressure of 100/60. Heart rate is 96 bpm. There is elevation in jugular venous pressure, with a large *a* wave and a prominent *v* wave. Lungs are clear. Cardiac examination reveals a nondisplaced PMI. Rhythm is regular. $S_1$ and $S_2$ (including $P_2$) are normal. A diastolic murmur is heard along the sternal border, which increases with inspiration. A pan systolic murmur is also heard in this area. Hepatomegaly is present, along with ascites and peripheral edema.

6. What is the most likely cause of this patient's signs and symptoms?

   a. rheumatic heart disease
   b. carcinoid
   c. primary pulmonary hypertension
   d. cirrhosis of the liver secondary to chronic hepatitis

## Case 4

A 60-year-old male presents to the emergency room with complaints of weakness, lethargy, and severe dyspnea. One week prior, his family notes that he complained of chest pressure that lasted for several hours. On physical examination, he appears to be in respiratory distress. Blood pressure is 80/50. Heart rate is 130 bpm. His oxygen saturation is 87% on room air. Chest exam reveals diffuse crackles. Cardiac examination reveals a nondisplaced PMI. A third and fourth heart sound are heard, as is an apical systolic murmur. No thrill is present. Electrocardiogram reveals inferior Q waves without ST segment elevation. He is urgently intubated and pressors are started. An intra-aortic balloon pump is placed. A surface echocardiogram reveals a normal sized left atrium and a mild jet of MR.

**7.** What test do you perform first?

   **a.** cardiac catheterization

   **b.** transesophageal echocardiography

   **c.** right heart catheterization with an oxygen saturation run

   **d.** administration of thrombolytic therapy

## Case 5

A 65-year-old female presents to your office for follow-up of a murmur she was told about several years prior. She denies any symptoms, but is not very active. Her past medical history is significant for hypertension and diabetes, both of which have been well controlled. On examination, she is in no acute distress. Blood pressure is 125/75 mm Hg, with a resting heart rate of 70 bpm. Lungs are clear. Cardiac examination reveals a displaced PMI. $S_1$ is soft. $S_2$ reveals an increased $P_2$ component. There is an RV lift. An $S_3$ is present. There is a grade III/VI holosystolic murmur heard at the apex radiating to the base. She has no peripheral edema. Chest x-ray demonstrated cardiomegaly with prominence of the central pulmonary vasculature.

**8.** An echocardiogram is performed on this patient (Fig. 2–1). Left ventricular systolic dimension is 4.7 cm. Ejection fraction is 45%. There is posterior leaflet prolapse. There is a very eccentric jet of MR, which is read out as 2+. Which of the following is most likely?

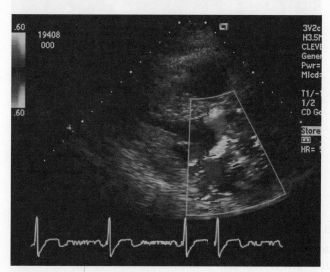

**FIGURE 2–1**  (See color plate)

   **a.** Mitral regurgitation is unlikely to account for her presentation.

   **b.** She likely has more severe MR than is evident on the echocardiogram.

   **c.** Her LV function is better than it appears on the echocardiogram.

   **d.** TEE is unlikely to be helpful here.

**9.** What do you recommend next?

   **a.** stress echo, to assess LV and PA pressures post stress

   **b.** mitral valve surgery

   **c.** start an ACEI and reassess in 3 months

   **d.** start a beta-blocker

## Case 6

A 75-year-old female with history of rheumatic fever presents for evaluation of significant progressive exertional dyspnea. She is no longer able to climb one flight of stairs without severe dyspnea.

### Physical Examination

Normotensive. Heart rate 70 bpm.

A malar flush is present. Jugular venous pressure is elevated with prominent CV waves. A right ventricular lift is present.

Rhythm is regular.

An opening snap is barely audible, which occurs 0.07 seconds after $S_2$. $P_2$ is increased. A pan diastolic rumble is heard. A high-pitched holosystolic murmur is heard at the lower sternal border, which increases with inspiration.

Chest x-ray reveals an enlarged left atrium with significant calcification seen of the mitral apparatus.

An echocardiogram is performed (Fig. 2–2).

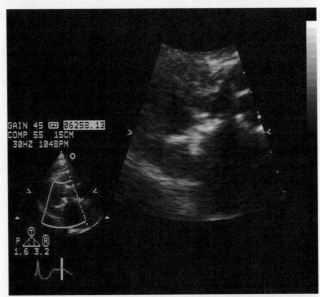

**FIGURE 2–2**

10. Which of the following would be appropriate management?

    **a.** mitral valve replacement
    **b.** mitral valve replacement with tricuspid annuloplasty
    **c.** percutaneous valvuloplasty
    **d.** digoxin and beta-blocker
    **e.** tricuspid annuloplasty

11. If she undergoes mitral valve replacement, what valve would you recommend?

    **a.** bioprosthetic valve
    **b.** mechanical valve
    **c.** mitral homograft

12. The above patient refuses surgical or percutaneous intervention. Which of the following would *not* be a possible indication to initiate anticoagulation therapy with warfarin?

    **a.** the development of paroxysmal atrial fibrillation
    **b.** a transient ischemic attack

c. left atrial size >55 mm
d. normal sinus rhythm, left atrial size 4.4 cm

## Case 7

A 28-year-old male is referred to your office for a second opinion regarding his hypertension. On physical examination, he is in no acute distress. Blood pressure is 160/90 mm Hg, symmetric in both arms. Pulse rate is 75 bpm. Cardiac examination reveals a nondisplaced PMI. $S_1$ is normal. It is followed by a high-pitched sound widely transmitted throughout the precordium. A short II/VI systolic ejection murmur is heard. $S_2$ is normal.

**13.** What is the most important diagnostic maneuver to perform next?
   a. check plasma catecholamines
   b. check serum potassium level
   c. check lower extremity blood pressure
   d. check plasma cortisol levels
   e. 24-hour blood pressure recording

**14.** The above patient is treated appropriately and does well. Three years later, he presents to the emergency room with acute chest pain radiating to the back. He is hypotensive on presentation. Electrocardiogram reveals T-wave inversions, no ST segment elevation. A quick bedside echocardiogram reveals normal LV function with a pericardial effusion. What is your next step?
   a. emergency coronary angiography
   b. CT scan
   c. start IV heparin and nitrates, admit to coronary care unit
   d. start IV heparin, IIbIIIa inhibitor, nitrates and admit to coronary care unit
   e. none of the above

## Case 8

A 59-year-old male presents for further evaluation of recurrent congestive heart failure. He appears to be in no acute distress on your evaluation. Blood pressure is 100/60 mm Hg. Carotid upstrokes are weak, but not delayed. Chest examination shows minimal bibasilar rales. PMI is displaced and sustained. A summation gallop is present. There is an increased $P_2$. There is mild peripheral edema. An echocardiogram reveals a dilated left ventricle with an ejection fraction of 25%. The aortic valve does have some calcification, with restricted leaflet excursion. Peak/mean gradients are 25/15 mm Hg. By the continuity equation, the aortic valve area is calculated at 0.7 cm². What is your next step?

**15.** What is your next step?
   a. immediate referral for aortic valve replacement
   b. referral for cardiac transplant
   c. dobutamine echocardiogram
   d. start an ACEI

**16.** With dobutamine echocardiography, the gradients across the valve increase to 50/35 mm Hg, and the calculated valve area stays at 0.7 cm². What do you recommend?
   a. aortic valve replacement
   b. continued medical management
   c. cardiac transplant evaluation

## Case 9

A 32-year-old male with known bicuspid aortic valve is referred to you for management of aortic insufficiency. He is completely asymptomatic and jogs 3 miles a day as well as doing other aerobic exercise for 30 minutes daily. An echocardiogram reveals a mildly dilated left ventricle (end diastolic dimension of 6.0 cm) with an ejection fraction of 65%. There is prolapse of the conjoined aortic leaflet with 3–4+ insufficiency.

**17.** What is your recommendation?

    **a.** referral for surgery
    **b.** addition of vasodilator therapy
    **c.** observation for now, return for follow-up in 3 years
    **d.** cardiac catheterization

**18.** What do you tell him is his yearly risk of sudden death?

    **a.** less than 1%
    **b.** 2%
    **c.** 3% to 5%
    **d.** >5%

**19.** If, in the above patient, echocardiographic evaluation revealed an ascending aortic dimension of 5.1 cm, what would you recommend?

    **a.** observation with echocardiography every 6 months
    **b.** start a beta-blocker and reassess in 6 months
    **c.** referral for surgery

## Case 10

A 45-year-old male with rheumatic mitral stenosis presents for further evaluation. In the past 2 to 3 years, he has noted progressive dyspnea with less than moderate activity. He was started on a beta-blocker 1 year ago, but remains symptomatic. Echocardiogram reveals a mean mitral gradient of 4 mm Hg with a valve area of 1.6 cm$^2$.

**20.** What would be a reasonable next step in the evaluation/management of this patient?

    **a.** stress echocardiogram
    **b.** referral for percutaneous intervention
    **c.** referral for mitral valve replacement
    **d.** reassurance and follow-up in 1 year

**21.** You decide to send this patient for percutaneous intervention. What is the most appropriate test to order at the time of or prior to the valvuloplasty procedure?

    **a.** transesophageal echocardiogram
    **b.** 24-hour electrocardiographic monitoring to assess for paroxysmal atrial fibrillation
    **c.** cardiac CT to assess for aortic calcification
    **d.** stress nuclear perfusion study

**22.** Which of the following is *not* true about ischemic MR?

    **a.** Revascularization alone may sometimes reduce the MR, but not often.
    **b.** Surgical repair or replacement of the valve is often needed.
    **c.** Prognosis is better than that of myxomatous MR.
    **d.** Vasodilator therapy in the setting of ischemic LV dysfunction may reduce severity of MR.
    **e.** Even with initial successful valve repair, MR often recurs.

## Case 11

A 65-year-old male is referred to you for evaluation of a heart murmur. He denies any symptoms at this time. On physical examination, he is in no acute distress. Blood pressure is 135/75 mm Hg, pulse is 82 bpm and regular. Carotid upstrokes are diminished. The PMI is sustained and displaced. A$_2$ is soft. A late peaking systolic murmur is heard at the base. You order an echocardiogram. This reveals left ventricular hypertrophy with moderate global impairment of left ventricular function, calculated ejection fraction of 35%. There is severe calcific aortic stenosis, with peak/mean gradients of 75/45 mm Hg. Aortic valve area is 0.5 cm$^2$.

**23.** What is the role of aortic valve replacement in this setting?

    **a.** It is absolutely indicated.

    **b.** It is absolutely not recommended.

    **c.** There is some evidence/opinion that would favor valve replacement.

**24.** A patient with asymptomatic AS presents for evaluation. Aortic valve area is calculated at 0.8 cm$^2$, with a mean gradient of 41 mm Hg. Mild hypertrophy is present with preserved LV function. The patient walks for 8 METs on a treadmill with a normal hemodynamic response and without any ectopy. He is very compliant with medical follow-up. Which of the following is *not* true regarding valve replacement for this patient?

    **a.** AVR is recommended to prevent sudden death.

    **b.** AVR is not recommended at this time.

    **c.** If he were found to have coronary artery disease that required bypass surgery, he should undergo AVR as well.

    **d.** If he were found to have a dilated ascending aorta (6.4 cm), he should undergo concomitant AVR and aortic conduit.

## Case 12

A 75-year-old gentleman is referred to you for evaluation of aortic regurgitation. He has no symptoms at this time. His past medical history is significant only for hypertension. On physical examination, he is in no acute distress. Blood pressure is 170/60 mm Hg. Arterial pulses are brisk. A bisferiens pulse is noted in the brachial artery. The apical impulse is displaced and hyperdynamic. S$_1$ is not loud, and no opening snap is heard. A high frequency holodiastolic murmur is heard, loudest along the right sternal border. A late diastolic apical rumble is heard as well.

**25.** You order an echocardiogram. Which of the following are you most concerned about?

    **a.** aortic valve commissural anatomy

    **b.** degree of aortic insufficiency

    **c.** aortic root dimension

    **d.** mitral valve

**26.** The above patient returns for follow-up 6 months later. He now reports symptoms of marked exertional dyspnea. An echocardiogram is read as 2+ central aortic regurgitation, with a left ventricular end-diastolic dimension of 6.9 cm and an ejection fraction of 50%. What do you do next?

    **a.** cardiac catheterization with aortography

    **b.** start an ACEI, reassess in 6 months

    **c.** continue observation

    **d.** start a beta-blocker, reassess in 6 months

## Case 13

A 56-year-old male presents to the emergency room with the sudden onset of chest pain. He is tachypneic on presentation. O$_2$ saturation is 82% on room air. Blood pressure is 80/60 mm Hg. Heart rate is 125 bpm. Lung exam reveals diffuse bilateral crackles. Cardiac examination reveals a nondisplaced PMI. S$_1$ is soft. P$_2$ is loud. An S$_3$ is present. A short decrescendo diastolic murmur is heard at the upper sternal border. Extremities are cool. ECG reveals inferior ST segment elevation. He is promptly intubated, and pressors are started. A brief echocardiogram is performed at the bedside. The study is difficult, but reveals premature closure of the mitral valve. There is hypokinesis of the inferoposterior walls.

**27.** Which of the following would be your next course of action?

    **a.** transesophageal echocardiogram, emergent cardiac surgical consultation

    **b.** intra-aortic balloon pump to stabilize hemodynamics, followed by emergent angiography

    **c.** administer thrombolytics

    **d.** send patient for an MRI

## Case 14

A 77-year-old patient is admitted to the hospital for urosepsis. His past medical history is significant only for having undergone aortic valve replacement 5 years prior. On examination, he is febrile to 102°. Heart rate is 106 bpm. Carotid upstrokes are full. Chest examination reveals clear lung fields. Cardiac examination reveals a hyperdynamic apical impulse, which is not displaced. $S_1$ and $S_2$ are normal. An early-peaking systolic murmur is heard at the sternal border. An echocardiogram is performed. Peak/mean gradients are 50/30 mm Hg. LVOT VTI (velocity time integral) is 36, aortic valve VTI is 78. The aortic valve itself is not well seen. An echocardiogram 2 years prior had revealed peak/mean gradients of 24/12 mm Hg. LVOT VTI was 19, aortic valve VTI 41.

**28.** What do you conclude about prosthetic aortic valve function?

    **a.** He has prosthetic valve stenosis.

    **b.** No evidence for dysfunction.

    **c.** He has severe prosthetic valve regurgitation.

    **d.** He likely has endocarditis in addition.

**29.** The above patient remains febrile despite 1 week of antibiotic therapy. Electrocardiogram reveals a new long first-degree AV block. The patient becomes progressively dyspneic. A short, regurgitant murmur is heard. What do you recommend?

    **a.** transesophageal echocardiography with surgical consultation

    **b.** transesophageal echocardiography

    **c.** change antibiotic regimen

## Case 15

A 56-year-old male with mitral stenosis presents for evaluation. He has class II-III symptoms.

### Physical Examination

    He is in no acute distress.

    JVP is mildly elevated.

    Pulse is regular at 80 bpm.

    Chest is clear.

    Cardiac: Nondisplaced PMI. Opening snap heard 0.09 milliseconds after $S_2$. Long diastolic rumble. No peripheral edema.

    Echocardiogram reveals a planimetered mitral valve area of 1.2 cm². Mean gradient 10 mm Hg. Pressure half-time of 185 milliseconds.

    He undergoes percutaneous valvuloplasty. The following morning, on exam, you note that he is comfortable. He has a 100% oxygen saturation on room air. Opening snap is 0.12 milliseconds after $S_2$. A shorter decrescendo diastolic rumble is heard. You obtain a predischarge echocardiogram. The report indicates a pressure half-time of 180 milliseconds.

**30.** What do you do next based on the echocardiogram?

    **a.** There was a less-than-optimal result from the valvuloplasty. No significant change in mitral valve area was achieved. You plan to send him for another procedure or surgery.

    **b.** There was an error in half-time measurement. You order a repeat assessment of pressure half-time later that day.

    **c.** Repeat echocardiogram with planimetry of mitral valve area.

**31.** The echocardiogram reveals a small left-to-right shunt at the atrial level by color. What do you recommend?

    **a.** observation

    **b.** referral for percutaneous closure

    **c.** referral for surgical closure

    **d.** indefinite anticoagulation

## Case 16

An 80-year-old gentleman underwent successful aortic valve replacement with a bio-prosthetic valve 4 months ago. He presents to your office for a routine follow-up visit. He is asymptomatic. He is in sinus rhythm. Echocardiogram reveals a normally functioning prosthetic valve. Chamber dimensions are normal with normal biventricular function. He has no clinical history of embolic events.

**32.** Which of the following should you recommend?

    **a.** antibiotic prophylaxis, office visits if he feels unwell

    **b.** antibiotic prophylaxis, with yearly office visits

    **c.** warfarin

## Case 17

A 67-year-old woman is referred to your office for evaluation of a heart murmur. She describes symptoms of significant and limiting exertional dyspnea. On examination, she is normotensive. Pulse rate is 67 bpm and regular. Cardiac examination reveals a sustained but nondisplaced PMI. $S_1$ and $S_2$ are normal. An $S_4$ is present. A loud III/VI systolic ejection murmur is heard throughout the precordium. Carotid upstrokes are delayed and diminished. An echocardiogram is performed (Fig. 2–3). Continuous wave Doppler evaluation reveals a 4.5-m/s jet across the LVOT.

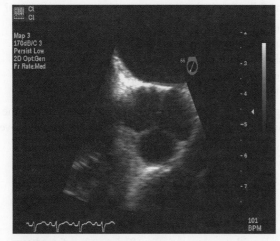

**FIGURE 2–3**  *(Continued)*

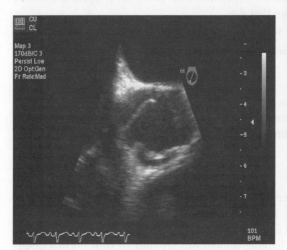

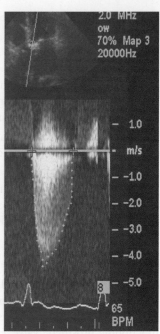

**FIGURE 2–3**

**33.** Which of the following would you do next to arrive at a diagnosis?

    **a.** transesophageal echocardiography
    **b.** repeat echocardiogram with amyl nitrate
    **c.** stress echocardiogram
    **d.** dobutamine echocardiogram

## Case 18

A 30-year-old woman presents to your office for a routine physical examination. She is asymptomatic. Blood pressure is 95/65 mm Hg, with a resting heart rate of 65 bpm. Physical examination is remarkable for a mild pectus deformity. On cardiac auscultation, a mid systolic click is heard. The click is heard earlier in systole with standing, and later in systole with squatting. No murmur is heard at rest, but a soft systolic murmur becomes audible with dynamic maneuvers.

**34.** Which of the following is the most appropriate course of action?

    **a.** recommend antibiotic prophylaxis
    **b.** follow-up examination in 5 years
    **c.** tell her she has no valve problems
    **d.** recommend beta-blockade
    **e.** none of the above

**35.** Echocardiography demonstrates no high-risk features. What is the role of aspirin therapy in such patients who have had no evidence of embolic events?

    **a.** Should be prescribed to all patients.
    **b.** May play a role, if a murmur is heard.
    **c.** There is no clear role for aspirin therapy in such patients.

## Case 19

A 50-year-old male with severe aortic insufficiency is referred to you for a second opinion. He is asymptomatic. An echocardiogram reveals a mildly dilated left ventricle (end-diastolic dimension of 6.2 cm, end-systolic dimension of 3.5 cm) with a normal ejection fraction. He has already undergone a stress echocardiogram. He exercised for 14 METs. No symptoms or electrocardiographic changes were noted. Resting ejection fraction was calculated at 65%. Post stress, the ejection fraction is 60%. No segmental wall motion abnormalities were seen.

**36.** What do you recommend?

    **a.** surgical intervention

    **b.** continue with vasodilator therapy, reassess in 6 months

    **c.** cardiac catheterization

    **d.** stress nuclear ventriculogram

## Case 20

A 70-year-old male presents to your office with complaints of exertional dyspnea. He is mildly hypertensive on examination. Carotid upstrokes are brisk, with a secondary upstroke. A loud III/VI systolic murmur is heard along the sternal border radiating to the neck. $S_1$ and $S_2$ are normal. An $S_4$ is heard. The murmur increases in intensity with Valsalva and decreases with handgrip.

**37.** An echocardiogram reveals a less than 2-m/s jet across the left ventricular outflow tract. What is your next step?

    **a.** Repeat the echocardiogram, but have Doppler interrogation performed in other views and with a nonimaging transducer. The degree of aortic stenosis has been underestimated.

    **b.** Repeat the echocardiogram with amyl nitrate.

    **c.** Transesophageal echocardiogram to better assess the valves.

    **d.** Coronary angiography.

## Case 21

A 62-year-old male with a history of rheumatic heart disease presents to your office with complaints of exertional dyspnea. No constitutional complaints are present. He had undergone a mitral valve replacement with a bileaflet tilting disk mechanical valve 11 years prior. He is normotensive with a heart rate of 73 bpm. On examination, you note a grade II/VI holosystolic murmur at the apex. An echocardiogram is performed, which reveals normal left and right ventricular function. Peak mitral gradient is 30 mm Hg. Mean transmitral gradient is 7 mm Hg. Pressure half-time is 80 milliseconds.

**38.** What is your next diagnostic step?

    **a.** fluoroscopy of the valve

    **b.** transesophageal echocardiogram

    **c.** invasive assessment of hemodynamics

    **d.** draw blood cultures

**39.** Which of the following would be the expected physical findings in this patient if the valve were functioning normally?

    **a.** prominent closing click, soft and brief diastolic rumble

    **b.** prominent opening and closing clicks, soft and brief diastolic rumble

    **c.** prominent opening click, long diastolic rumble

    **d.** prominent closing click, systolic murmur

**40.** If the patient had a ball and cage valve instead, what would you expect to hear?

    **a.** prominent closing click, soft and brief diastolic rumble

    **b.** prominent opening and closing clicks, soft and brief diastolic rumble

    **c.** prominent opening click, long diastolic rumble

    **d.** prominent closing click, systolic murmur

## Case 22

A 65-year-old male presents to your office for evaluation of valvular heart disease. He is asymptomatic. He walks 5 miles a day without difficulty. An echocardiogram reveals severe aortic stenosis, with a maximum aortic jet velocity of 4.7 m/s by Doppler echocardiography. Left ventricular systolic function is preserved. There is mild left ventricular hypertrophy (wall thickness 1.4 cm). He walks on a treadmill for 9 minutes, with a normal hemodynamic response.

**41.** Continued observation is recommended. What do you tell him is his yearly risk of sudden death, provided he remains asymptomatic?

    **a.** less than 2%
    **b.** 5%
    **c.** 5% to 10%
    **d.** >10%

**42.** What is the likelihood that he will become symptomatic, or come to surgery, within the next 3 years?

    **a.** 10%
    **b.** 10% to 25%
    **c.** 25% to 50%
    **d.** >50%

**43.** What is the role for balloon valvuloplasty in this patient?

    **a.** no indication in this setting
    **b.** may result in a survival benefit, albeit with a higher procedural risk than for AVR
    **c.** would be a good choice as a bridge to surgery
    **d.** would definitely be indicated if he were to need urgent noncardiac surgery

## Case 23

A 52-year-old male who previously underwent aortic valve replacement with a tilting disk valve presents to you several months following a documented TIA. He presently has no symptoms. Workup at the time of his TIA included carotid Dopplers, and transthoracic and transesophageal echocardiogram. These were unremarkable. The valve was well seated and was functioning normally. No thrombus was seen. Only minimal aortic atheroma was seen. No intracardiac shunt was identified. He has been on warfarin throughout, and has maintained an INR between 2 and 3. INR was 2.2 at the time of his TIA. On examination, he is in no acute distress. Blood pressure is 120/80 mm Hg; pulse is 68 and regular. Carotid upstrokes are full and not delayed. Crisp valve closure sound is heard along with a short, early peaking systolic ejection murmur at the base. No S$_3$ is heard. P$_2$ is normal. No peripheral edema is noted.

**44.** Which of the following would you recommend?

    **a.** start ASA, 325 mg/day
    **b.** increase warfarin, to achieve an INR of 3.5 to 4.5
    **c.** increase warfarin, to achieve an INR of 4.0 to 5.0
    **d.** Start ASA, 81 mg/day, and increase warfarin, to achieve an INR of 2.5 to 3.5

**45.** If his transesophageal study had revealed a small (1 to 2 mm) echodensity on the valve strut—suggestive of thrombus—but no obstruction to valve function, what should have been done?

    **a.** intravenous heparin
    **b.** bolus thrombolytic therapy
    **c.** reoperation
    **d.** intravenous IIb/IIIa inhibitors

## Case 24

You are following a 50-year-old male with moderate mitral stenosis, who had been asymptomatic. He presents to the emergency room with complaints of mild exertional dyspnea and palpitations, present for the past 3 to 4 days. On arrival, he appears comfortable, with an $O_2$ saturation of 99% on room air. His pulse rate is 140 and irregular. Blood pressure is 130/75 mm Hg. ECG reveals atrial fibrillation.

**46.** Which of the following is *not* appropriate in the treatment of this patient?

    **a.** intravenous beta-blocker

    **b.** intravenous heparin

    **c.** immediate electrical cardioversion

    **d.** intravenous digoxin

    **e.** TEE-guided cardioversion following initiation of anticoagulation with intravenous heparin

**47.** The above patient spontaneously converts to sinus rhythm. Which of the following are you *most* likely to recommend?

    **a.** therapy with warfarin

    **b.** percutaneous valvuloplasty

    **c.** mitral valve replacement

    **d.** no change in therapy

## Case 25

A 34-year-old woman presents to your office for evaluation because she had been on treatment with anorectic agents 5 years ago. She is asymptomatic at this time. She is now at her ideal body weight. On examination, she is in no acute distress. Blood pressure is 107/68 mm Hg. Jugular venous pulsations appear normal. Chest is clear. Cardiac examination reveals a nondisplaced PMI. $S_1$ and $S_2$ are normal, with an appropriate physiological split of $S_2$. $P_2$ is not loud. No $S_3$ or $S_4$ is heard. Auscultation is performed with the patient sitting, supine, and in the left lateral decubitus position. No murmur is heard.

**48.** What do you *most* likely recommend for this patient?

    **a.** reassurance, with a repeat physical examination in 6 months

    **b.** echocardiogram

    **c.** stress test

## Case 26

A 50-year-old male presents for his first physical examination in several years. He notes that a murmur had been documented a number of years ago. He is entirely asymptomatic. On examination, he has a blood pressure of 120/70 mm Hg with a pulse rate of 58 bpm. Neck veins are not distended. Carotid upstrokes are brisk. Lungs are clear. Cardiac examination reveals a nondisplaced PMI. $S_1$ is soft; $S_2$ is normal (with a preserved $A_2$). An $S_3$ is heard. A III/VI holosystolic murmur is heard at the apex radiating to the base and carotids, which increases with handgrip.

**49.** Of the four echocardiographic panels shown, which most likely represents the pathology in this particular patient?

    **Panel a.** Figure 2–4

    **Panel b.** Figure 2–5A,B

    **Panel c.** Figure 2–6A,B

    **Panel d.** Figure 2–7A,B

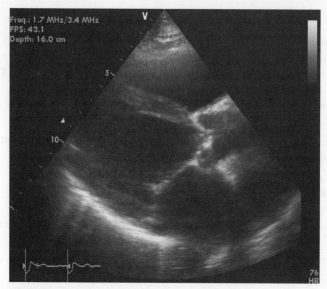

**FIGURE 2–4**

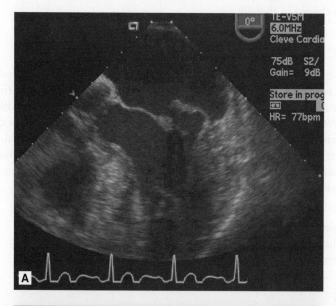

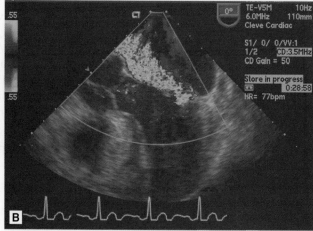

**FIGURE 2–5** (See color plate)

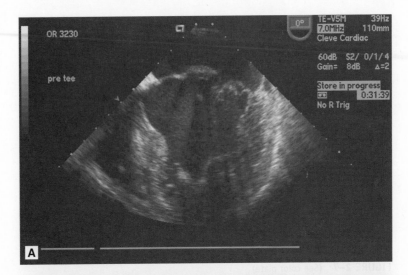

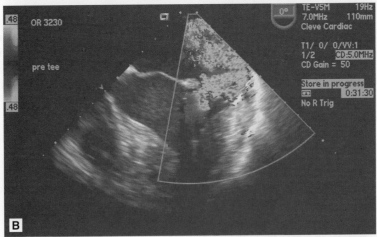

**FIGURE 2–6**  (See color plate)

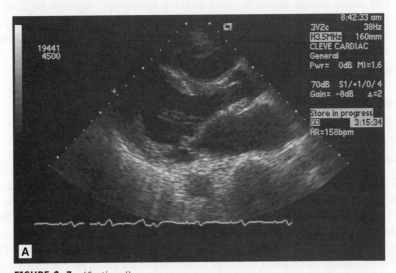

**FIGURE 2–7**  (Continued)

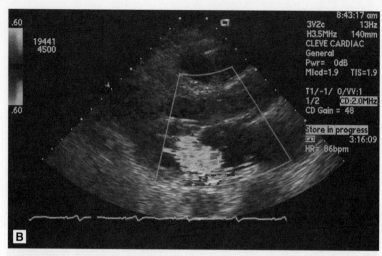

**FIGURE 2–7**   (See color plate)

50. Echocardiogram confirms your clinical suspicion. There is myxomatous mitral valve disease with posterior leaflet prolapse and severe MR. End-systolic dimension is 3.0 cm; end-diastolic dimension is 5.6 cm. Ejection fraction is 65%. TR velocity is 2.9 m/s. Which of the following would be most appropriate at this time?

    a. a stress echocardiogram, to assess PA pressures with stress
    b. immediate referral for mitral valve replacement
    c. the addition of an ACEI and follow-up in two years
    d. the addition of amiodarone to prevent atrial fibrillation
    e. follow-up in 2 years without an echocardiogram

51. The above patient undergoes a stress echo, and the PA pressures do not increase significantly with stress. What are you *least* likely to recommend?

    a. referral for mitral valve replacement
    b. reassess in 6 months with an echocardiogram
    c. referral for mitral valve repair

52. The above patient agrees to close medical follow-up. However, he does not present back to your office until 2 years later, now with complaints of dyspnea. A repeat echocardiogram reveals an ejection fraction of 45% with an end-systolic dimension of 4.7 cm. What do you recommend?

    a. referral for mitral valve repair
    b. start an ACEI and reassess in 3 months
    c. mitral valve replacement
    d. start a beta-blocker and reassess in 3 months

## Case 27

A 37-year-old male with history of rheumatic fever as a child presents to establish regular cardiology follow-up. His past medical history is otherwise unremarkable. He is active and jogs 5 miles a day without any symptoms. On examination, he is in no acute distress. Blood pressure is 150/85 mm Hg. Pulse is 52 bpm and regular. Lungs are clear. Cardiac examination reveals a nondisplaced PMI. $S_1$ and $S_2$ are normal. No opening snap is heard. There is a holosystolic murmur heard at the apex, radiating to the axilla. He has no peripheral edema. Chest x-ray demonstrates calcified mitral apparatus. The cardiac silhouette and pulmonary vasculature appear within normal limits. Echocardiogram reveals a rheumatic-appearing mitral valve with minimal stenosis but severe regurgitation. The mitral leaflets are calcified but have good mobility. Left ventricular dimensions are normal and ejection fraction is 70%. Right ventricular systolic pressure is estimated at 25 mm Hg.

53. Which of the following are you *least* likely to recommend?
    a. follow-up in 6 months with a physical examination and an echocardiogram
    b. referral for surgery
    c. initiation of an ACEI

54. The above patient does not seek follow-up for another 3 years. At this time, he complains of mild dyspnea with climbing four flights of stairs. He stopped jogging a year ago and he has gained 40 lb. What is the best course of action at this time?
    a. referral for surgery
    b. increase ACEI
    c. start a diuretic
    d. stress echocardiography

55. A 42-year-old male presents to you for a second opinion. He is asymptomatic with good functional capacity, but has been diagnosed with mitral valve prolapse with severe MR. His LVEF is 70% and dimensions are normal. Which of the following is *not* true?
    a. There is a consensus of opinion that he needs surgery now.
    b. There are data that in patients like him, there is a very high likelihood of requiring surgery in the next 10 years.
    c. There are some data that he may face a risk of sudden death in the absence of intervention, between 0% and 4% per year.

## Case 28

A 35-year-old male presents to your office for evaluation of valvular heart disease. He complains of shortness of breath with only modest amounts of exertion, as well as two-pillow orthopnea. He also complains of easy fatigability, as well as lower extremity edema and abdominal fullness. On examination, he is in no acute distress. He is normotensive. Jugular venous pressure is elevated, with a prominent *a* wave. The *v* wave is not easily discerned. $S_1$ is loud. $S_2$ is normal. A sound is heard in diastole, 0.07 milliseconds after $S_2$. A diastolic rumble is heard at the apex. A diastolic murmur is also heard along the left sternal border, which increases with inspiration. Mild hepatomegaly is present. There is 2+ peripheral edema.

56. What is your diagnosis?
    a. mitral stenosis
    b. mitral stenosis with tricuspid insufficiency
    c. mitral and tricuspid stenosis
    d. mitral and aortic stenosis

## Case 29

An 80-year-old male presents to your office with complaints of chest tightness when climbing up a flight of stairs. His past medical history is unremarkable. On physical examination, he is in no acute distress. Blood pressure is 140/80 mm Hg; pulse is 78 bpm and regular. Chest is clear. Carotid upstrokes are diminished. The PMI is sustained, but not displaced. A fourth heart sound is present. The second heart sound is diminished and single. A loud late-peaking systolic murmur is heard, loudest at the second intercostal space, radiating to the neck.

57. Which of the following would be your next step?
    a. stress sestamibi
    b. stress electrocardiogram
    c. cardiac catheterization
    d. prescribe prn SL NTG and see how he does

**NOTES**

58. The above patient is found to have an aortic valve area of 0.7 cm² with a mean gradient of 60 mm Hg. Following catheterization, he develops massive upper GI bleeding. Endoscopy reveals a gastric ulcer with a bleeding vessel at its base. Cauterization is performed, which temporarily stops the bleeding. However, the bleeding recurs and urgent partial gastrectomy is recommended. He complains of chest pain during these bleeding episodes. What is the best course of action?

    **a.** Proceed to aortic valve replacement first.
    **b.** Refer for percutaneous balloon valvuloplasty, followed by gastrectomy.
    **c.** Start nitroprusside and proceed with gastric surgery.
    **d.** Proceed with gastric surgery directly.

59. What valve would you recommend to an 80-year-old patient with aortic stenosis?

    **a.** bovine pericardial valve
    **b.** ball and cage mechanical valve
    **c.** bileaflet mechanical valve
    **d.** aortic homograft

## Case 30

A 65-year-old gentleman with a history of rheumatoid arthritis (well controlled) presents for evaluation of a heart murmur. He notes some increase in fatigue and decrease in activity level over the past 2 years, but denies any specific complaints of dyspnea. He leads a rather sedentary lifestyle. On examination, he is 6-ft, 1-in tall. Blood pressure is 150/50 mm Hg. Heart rate is 80 bpm and regular. Carotid upstrokes are brisk with a rapid upstroke and decline. Apical impulse is displaced and hyperdynamic. $S_1$ and $S_2$ are normal. A decrescendo, nearly holodiastolic murmur is heard along the left sternal border, loudest with the patient sitting up. An echocardiogram is performed, which reveals a dilated left ventricle (end-diastolic dimension of 6.8 cm, end-systolic dimension of 3.5 cm). Ejection fraction is 55%. There is significant aortic regurgitation.

60. What do you most likely recommend?

    **a.** stress test
    **b.** reassess with repeat echocardiogram in 6 months
    **c.** start vasodilator therapy and reassess in 2 years
    **d.** refer to surgery

61. He is started on a vasodilator and is seen back in 6 months. He reports no change in symptoms. A repeat echocardiogram demonstrates an end-diastolic dimension of 7.6 cm. Ejection fraction remains normal. What do you recommend now?

    **a.** stress test
    **b.** surgical intervention
    **c.** increase vasodilators and reassess in 6 months
    **d.** MRI to assess LV volumes

## Case 31

A 42-year-old woman, who underwent mitral valve replacement with a bileaflet tilting disk valve for rheumatic disease, presents to the emergency room with complaints of severe dyspnea. On exam, she has a blood pressure of 120/60 mm Hg. Heart rate is 83 bpm. Chest reveals bilateral crackles, one third up. Cardiac examination reveals a nondisplaced PMI. Prosthetic clicks are muffled. A long diastolic rumble is heard at the apex. Her past medical history is otherwise unremarkable.

62. An echocardiogram is ordered on the above patient. Which of the following would you expect to see?

    **a.** severe mitral regurgitation
    **b.** mean gradient 17 mm Hg
    **c.** pressure half-time of 80 milliseconds
    **d.** ejection fraction of 20%

**63.** The above patient undergoes atransesophageal echocardiogram (Fig. 2–8). A large echodensity consistent with thrombus is seen extending from the atrial wall onto the prosthesis, causing significant restriction in leaflet mobility. What do you recommend?

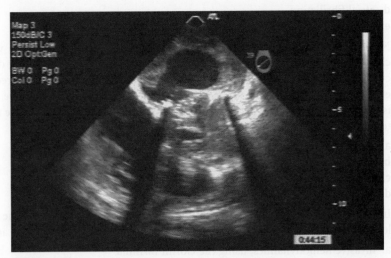

**FIGURE 2–8**

   **a.** urgent reoperation
   **b.** thrombolytic therapy
   **c.** intravenous heparin and glycoprotein IIB/IIIA inhibitor
   **d.** increase warfarin dose, aiming for a higher INR

## Case 32

A 26-year-old woman presents to your office for evaluation. She was told she had a murmur many years ago. She has a history of palpitations, but is otherwise asymptomatic. On examination, she is in no acute distress. Prominent *v* waves are noted in the JVP. Carotid upstrokes are normal. Chest is clear to auscultation. Cardiac examination reveals a nondisplaced PMI. Auscultation reveals a widely split first heart sound, with a loud second component that sounds like a click. A holosystolic murmur is heard at the right sternal border, which increases with inspiration. Hepatomegaly is present. An echocardiogram is performed (Fig. 2–9).

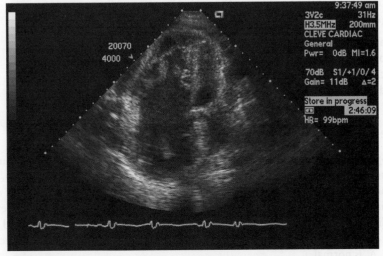

**FIGURE 2–9**

**64.** What is the most likely cause for her palpitations?

   **a.** arrhythmias secondary to an accessory pathway
   **b.** AV nodal reentrant tachycardia
   **c.** ventricular tachycardia
   **d.** atrial fibrillation
   **e.** anxiety

**65.** No intervention is performed for the above patient. She returns to your clinic 3 months later. She describes an episode of transient word-finding difficulty, which lasted for a number of seconds. This occurred while she was recovering from a fractured tibia. A CT scan was performed, which was negative. She is concerned that she may have a recurrence. What is the most appropriate next test for her?

   **a.** echocardiography with saline contrast study
   **b.** carotid Dopplers
   **c.** 24-hour ambulatory electrocardiographic monitoring
   **d.** right heart catheterization with oxygen saturation run

**66.** In the setting of aortic stenosis with moderate insufficiency, which of the following methods would provide the most accurate estimate of aortic valve area?

   **a.** invasive hemodynamics, using the Gorlin formula
   **b.** Doppler echocardiography, using the continuity equation
   **c.** pressure half-time
   **d.** Bernoulli equation

**67.** Which of the following valves has the lowest incidence of endocarditis?

   **a.** mechanical valve
   **b.** bioprosthetic valve
   **c.** aortic homograft
   **d.** stentless mitral valve

## Case 33

A 75-year-old gentleman is transferred to the coronary intensive care unit for refractory heart failure. He arrives intubated, on mechanical ventilatory support. Blood pressure is 95/40 mm Hg. Extremities are cool. Carotid upstrokes are delayed and very weak. Coarse rales are present bilaterally. A systolic murmur is present. He is making 30 cc of urine per hour on arrival. Echocardiogram reveals moderate left ventricular dysfunction, ejection fraction of 30%. There is severe aortic stenosis, valve area of 0.6 cm$^2$. Laboratory evaluation reveals a BUN of 80, creatinine of 2.2 (documented to be normal 6 months ago). Albumin is 2.0.

**68.** Which of the following would you *least* likely recommend?

   **a.** percutaneous valvuloplasty
   **b.** emergency surgery
   **c.** intraaortic balloon pump
   **d.** urgent dialysis

## Case 34

A 21-year-old man presents to your office for evaluation. He tells you that a murmur was noted a few days after birth. He is presently asymptomatic. On examination, he is normotensive. Pulse is 65 and regular. Carotid upstrokes are normal. Chest is clear. Cardiac examination reveals a nondisplaced PMI. A right ventricular lift is present. A systolic thrill is present in the suprasternal notch. A high-pitched sound is heard after $S_1$. A crescendo-decrescendo systolic murmur is heard at the left second intercostal space. $A_2$ is normal.

**69.** Which of the following would you expect to find on echocardiography?

   **a.** $V_{max}$ across the aortic valve of 4 m/s
   **b.** $V_{max}$ across the pulmonic valve of 4 m/s
   **c.** a wide jet of mitral insufficiency
   **d.** flow reversal in the hepatic veins

**70.** The above patient returns 1 year later for follow-up. Which of the following is a definite indication for intervention?

   **a.** He tells you of an episode of syncope.
   **b.** No symptoms, but right ventricular to pulmonary artery peak gradient 30 to 39 mm Hg.
   **c.** No symptoms, but right ventricular to pulmonary artery peak gradient 20 to 29 mm Hg.

**71.** If intervention is recommended, what is the preferred treatment approach?

   **a.** percutaneous valvuloplasty
   **b.** Ross procedure
   **c.** mechanical valve
   **d.** bioprosthetic valve

**72.** What is the most common cause of tricuspid regurgitation in an adult population?

   **a.** rheumatic tricuspid disease
   **b.** carcinoid
   **c.** congenital abnormalities
   **d.** pulmonary hypertension resulting from primary left-sided disease
   **e.** myxomatous disease of the tricuspid valve

**73.** Which of the following statements is true regarding treatment of tricuspid valvular disease?

   **a.** In patients with mitral stenosis and pulmonary hypertension who develop severe tricuspid insufficiency, but have normal tricuspid leaflets, placement of an annuloplasty ring is usually inadequate to treat the regurgitation.
   **b.** Mechanical valves are the preferred option when valve replacement becomes necessary.
   **c.** Bioprosthetic valves are the preferred option when valve replacement is necessary.

**74.** The most common organism seen in native valve endocarditis is what?

   **a.** *Streptococcus viridans*
   **b.** *Enterobacter faecalis*
   **c.** *Staphylococcus aureus*
   **d.** *Chlamydia pneumoniae*
   **e.** HACEK organisms

**75.** A patient presents with systemic embolic events 1 month after uncomplicated mitral valve replacement. He has been febrile for the past week. TEE demonstrates multiple echodensities on the valve ring. Blood cultures that are drawn are most likely to grow which of the following?

   **a.** *Streptococcus viridans*
   **b.** *Staphylococcus aureus*
   **c.** *Staphylococcus epidermidis*
   **d.** *Enterobacter faecalis*
   **e.** *Candida albicans*

**76.** Which of the following is *not* a class I indication for surgery in patients with native valve endocarditis?

   **a.** acute MR or AR with heart failure
   **b.** fungal endocarditis

**NOTES**

c. development of heart block

d. recurrent embolic events and persistent vegetations despite appropriate antibiotic therapy

77. Which of the following are *not* considered high risk for development of endocarditis?

   a. presence of prosthetic valve
   b. prior episode of endocarditis
   c. cyanotic congenital heart disease
   d. surgically repaired ASD

78. In an at-risk patient, which of the following procedures *definitely* requires prophylactic antibiotics?

   a. dental procedures involving manipulation of gingival tissue or perforation of oral mucosa
   b. GI endoscopy
   c. flexible bronchoscopy, without incision of the respiratory tract mucosa
   d. cardiac catheterization
   e. all of the above

79. Prophylactic regimens for appropriate dental procedures include all of the following *except*

   a. amoxicillin (2 g PO) 1 hour prior to the procedure
   b. ampicillin (2 g IV) 30 to 60 minutes prior to the procedure
   c. clindamycin (600 mg) 30 to 60 minutes prior to the procedure
   d. vancomycin (1 g IV) 30 minutes prior to procedure

80. A 35-year-old woman is referred to your office by her internist. She desires to become pregnant. Her past medical history is significant for congenital mitral stenosis, for which she underwent mitral valve replacement with a Starr-Edwards valve. Her physical examination is consistent with a normally functioning mechanical prosthesis. Which of the following is *not* true?

   a. Anticoagulation for mechanical prosthesis in pregnancy carries both maternal and fetal risk. The use of warfarin in the first trimester has been associated with an embryopathy in 4% to 10% of cases. Heparin is probably safer for the fetus, but is associated with an increased risk of thrombosis in the mother.
   b. If this patient chooses not to be on warfarin in the first trimester, you would recommend intravenous heparin to prolong aPTT to at least 2 times control.
   c. If this patient chooses not to be on warfarin in the first trimester, and low-molecular-weight heparin (LMWH) is used, the LMWH should be dosed twice daily, to achieve an anti–factor Xa level of 0.7 to 0.12, as tested 4 hours post administration.
   d. Dipyridamole can be used as an adjunct antiplatelet agent during pregnancy.

81. Which of the following would have the least risk for a patient contemplating pregnancy?

   a. congenital heart disease with Eisenmenger's physiology
   b. asymptomatic aortic stenosis, with a mean gradient of 60 mm Hg
   c. severe mitral regurgitation, with functional class I
   d. severe aortic regurgitation in a patient with Marfans disease.
   e. mitral stenosis, asymptomatic, valve area 1.0 cm$^2$

# ANSWERS

1. **b.** Exercise. The most likely diagnosis is mitral stenosis, based on the increased $S_1$ and the presence of the opening snap (high-pitched diastolic sound). The clinical history of febrile illness as a child is also suggestive. With exercise, flow is increased across the valve and the diastolic rumble may be evident.

2. **a.** A mitral pressure half-time of 230 milliseconds. The presence of the opening snap 0.12 milliseconds after $S_2$, a brief duration of the murmur, suggests that the degree of stenosis is mild. A pressure half-time of 230 milliseconds would suggest a mitral valve area of $<1.0$ cm$^2$—consistent with severe MS.

3. **e.** None of the above. The patient has mild mitral stenosis with good functional capacity. No further evaluation is necessary at this time. Her left atrial size is normal and she has no history of atrial fibrillation or other embolic events. She has no indication for warfarin. Her MS is only mild, so she has no indication for consideration for percutaneous valvotomy (class III indication by ACC/AHA practice guidelines). Thus there is no need for a stress echocardiogram. In addition, she has good functional capacity (jogs 2 to 3 miles per day without symptoms). There is no role for digoxin with normal biventricular function and normal sinus rhythm. By 2007 AHA guidelines for endocarditis prophylaxis, mitral stenosis without prior cardiac repair is no longer an indication for SBE prophylaxis.

4. **c.** Stress echocardiogram. The fact that she has stopped exercising may be a clue to the onset of symptoms. An assessment of functional capacity and post-stress mitral and PA pressures would be useful in management and assessment of true hemodynamic state. There is insufficient data for immediate referral for intervention. Follow-up in a short period of time may not be unreasonable, however 5 years is too long a period.

5. **a.** Consideration for percutaneous valvuloplasty. Her functional capacity is below average for her age. Her valve is favorable for percutaneous valvuloplasty (splittability score of six) and she had a significant rise in PA pressures post stress. This is a class I indication by the ACC/AHA guidelines. A beta-blocker would not be an unreasonable addition, but she should be followed more frequently than every 2 years. In addition, she does have class I indication for intervention. She has normal LV function and is in sinus rhythm—there is no role for digoxin in this setting. Valve replacement is considered only if the valve is deemed unsuitable for percutaneous valvuloplasty or surgical repair.

6. **b.** Carcinoid. The history and examination is consistent with tricuspid stenosis and regurgitation. (She has symptoms of fatigability from decreased cardiac output, signs and symptoms of systemic venous congestion–hepatic distension and right upper quadrant pain, peripheral edema, and ascites. There is a diastolic murmur along the sternal border, which increases with inspiration, along with a prominent *a* wave in the JVP. In addition, she has a pan systolic murmur and a prominent *v* wave). However, no evidence for mitral stenosis is noted on examination. Isolated rheumatic tricuspid stenosis is very rare. Thus, other causes for tricuspid stenosis should be considered. The second most common cause of tricuspid stenosis is the carcinoid syndrome. She also has brochospasm and diarrhea, which go along with this diagnosis. She has a normal $P_2$, making primary pulmonary hypertension unlikely. Liver disease in and of itself would not produce elevation in the JVP.

7. **b.** Transesophageal echocardiography. The clinical history is of a patient who had an inferior wall myocardial infarction approximately 1 week ago. He now presents in shock with acute congestive heart failure. Mechanical complication of myocardial infarction is first on the differential. The presence of a ventricular gallop and an apical murmur without a thrill makes papillary muscle rupture

the leading diagnosis (as opposed to VSD). Transthoracic echocardiography may miss eccentric jets in this setting. Transesophageal echocardiography should be performed to make the diagnosis. He will certainly need a cardiac catheterization (at which time a saturation run may be performed), but a TEE should be done quickly at the bedside to confirm the diagnosis so that the surgical team can be mobilized.

8. **b.** Her exam is suggestive of severe MR. The echo confirms LV dilation and mitral leaflet pathology, which could be consistent. The eccentric nature of the jet suggests that it may have been underestimated by transthoracic imaging. A more definitive imaging procedure such as TEE will be helpful here.

9. **b.** Mitral valve surgery. The presence of mild LV dysfunction with LV dilatation is a class I indication for surgery.

10. **b.** Mitral valve replacement with tricuspid annuloplasty. She has severe MS (increased PA pressure, opening snap less than 0.08 milliseconds after $S_2$, holodiastolic murmur—suggesting persistent pressure gradient) and is quite symptomatic. She does not appear to be a candidate for percutaneous intervention. A soft opening snap suggests that the valve is not pliable. The presence of valvular calcification on CXR would likewise suggest this. The echocardiogram confirms this, with extensive leaflet as well as subvalvular thickening and calcification. In addition, she has significant TR. She may benefit from an annuloplasty ring at the time of surgery.

11. **a.** Bioprosthetic valve. She is in an age group (>70 years) in whom the risk–benefit ratio would favor a biologic valve. Durability in this age group is reasonable. She has no other clinical indications for anticoagulation (in sinus rhythm, no history of embolic events). A homograft may prove to be a reasonable option, but there is not widespread availability or use as of yet.

12. **d.** Atrial fibrillation (paroxysmal or persistent) and a prior embolic event are class I indications for anticoagulation in a patient with mitral stenosis. Anticoagulation based on atrial size alone is controversial—the guidelines list a size >55 mm in the setting of severe mitral stenosis as a IIb indication. There is no established role for anticoagulation in the absence of above.

13. **c.** Check lower extremity blood pressure. He has a bicuspid aortic valve (an ejection sound is heard, along with a short systolic ejection murmur). There is an association between bicuspid aortic valves and coarctation of the aorta. Therefore, looking for discrepancy between upper and lower extremity blood pressure would be paramount.

14. **b.** CT Scan. Patients with bicuspid aortic valves (and in this case, aortic coarctation) have an associated aortopathy. They are thus at risk for aortic dissection. In this patient, a CT scan (or TEE or MRI) should be performed to look for this. Anticoagulant therapy should not be initiated until this possibility is ruled out, especially with a pericardial effusion.

15. **c.** Dobutamine echocardiogram. This is a patient presenting with low gradient aortic stenosis in the setting of left ventricular dysfunction. It may be that the patient has severe aortic stenosis, but the gradients are now low secondary to decreased stroke volume. However, the degree of aortic stenosis may not be that significant, but because of decreased cardiac output, the continuity equation overestimates aortic stenosis severity. In this setting, low dose dobutamine echocardiography may be useful. With inotropic stimulation, an improvement in stroke volume and cardiac output may help to differentiate true severe aortic stenosis from what has been labeled pseudo aortic stenosis. If true severe aortic stenosis is not present, then valve area will increase. It would not be prudent to send such a patient to aortic valve surgery without performing such an evaluation. It would be necessary to exclude severe stenosis before proceeding with transplant evaluation. ACEI may be beneficial, but it would be important

to proceed with the workup as above first. Afterload reduction would need to be introduced with very careful hemodynamic monitoring if true severe aortic stenosis were in fact present. The use of dobutamine echocardiographic testing to evaluate low gradient AS in setting of LV dysfunction is a class IIa indication by ACC/AHA guidelines.

16. **a.** Aortic valve replacement. The patient has true, severe aortic stenosis. The fact that he can generate a mean gradient of greater than 30 mm Hg suggests he has some contractile reserve.

17. **b.** Addition of vasodilator therapy. The patient is asymptomatic with good functional capacity. He has a normal ejection fraction with a mildly dilated left ventricle. Surgery is a class III indication in this setting. Vasodilator therapy may have some benefit in this asymptomatic population with preserved ejection fraction and left ventricular dilatation, although this is not definite. This is a class IIb indication. Observation alone would be reasonable, and would have been the best answer if the follow-up were closer than 3 years. There is no role for cardiac catheterization at this juncture.

18. **a.** From the available published literature, as summarized in the ACC/AHA consensus guidelines, the risk is about 0.2% per year in those asymptomatic patients with preserved left ventricular function.

19. **c.** Referral for surgery. An aortic dimension >5.0 cm (or growth >0.5 cm per year) in a patient with a bicuspid aortic valve is a class I indication for surgery.

20. **a.** Stress echocardiogram. There appears to be a discrepancy between the degree of symptoms and resting hemodynamics. Further workup is warranted. A stress echocardiogram revealed a post stress PA pressure of 70 mm Hg and a mean transmitral gradient of 17 mm Hg. Follow-up in 1 year without further workup is inappropriate given the degree of symptoms. There is insufficient information as of yet to proceed directly with intervention.

21. **a.** Transesophageal echocardiogram. Left atrial and appendage thrombus should be excluded prior to proceeding with percutaneous valvuloplasty, and is recommended by ACC/AHA guidelines to be performed prior to the procedure. Transthoracic echocardiography does not have sufficient sensitivity for this purpose. Documentation of atrial fibrillation by ambulatory monitoring may make the likelihood of finding a thrombus higher, but the transesophageal echocardiogram should be performed regardless. Routine surveillance for aortic calcification has no role in this setting. A nuclear perfusion study would not be necessary here (angiography can be performed if needed at the time of the procedure).

22. **c.** Generally, patients with ischemic MR, owing to concomitant coronary disease and LV dysfunction, have a worse prognosis than those with primary valvular MR. The most optimal treatment for ischemic MR is a matter of debate. If MR results transiently from papillary muscle dysfunction due to ischemia, then revascularization alone may be sufficient to treat the MR. If there are regional wall motion abnormalities, with annular dilatation and papillary muscle retraction, then direct intervention on the valve may be required. In those with significant impairment of left ventricular function, vasodilator therapy to reduce afterload and favorably influence left ventricular geometry can reduce MR severity.

23. **a.** Given LV dysfunction (EF <50%), this is a class I indication for surgery.

24. **a.** There is no indication for aortic valve surgery for the prevention of sudden death in this patient population without LV dysfunction (class I), exercise induced hypotension, or symptoms (class IIb). Since he is compliant with medical follow-up, it is unlikely that surgery would be delayed at time of symptom onset. If his AS were extremely severe (AVA <0.6 cm², mean gradient >60 mm Hg), surgery would be a IIb indication, if expected operative mortality ≤1.0%.

25. **c.** Aortic root dimension. The patient clinically has severe AI. The murmur is loudest at the right sternal border, suggesting aortic root dilation as a potential cause of his AI. The presence of root dilatation ($>$ or $=$ to 5.0 cm) may lead to earlier surgery, hence is vital to know. The diastolic rumble is most likely an Austin Flint murmur, and not concomitant mitral stenosis (no opening snap, $S_1$ not loud).

26. **a.** Cardiac catheterization with aortography. Clinically, the patient has severe aortic regurgitation. He is symptomatic. Consistent with this, the echocardiogram reveals a dilated left ventricle with low normal systolic function. The degree of aortic regurgitation must be underestimated by this study. When there is such discrepancy, proceed with aortography to confirm aortic regurgitation severity and to assess coronaries prior to surgical referral. As he is symptomatic, continued observation and/or medical therapy is not the preferred treatment approach. Beta-blockers, by prolonging the diastolic filling period, could actually increase regurgitant volume.

27. **a.** Transesophageal echocardiogram, emergent cardiac surgical consultation. The patient has a clinical presentation of severe acute aortic insufficiency (short diastolic murmur, soft $S_1$ from premature mitral valve closure, low output state, and pulmonary edema). In the context of chest pain, this scenario suggests aortic dissection until proven otherwise. The dissection flap likely involves the ostium of the right coronary artery, producing the inferior ST segment elevation. Thrombolytics should not be used until dissection is ruled out. Even if there is no dissection, balloon pumps should not be used with severe aortic insufficiency. The augmented diastolic pressure worsens the severity of the insufficiency. MRI would also provide the diagnosis, but given the hemodynamic instability of the patient, a bedside TEE would be a safer and quicker option to arrive at the diagnosis.

28. **b.** No evidence for dysfunction. The physical examination does not suggest either stenosis or insufficiency. He appears to be in a high-output state, secondary to his febrile illness. As a result, the gradients are increased. The LVOT VTI is also increased, secondary to the increased cardiac output. The LVOT/aortic valve VTI ratio is the same in the two echocardiograms, which would speak against any significant obstruction.

29. **a.** The clinical scenario, with a new first-degree AV block and acute aortic regurgitation, is highly suspicious for prosthetic valve abscess and possibly even partial dehiscence. A transesophageal echocardiogram should be performed, but prompt surgical consultation should also be requested. The patient is developing heart failure and is persistently febrile despite 1 week of antibiotic therapy.

30. **c.** With acute changes in atrial and ventricular compliance (as with valvuloplasty), the half-time is unreliable. Usually 72 hours or more is required after the procedure before the half-time can be used with reasonable reliability. Planimetry, if performed correctly, would provide a good estimate of stenosis severity. Clinically, the patient seems to have had a good result (longer $S_2$-OS interval, shorter murmur).

31. **a.** Observation. Most of these small shunts will close over the next 6 months without any intervention. The shunt is left to right by color. He has good $O_2$ saturation on room air, making any significant right-to-left shunting unlikely. Anticoagulation with an ASD/PFO may be recommended in certain settings, however not indefinitely, given the good chance that the defect will close.

32. **b.** He requires antibiotic prophylaxis with a prosthetic valve (by 2007 guidelines, prosthetic cardiac valves are an indication for SBE prophylaxis prior to dental procedures). These patients still require close follow-up with complete evaluations on a yearly basis. Some advocate a 3-month period of warfarin therapy

after bioprosthetic valve placement. He is now 4 months out, and has no other indications or a high-risk profile (LV dysfunction, prior embolic event, atrial fibrillation), thus warfarin is no longer needed at this time.

**33. a.** Transesophageal echocardiography. The echocardiogram reveals a normal-appearing aortic valve. Yet, the profile of the continuous wave Doppler jet is more consistent with a fixed obstruction, as opposed to the dagger shape of dynamic obstruction. These findings are suggestive of the presence of a subvalvular membrane. Transesophageal echocardiography would be useful to better delineate this area and identify the membrane. The patient already has a 5-m jet in the absence of systolic anterior motion; therefore, it would not be prudent to use provocation with amyl nitrate. A stress echocardiogram would have no diagnostic value, and may have some risk in the setting of symptomatic LVOT obstruction.

**34. e.** None of the above. By 2007 AHA guidelines, mitral valve prolapse is no longer a condition for which endocarditis prophylaxis is recommended. She should have follow-up sooner than 5 years. No documented role for beta-blockers, given her clinical presentation.

**35. c.** If there is echocardiographic evidence for high-risk MVP (leaflet thickening, elongated chordae, left atrial enlargement, LV dilatation), aspirin therapy is considered a class IIb indication. Therapy is clearly recommended if there have been documented stroke or transient ischemic events.

**36. b.** Continue vasodilator therapy and reassess. By ACC/AHA guidelines, decline in ejection fraction following stress echocardiography by itself is not an accepted indication for referral to surgical intervention. Owing to the high afterload and the increase in afterload on exercise, a small to modest decline in ejection fraction (<10%) may still be consistent with well-compensated aortic insufficiency. This patient has normal resting ejection fraction and mildly dilated left ventricle with excellent functional capacity.

**37. b.** Repeat echocardiogram with amyl nitrate (Fig. 2–10A–C). The physical examination is highly suggestive of hypertrophic cardiomyopathy (brisk, bisiferiens carotid pulse, normal $S_2$, murmur increasing with Valsalva and decreasing with handgrip). The patient may not have a significant resting tract gradient, but may have a significant provokable gradient. Generally, a transesophageal echocardiogram is not needed to make the diagnosis. Invasive hemodynamics with provocation would be useful, but angiography alone would not be sufficient.

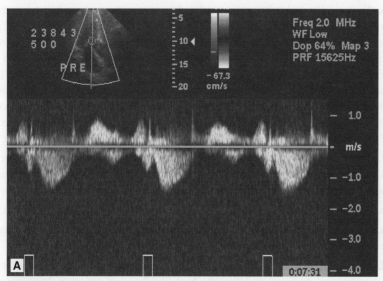

**FIGURE 2–10** *(Continued)*

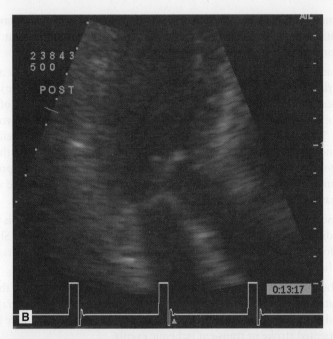

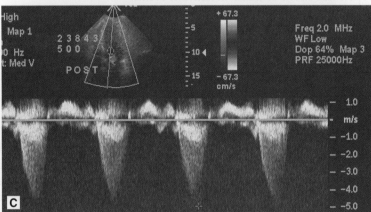

**FIGURE 2-10** **A.** Resting LVOT gradient; **B.** Post amyl, SAM evident; **C.** Post amyl LVOT gradient

**38. b.** Transesophageal echocardiography. By examination, the patient has mitral insufficiency. The echocardiogram is consistent with this, with an elevated peak transmitral gradient. Pressure half-time is not prolonged, thus there does not appear to be any significant stenosis (gradients elevated owing to increased flow from regurgitant volume). A TEE would be the most useful to confirm the diagnosis. Fluoroscopy may identify partial dehiscence, but would not be helpful if there were a leak in the setting of a well-seated valve. There is no evidence for stenosis, where fluoroscopic evaluation of leaflet motion could be diagnostic. There is no clinical evidence for endocarditis.

**39. a.** The bileaflet mechanical valves do not typically produce a loud opening sound, but do have prominent closing sounds. A brief diastolic rumble may be heard in a normally functioning prosthetic valve in the mitral position.

**40. b.** With the ball and cage valves, one would expect to hear the opening click as well.

**41. a.** Less than 2%. In the absence of symptoms, natural history studies would suggest a relatively low risk of sudden death.

**42. d.** More than 50%. He has a velocity across the aortic valve of greater than 4 m/s. Observational studies would suggest a high likelihood of symptom development in the next 3 years.

**43. a.** There is no indication for percutaneous valvuloplasty in this asymptomatic patient. This procedure has been advocated as a bridge to surgery in patients with symptomatic AS who are at the time considered too high risk for aortic valve replacement, or as palliation for symptomatic patients who are not surgical candidates (both class IIb indications). If preoperative intervention is required for noncardiac surgery, these patients should be evaluated for AVR.

**44. d.** ACC/AHA guidelines recommended an INR of 2.5 to 3.5 for patients with bileaflet tilting disk mechanical valves in the aortic position who have had a thromboembolic event, and who have atrial fibrillation, LV dysfunction, or a hypercoagulable state. Addition of low-dose ASA (75 to 100 mg) is a class I indication for all patients with mechanical heart valves, and those with the above risk factors and bioprosthetic valves.

**45. a.** Intravenous heparin. Since a small clot was present (without any obstruction to valve function) the patient would benefit from increased anticoagulant therapy. If he were to fail this, then the other alternatives could be considered, such as continuous infusion thrombolytic therapy. Such continuous therapy (although not bolus) could also be used as primary treatment. No established indications exist at this time for glycoprotein IIb/IIIa inhibitors in this clinical setting. It would not be advisable to proceed to reoperation just yet, in the absence of a large clot burden or obstruction to inflow. If treatment with heparin leads to clot resolution, then subsequent warfarin dosing should be increased to maintain INR in the 3.0 to 4.0 range.

**46. c.** Immediate electrical cardioversion. Primary treatment includes the initiation of anticoagulation and rate control measures. This patient is not hemodynamically unstable, so immediate cardioversion is not needed. Furthermore, the clinical history suggests that he has been in atrial fibrillation for greater than 24 to 48 hours. He is thus at increased risk for embolic events. Options include TEE-guided cardioversion with adequate anticoagulation, or anticoagulation with warfarin for at least 3 weeks followed by electrical cardioversion.

**47. a.** He should be on warfarin. Valvuloplasty in this setting (onset of atrial fibrillation, in an otherwise asymptomatic patient) is a class IIb indication by current guidelines.

**48. a.** If a thorough physical examination reveals no signs of cardiopulmonary disease and the patient has no symptoms, then reassurance and follow-up are all that are required. Echocardiography should be performed if obesity limits the physical examination or if signs or symptoms are present.

**49. b.** Fig. 2–5 A, B. Posterior leaflet prolapse with severe MR. Panel A demonstrates aortic stenosis; panel B is an example of predominant posterior leaflet prolapse with severe MR; panel C is an example of predominant anterior leaflet prolapse with severe MR; and panel D is an example of a posterior leaflet that is restricted with posteriorly directed MR. The presence of a soft $S_1$, normal carotid upstrokes, a holosystolic murmur that increases with handgrip, and an $S_3$ makes mitral regurgitation and not aortic stenosis the diagnosis. The radiation of the jet toward the base suggests an anterior jet direction, which is what would be expected with posterior leaflet prolapse. Both anterior leaflet prolapse and posterior leaflet restriction would produce a posteriorly directed jet.

**50. a.** A stress echo cardiogram. The patient does have evidence for mild resting pulmonary hypertension. If PA pressures increased significantly with exercise (to >60 mm Hg), referral for mitral valve surgery could be considered (class IIa indication by ACC/AHA guidelines). Referral for surgery is reasonable (class IIa indication) if chance of repair is greater than 90%. However, it would not be appropriate to refer for valve replacement in this situation. There are no data to suggest a beneficial role for the addition of afterload-reducing agents in the absence of systemic hypertension (again, by ACC/AHA guidelines). There is absolutely no role for the prophylactic use of amiodarone. Close clinical follow-up is reasonable, but repeat evaluation should not be deferred for 2 years. Guidelines use LV dimensions and ejection fraction to guide surgical intervention, even in the absence of symptoms. As such, these patients should have clinical re-evaluation and echo every 6 months.

51. **a.** Centers experienced in valve repair are increasingly moving to recommend surgery for asymptomatic patients with preserved LV function, and it is a class IIa indication by most recent guidelines. However, valve replacement is not recommended. In fact, in situations where there is significant doubt about the feasibility of repair, referral for surgery is a class III indication, in the absence of symptoms, LV dysfunction (EF <60%), LV dilatation (end-systolic dimension ≥4.0 cm), onset of atrial fibrillation, or presence of pulmonary hypertension (>50 mm Hg at rest, >60 mm Hg with exercise).

52. **a.** He is now symptomatic with depressed ejection fraction and a dilated left ventricle. This is a class I indication for surgery. Valve repair as opposed to replacement is the preferred surgical treatment. Medical therapy may be needed as an adjunct, but is insufficient as the sole treatment.

53. **b.** Referral for surgery. This is an asymptomatic patient with preserved LV function. The presence of a rheumatic etiology with calcification makes repair significantly less likely. This is a class III indication. This patient is hypertensive, so addition of an ACEI is reasonable.

54. **d.** Stress echocardiography. His symptoms are equivocal, and may just be related to deconditioning. A stress echocardiogram to assess PA pressures and LV response may be useful here. There is insufficient data to refer directly to surgery at this point.

55. **a.** There are data from the Mayo Clinic suggesting increased incidence of sudden death in such patients. However, data from Rosenhek et al., which was a prospective study following patients closely and referring only when guidelines were met, suggested a low event rate. Surgery in this setting is a class IIa indication, not a class I indication. There are numerous series that suggest that patients with severe MR will come to intervention within the next 10 years.

56. **c.** Mitral and tricuspid stenosis. The loud $S_1$, opening snap, and apical diastolic rumble are features of mitral stenosis. The presence of the diastolic rumble along the sternal border, which increases with inspiration, along with the prominent *a* wave in the JVP and evidence of systemic venous congestion (hepatomegaly, peripheral edema) suggests that concomitant tricuspid stenosis is present as well.

57. **c.** Cardiac catheterization. By physical examination, the patient has severe aortic stenosis (no $A_2$ of second heart sound, late-peaking murmur, and diminished carotid upstrokes). A stress test would not be appropriate in a patient with symptomatic aortic stenosis. An echocardiogram would usually be the first step, but proceeding directly to catheterization to measure transvalvular gradients and assess coronary anatomy would be reasonable. SL NTG could have disastrous consequences in this setting. By reducing preload, it may precipitate syncope.

58. **b.** Refer for balloon valvuloplasty. He has symptomatic critical aortic stenosis. Aortic valve replacement, with concomitant need for anticoagulation while on cardiopulmonary bypass, is not an attractive first option. Proceeding directly to gastric surgery would carry high risk, given the ongoing symptoms. Valvuloplasty would be a reasonable bridge to lower risk from the noncardiac surgery.

59. **a.** Bovine pericardial valve. He is at an age where there is substantial durability of the bioprosthetic valve. He is at increased risk for anticoagulation, thus mechanical valves would not be the valve of first choice. By history, he would not appear to need anticoagulation for any other indication. Homograft is not unreasonable, but there would not appear to be any hemodynamic or durability benefits for an 80-year-old patient, and its insertion requires a more difficult operation.

**60. a.** Stress test. The patient has significant aortic regurgitation with a dilated left ventricle (although not yet at the dimensions that would be indicative of surgery in the absence of symptoms, either class I or II: His end-systolic dimension is less than 5.0 cm and end-diastolic dimension is less than 7.0 cm). He leads a sedentary lifestyle, and although he has no dyspnea, he does relate some equivocal symptom. A stress test would be useful to assess functional capacity and to objectively assess symptoms. If he were to develop symptoms at a low level of exercise, this may be an indication for surgical intervention. A vasodilator may be useful (class IIb indication with dilated LV), but he would need more frequent follow-up, given the LV dilatation.

**61. b.** Surgical Intervention (Refer for surgery). His ventricle has dilated even further. An end-diastolic dimension of greater than 7.5 cm is a class IIa indication for surgery and is associated with an increased risk of sudden death, even in the absence of symptoms.

**62. b.** Mean gradient 17 mm Hg. The clinical presentation and examination are suggestive of prosthetic mitral stenosis (long diastolic rumble, muffled closing click, clinical heart failure). The PMI is not displaced, so it is unlikely that she has significant left ventricular dysfunction. There are no clinical signs of severe MR.

**63. a.** Urgent reoperation. She appears to have significant thrombus burden leading to valvular obstruction and has significant congestive heart failure. By ACC/AHA guidelines, reoperation would be the preferred treatment approach in this setting. If other comorbidities were prohibitive, thrombolytic therapy could be considered.

**64. a.** The examination is highly suggestive of Ebstein's anomaly (presence of TR, widely split first heart sound with sail-like second component). The echocardiogram confirms this. Accessory pathways are frequently associated with this condition.

**65. a.** Echocardiography with saline contrast. Ebstein's anomaly is frequently associated with cardiac shunts (either patent foramen ovale, or atrial or ventricular septal defect). The setting of a TIA in someone who has been immobilized (such as with a fracture) raises the concern of paradoxical embolism of a venous thrombus to the systemic circulation.

**66. b.** Doppler echocardiography using the continuity equation. With significant insufficiency, the Gorlin formula becomes less reliable. Pressure half-time is not used to calculate aortic valve area, but does give a clue to the severity of the aortic insufficiency.

**67. c.** Aortic homograft. Mechanical and bioprosthetic valves have a similar incidence of endocarditis, which is higher than that seen for homografts. In the setting of acute bacterial endocarditis of a prosthetic aortic valve, homografts are the valve of first choice when surgery is indicated.

**68. d.** The patient has severe aortic stenosis with clinical evidence of heart failure and hypoperfusion. His low albumin suggests a chronically ill state. This is a case where percutaneous valvuloplasty may be useful, as a bridge to more definitive surgical therapy. Improved perfusion post valvuloplasty may allow for improved overall status and a lower risk for aortic valve replacement. Surgery may also be considered at this point. A balloon pump may be helpful, and some centers may opt for these approaches. Dialysis is unlikely to help in that it does not address the most likely cause of renal dysfunction, which is impaired renal perfusion.

**69. b.** The physical examination is consistent with pulmonic stenosis (presence of thrill, right ventricular heave, ejection click, crescendo-decrescendo murmur loudest over the pulmonic area). Normal carotid upstrokes and preserved $A_2$ makes significant aortic stenosis unlikely. The murmur is not consistent with a regurgitant murmur.

**70. a.** The presence of exertional dyspnea, angina, syncope, or near-syncope are class I indications for intervention. For gradients between 30 and 39 mm Hg, there is some divergence of opinion about the role of intervention (class IIb for gradients 30 to 39). There is no role for intervention in those with gradients less than 30 mm Hg who have no symptoms. A peak-to-peak gradient >40 mm Hg by catheterization is a class I indication for intervention, even in an asymptomatic patient.

**71. a.** Percutaneous valvuloplasty. This is the preferred treatment for young adults with pulmonic stenosis.

**72. d.** The most common cause of tricuspid insufficiency is pulmonary hypertension that results from primary pathology on the left side of the heart. This includes aortic and mitral valvular disease, as well as left ventricular dysfunction from coronary artery disease or other cardiomyopathies.

**73. c.** There is a greater risk of thrombosis with mechanical valves at the tricuspid position than at other valve positions, hence bioprosthetic valves are generally preferred. In secondary TR, resulting from RV and annular dilatation from left-sided disease and pulmonary hypertension, annuloplasty is usually successful in alleviating the regurgitation, in conjunction with treatment of the left-sided valve disease.

**74. a.** *Streptococcus. viridans* accounts for up to 50% of cases. *Staphylococcus. aureus* is the next most common pathogen.

**75. c.** *Staphylococcus epidermidis.* This patient presents with early prosthetic valve endocarditis (within 2 months of surgery). This is usually acquired during the operation, and the skin species *S. epidermidis* is the most frequent pathogen encountered. Late prosthetic valve endocarditis is similar to native valve endocarditis in terms of the spectrum of pathogens involved.

**76. d.** Recurrent embolic events and persistent vegetations despite appropriate antibiotic therapy. By recent ACC/AHA guidelines, this is a class IIa indication. All the others listed are class I indications.

**77. d.** Surgically repaired ASD. This is considered to have a negligible risk, by recent ACA/AHA guidelines. All the others listed, along with surgically constructed systemic-pulmonary shunts, are considered high-risk populations.

**78. a.** Dental procedures involving manipulation of gingival tissue or perforation of oral mucosa. Respiratory tract procedures in which prophylaxis is reasonable are those involving incision of the respiratory tract mucosa (such as tonsillectomy, adenoidectomy, and bronchoscopy only if there will be incision of the mucosa), or procedures done to treat active infections. By the latest guidelines, antibiotics solely to prevent endocarditis is no longer recommended for GI or GU tract procedures, including EGD and colonoscopy.

**79. d.** All the other regimens listed are current guidelines.

**80. d.** Dipyridamole should not be used because of harmful effects to the fetus. It is imperative that the physicians discuss thoroughly these issues of anticoagulation with any patients considering pregnancy.

**81. c.** Severe mitral regurgitation with functional class I. Generally, regurgitant lesions are better tolerated than stenotic lesions, as pregnancy is associated with decreased systemic vascular resistance. Cardiac output and blood volume are increased, usually compounding stenotic lesions. Eisenmenger's and aortic stenosis with a mean gradient >50 mm Hg are both associated with significant maternal and fetal risk. The aortic regurgitation in and of itself could likely be tolerated, but in the setting of Marfan's syndrome, the concern is for aortic root dilatation as the etiology for the aortic regurgitation. There is a risk of aortic dissection and rupture in these patients, particularly if the root size is greater than 4.0 cm.

# Suggested Reading

Bonow RO, Carabello BA, Chatterjee K, et al. ACC/AHA 2006 guidelines for the management of patients with valvular heart disease: a report of the American College of Cardiology/ American Heart Association Task Force on Practice Guidelines (Writing Committee to Develop Guidelines for the Management of Patients with Valvular Heart Disease). American Heart Association Web Site. Available at: http://www.americanheart.org. *Circulation.* 2006 Aug 1;114(5):e84–231.

Bonow RO, Lakatos E, Maron BJ, et al. Serial long-term assessment of the natural history of asymptomatic patients with chronic aortic regurgitation and normal left ventricular systolic function. *Circulation.* 1991 Oct;84(4):1625–1635.

Centers for Disease Control and Prevention. Cardiac valvulopathy associated with exposure to fenfluramine and dexfenfluramine: US Department of Health and Human Services interim public health recommendations, November 1997. *JAMA.* 1997;278:1729–1731.

Enriquez-Sarano M, Avierinos JF, Messika-Zeitoun D, et al. Quantitative determinants of the outcome of asymptomatic mitral regurgitation. *N Engl J Med.* 2005 Mar 3;352(9):875–883.

Grigioni F, Enriquez-Sarano M, Ling LH, et al. Sudden death in mitral regurgitation due to flail leaflet. *J Am Coll Cardiol.* 1999 Dec;34(7):2078–2085.

Ling LH, Enriquez-Sarano M, Seward JB, et al. Clinical outcome of mitral regurgitation due to flail leaflet. *N Engl J Med.* 1996 Nov 7;335(19):1417–1423.

Otto CM, Burwash IG, Legget ME, et al. Prospective study of asymptomatic valvular aortic stenosis. Clinical, echocardiographic, and exercise predictors of outcome. *Circulation.* 1997 May 6;95(9):2262–2270.

Rosenhek R, Rader F, Klaar U, et al. Outcome of watchful waiting in asymptomatic severe mitral regurgitation. *Circulation.* 2006 May 9;113(18):2238–2244.

Wilson W, Taubert KA, Gewitz M, et al. American Heart Association. Prevention of infective endocarditis: guidelines from the American Heart Association: a guideline from the American Heart Association Rheumatic Fever, Endocarditis, and Kawasaki Disease Committee, Council on Cardiovascular Disease in the Young, and the Council on Clinical Cardiology, Council on Cardiovascular Surgery and Anesthesia, and the Quality of Care and Outcomes Research Interdisciplinary Working Group. *Circulation.* 2007 Oct 9; 116(15):1736–1754.

**NOTES**

# chapter 3

# Acute Myocardial Infarction

DEEPAK L. BHATT

## QUESTIONS

1. A 54-year-old man comes into the emergency department reporting worsening chest pain and dyspnea on exertion. His vital signs are stable. An ECG shows T-wave inversion anterolaterally. Which of the following should be your next step?

   **a.** give aspirin
   **b.** start heparin
   **c.** start nitroglycerin
   **d.** TTE
   **e.** cardiac catheterization

2. The patient is given an aspirin and started on IV heparin and nitroglycerin. The patient's chest pain worsens, and he becomes hypotensive. Which of the following is an unlikely explanation for this clinical scenario?

   **a.** RV infarction
   **b.** aortic stenosis
   **c.** pulmonary embolus
   **d.** esophageal spasm
   **e.** vagal episode

3. A 68-year-old woman comes into the emergency room with worsening chest pain at rest for the past 24 hours. The troponin level is elevated. An ECG shows 1- to 2-mm ST depression in leads II, III, and aVF. Which of the following is the *least* appropriate treatment?

   **a.** aspirin
   **b.** heparin
   **c.** glycoprotein (GP) IIb/IIIa inhibitors
   **d.** LMWH
   **e.** ticlopidine

4. During catheterization, the patient's pain continues. She has received aspirin and heparin and is on eptifibatide. What should your next step be?

   **a.** add tirofiban and recatheterize in 2 days
   **b.** emergent bypass surgery
   **c.** dipyridamole (Persantine) nuclear stress test
   **d.** IABP placement
   **e.** angioplasty and stenting

5. Because of his hemodynamic deterioration, he is taken to the catheterization laboratory emergently. The right coronary artery (RCA) is normal. Left ventriculography is shown in systole and diastole. What is the abnormality (Fig. 3–1)?

**NOTES**

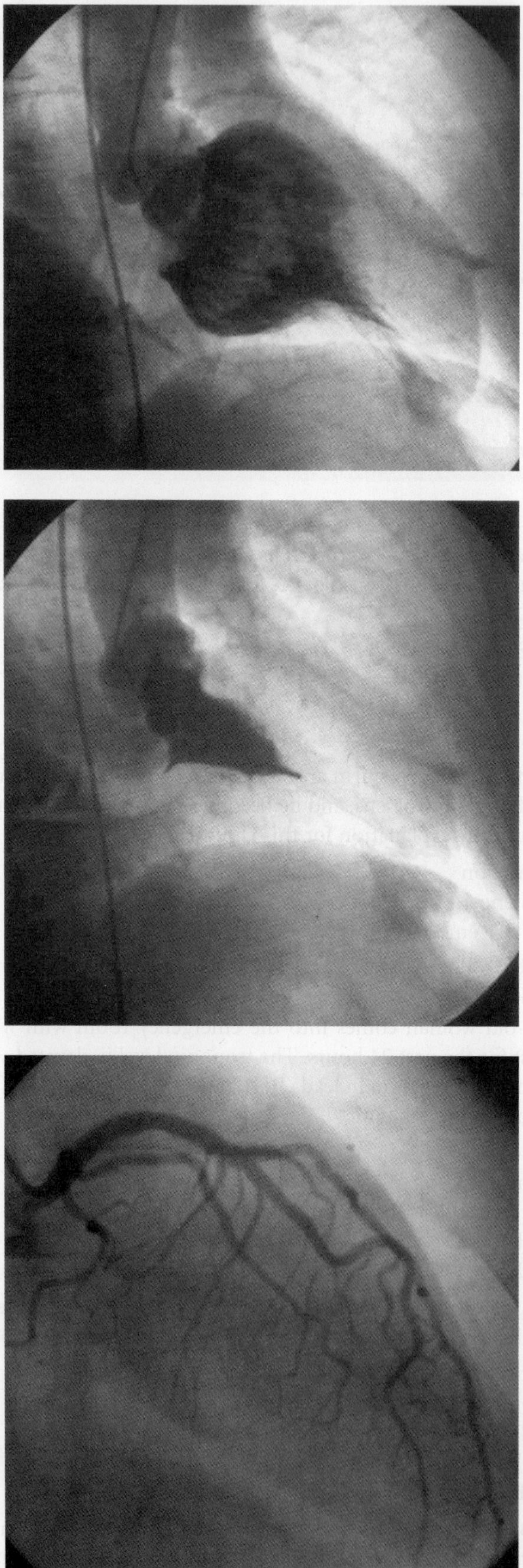

**FIGURE 3–1** From Bhatt DL, Heupler FA. Coronary angiography. In: Topol EJ, Prystowsky EN, Califf RM, et al., eds. *Textbook of Cardiovascular Medicine*, 2nd ed. Philadelphia: Lippincott Williams & Wilkins, 2002: eFigure 78.3.5E, with permission.

**a.** anomalous left anterior descending artery (LAD) with severe stenosis

**b.** hypertrophic cardiomyopathy

**c.** aortic stenosis

**d.** LV aneurysm

**e.** LV pseudoaneurysm

**6.** What abnormality does the arrow indicate (Fig. 3–2)?

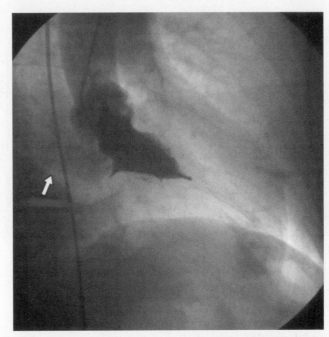

**FIGURE 3–2**    From Bhatt DL, Heupler FA. Coronary angiography. In: Topol EJ, Prystowsky EN, Califf RM, et al., eds. *Textbook of Cardiovascular Medicine*, 2nd ed. Philadelphia: Lippincott Williams & Wilkins, 2002: eFigure 78.3.5E, with permission.

**a.** VSD

**b.** aortic dissection

**c.** MR

**d.** anomalous pulmonary venous return

**e.** bicuspid aortic valve

**7.** Appropriate methods to treat RV infarction might include all of the following *except*

**a.** aggressive hydration

**b.** AV pacing

**c.** IABP placement

**d.** reperfusion

**e.** diuresis

**8.** Which of the following has been shown to potentially trigger acute MI?

**a.** earthquakes

**b.** stress

**c.** anger

**d.** sexual activity

**e.** all of the above

**9.** Which of the following is the mechanism of action of clopidogrel?

**a.** thromboxane inhibition

**b.** GP IIb/IIIa receptor blockade

**c.** adenosine diphosphate blockade

**d.** increase in cyclic adenosine monophosphate production
**e.** free radical scavenger

**10.** A 64-year-old man comes into a rural emergency department reporting worsening chest pain. His vital signs are stable. The ECG is shown in Figure 3–3. What should your next step be?

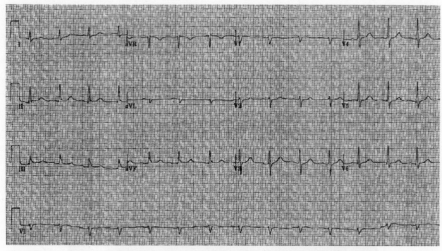

**FIGURE 3–3**

**a.** give aspirin
**b.** give aspirin, heparin, and fibrinolytics
**c.** give sublingual nitroglycerin and reassess
**d.** move to the waiting area and observe symptoms
**e.** discharge to home

**11.** In which of the following has the high-sensitivity C-reactive protein (CRP) been shown to be predictive of risk?

**a.** acute MI
**b.** acute coronary syndromes (ACSs)
**c.** chronic stable angina
**d.** peripheral vascular disease
**e.** all of the above

**12.** Which of the following has been shown to decrease the level of the high-sensitivity CRP?

**a.** unopposed estrogen
**b.** amlodipine besylate (Norvasc)
**c.** simvastatin
**d.** all of the above
**e.** none of the above

**13.** The patient has hypotension. To which of the following is this most likely due?

**a.** volume depletion
**b.** RV infarction
**c.** pulmonary embolism
**d.** aortic dissection
**e.** pericarditis

**14.** The patient is given nitroglycerin with no response and a GI cocktail with partial resolution of symptoms. He is sent to the waiting area. While there, his wife sees him slump over, and he is found to be in VF. After several shocks, he is successfully defibrillated. His next ECG is shown in Figure 3–4. What should your next step be?

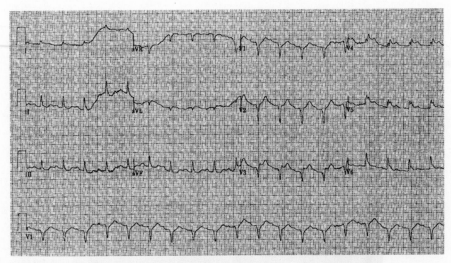

**FIGURE 3–4**

    **a.** aspirin, heparin, and full-dose tissue plasminogen activator (tPA)
    **b.** aspirin, heparin, and abciximab
    **c.** aspirin, low-molecular-weight heparin (LMWH), and abciximab
    **d.** aspirin, LMWH, abciximab, and full-dose t-PA
    **e.** aspirin and heparin; transfer the patient to a tertiary care center (3 hours away) for primary percutaneous coronary intervention (PCI)

**15.** Which of the following is an effective adjunct to increase the rate of smoking cessation?

    **a.** aldosterone
    **b.** bupropion
    **c.** buspirone
    **d.** cimetidine
    **e.** allopurinol

**16.** Bupropion hydrochloride (Zyban) is contraindicated in patients with a history of which of the following?

    **a.** seizures
    **b.** insulin-dependent diabetes mellitus
    **c.** severe chronic obstructive pulmonary disease (with reversible component)
    **d.** longer than 40-year history of tobacco use
    **e.** recent MI

**17.** Which of the following is *true* for management of acute ST segment–elevation MI?

    **a.** Aspirin has a much larger effect than streptokinase.
    **b.** Streptokinase has a much larger effect than aspirin.
    **c.** Streptokinase and aspirin each have a similar effect on outcome.
    **d.** When streptokinase and aspirin are used together, their effects are blunted.

**18.** Currently recommended therapies in the emergency department for acute MI include all of the following *except*

    **a.** aspirin
    **b.** tPA
    **c.** prasugrel
    **d.** heparin

**19.** Which of the following is *least* predictive of mortality in patients presenting with acute MI who are treated with fibrinolytics?

    **a.** location of MI (i.e., anterior vs. inferior)
    **b.** age
    **c.** heart rate

**d.** BP

**e.** presence or absence of diabetes

**f.** Killip class

**20.** The patient receives aspirin, heparin, and t-PA. He is transferred for catheterization. On arrival, he is sedated, intubated, and hemodynamically stable. The patient is taken to the catheterization laboratory. What do you see in Figures 3–5 and 3–6?

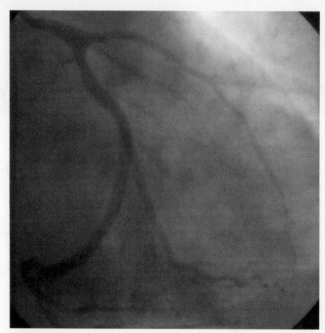

**FIGURE 3–5**

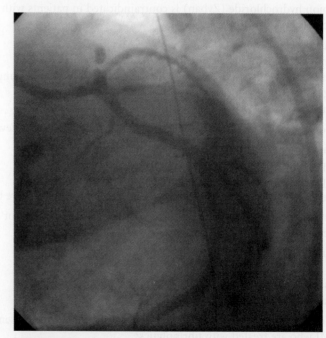

**FIGURE 3–6**

**a.** severe left main disease
**b.** LAD occlusion
**c.** diagonal occlusion
**d.** left circumflex artery (LCx) occlusion
**e.** mild LAD stenosis with thrombus

21. The patient is taken to the catheterization laboratory. What is the abnormality (Fig. 3–7)?

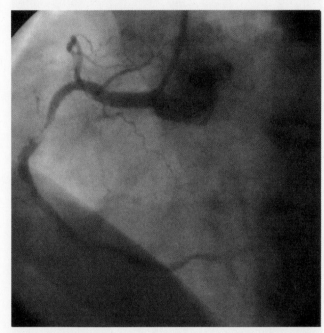

**FIGURE 3–7**

**a.** spontaneous dissection
**b.** coronary spasm
**c.** anomalous origin of severely stenosed vessel
**d.** severe stenosis with thrombus
**e.** coronary aneurysm

22. Which of the following have oral beta-blockers for acute MI been shown to do?

**a.** decrease the rate of intracranial hemorrhage from fibrinolysis
**b.** decrease ventricular arrhythmias
**c.** improve mortality
**d.** all of the above
**e.** none of the above

23. In the setting of primary angioplasty for acute MI, which of the following have stents been convincingly shown to do?

**a.** decrease subsequent repeat target vessel revascularization (TVR)
**b.** decrease long-term mortality
**c.** decrease long-term MI risk
**d.** decrease the incidence of heart failure

24. A 70-year-old woman comes into the emergency department reporting 3 hours of crushing chest pain. The initial ECG shows NSR with nonspecific ST-T–wave changes. Initial troponin is borderline positive. Because of the patient's severe chest pain, she is taken to the catheterization laboratory. What do the angiograms (Fig. 3–8) demonstrate?

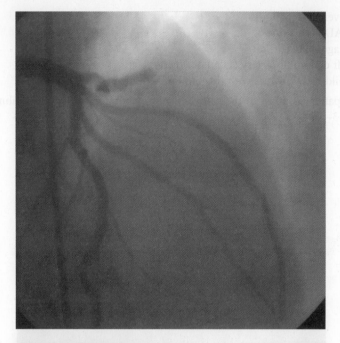

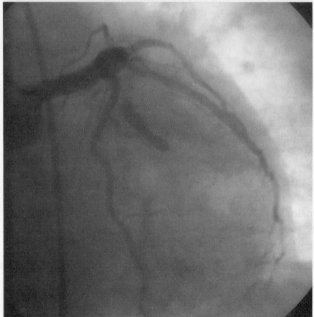

**FIGURE 3–8**

    **a.** severe LAD stenosis
    **b.** normal coronary arteries
    **c.** occluded LAD
    **d.** occluded LCx
    **e.** occluded RCA

**25.** Factors believed to be important in the pathogenesis of plaque rupture include which of the following?

    **a.** matrix metalloproteinases
    **b.** shear stress
    **c.** macrophages
    **d.** all of the above
    **e.** none of the above

**26.** The angiogram (Fig. 3–9) shows the result after PCI. What do you see?

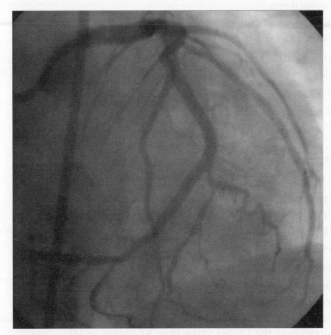

**FIGURE 3–9**

    **a.** residual stenosis
    **b.** propagation of thrombus
    **c.** procedural dissection flap
    **d.** patent vessel with thrombolysis in myocardial infarction (TIMI)-3 flow
    **e.** patent vessel with TIMI-1 flow

**27.** What physical examination findings may be present in a patient with the following findings at catheterization (Fig. 3–10)?

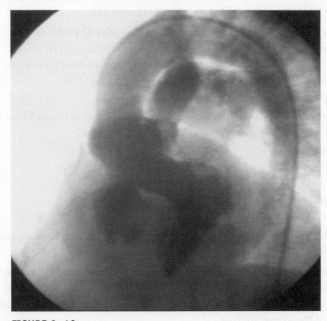

**FIGURE 3–10**

**a.** $S_3$
**b.** systolic and diastolic murmur
**c.** pericardial rub
**d.** crescendo-decrescendo systolic murmur
**e.** diastolic rumble

28. The rate of stroke seen in the Global Utilization of Streptokinase and tPA for Occluded Coronary Arteries (GUSTO)-III trial was approximately which of the following?

    **a.** 0.01%
    **b.** 0.1%
    **c.** 1%
    **d.** 10%

29. Which of the following is *true* about reteplase in GUSTO-III?

    **a.** It had a significantly higher rate of stroke than alteplase.
    **b.** It significantly reduced mortality compared with alteplase.
    **c.** It significantly reduced mortality, but increased stroke compared with alteplase.
    **d.** It had similar rates of mortality to alteplase.

30. Which of the following statements is *not* true?

    **a.** Vitamin E is beneficial for acute MI patients.
    **b.** Fibrinolysis leads to platelet activation.
    **c.** Unstable angina and non–ST-elevation MI are more common causes of hospitalization in the United States than ST-elevation MI.
    **d.** Troponin levels are useful for risk stratification of acute MI.

31. The Antiarrhythmics Versus Implantable Defibrillators study showed that which of the following is true for patients with acute MI who survive VF or sustained, symptomatic VT with an EF less than or equal to 40%?

    **a.** They benefit from an ICD more than antiarrhythmic therapy.
    **b.** They benefit from EP testing to decide whether an ICD is indicated.
    **c.** They should receive an ICD and concomitant amiodarone.
    **d.** All of the above are true.
    **e.** None of the above is true.

32. The Survival and Ventricular Enlargement study demonstrated which of the following regarding captopril among patients with MI?

    **a.** It decreased mortality if patients did not receive fibrinolysis.
    **b.** It decreased mortality in patients with symptomatic CHF.
    **c.** It decreased the need for subsequent CHF-related hospitalization.
    **d.** All of the above are true.
    **e.** None of the above is true.

33. With which of the following is sildenafil acetate (Viagra) most likely to interact adversely?

    **a.** fibrinolytic therapy
    **b.** primary PCI
    **c.** nitrates
    **d.** aspirin
    **e.** beta-blockers

34. The GUSTO-I trial showed which of the following regarding accelerated tPA for acute MI?

    **a.** It reduced mortality compared with streptokinase and IV heparin.
    **b.** It reduced mortality compared with streptokinase and SC heparin.
    **c.** It increased the rate of hemorrhagic stroke compared with streptokinase.
    **d.** All of the above are true.
    **e.** None of the above is true.

**35.** For patients presenting with cardiogenic shock, which of the following was demonstrated in the SHOCK trial?

 **a.** There is a statistically significant reduction in mortality at 30 days with early revascularization.

 **b.** In the patients randomized to medical therapy, the rate of mortality at 30 days was almost 100%.

 **c.** At 6 months, mortality was reduced by over 50% in patients randomized to emergency revascularization.

 **d.** All of the above are true.

 **e.** None of the above is true.

**36.** Which of the following statements is *true* regarding patients who develop VF after admission for acute MI?

 **a.** VF in the first 48 hours is generally benign.

 **b.** VF in the first 48 hours is associated with a worse prognosis.

 **c.** Only VF developing after 48 hours affects prognosis.

 **d.** None of the above is true.

**37.** Which of the following supports the routine use of type 1 antiarrhythmics in patients with PVCs who have had an MI?

 **a.** the Cardiac Arrhythmia Suppression Trial (CAST) study

 **b.** the Basal Antiarrhythmic Study of Infarct Survival (BASIS) study

 **c.** the Multicenter Unsustained Tachycardia Trial (MUSTT) study

 **d.** all of the above

 **e.** none of the above

**38.** The MADIT-I trial showed which of the following in patients with prior MI?

 **a.** ICD implantation decreased mortality in patients with an EF ≤35%.

 **b.** ICD implantation reduced mortality in patients with an abnormal signal-averaged ECG.

 **c.** ICD implantation in patients with suppressible VT on EP testing had decreased mortality.

 **d.** ICDs decreased mortality in patients, irrespective of their baseline LV function.

**39.** In patients with acute MI who undergo angiography, which of the following statements is *true* regarding TIMI flow?

 **a.** TIMI-3 flow is associated with a higher mortality than TIMI-2 flow.

 **b.** TIMI-2 or -3 flow is associated with a patent artery.

 **c.** TIMI-2 and -3 flows are associated with similar rates of mortality.

 **d.** All of the above are true.

 **e.** None of the above is true.

**40.** In diabetic patients with acute MI, the rate of mortality compared with nondiabetic patients is approximately which of the following?

 **a.** the same

 **b.** twice as high

 **c.** five times as high

 **d.** ten times as high

**41.** Which of the following statements about acute MI is *false*?

 **a.** An elevated white blood cell count is associated with a greater risk of mortality.

 **b.** Aspirin, beta-blockers, and ACE inhibitors remain underused.

 **c.** Passive smoking is a risk factor for lung cancer as well as for heart disease.

 **d.** Patients with a history of heart failure should not receive beta-blockers.

**42.** For acute MI, which of the following is *true*?

 **a.** Large, randomized studies have found that nitrates reduce long-term mortality.

 **b.** ACE inhibitors have been shown to reduce mortality.

**NOTES**

c. Multiple randomized studies have found that heparin reduces mortality.
d. All of the above are true.
e. None of the above is true.

43. Which of the following is a true statement about the class III antiarrhythmic dofetilide in acute MI?

    a. It decreases the rate of death compared with placebo.
    b. It increases the rate of death compared with placebo.
    c. It is effective for the treatment of AFib and flutter.
    d. It decreases the risk of torsades de pointes.
    e. A, C, and D are true.

44. In acute MI, which of the following is *true* about IV lidocaine?

    a. When used prophylactically, it reduces mortality by more than 50%.
    b. It should not be used prophylactically.
    c. It should be administered routinely in patients with an EF of less than 35%.
    d. It should be given to all patients who receive streptokinase.

45. During acute MI, which of the following is *true* about IV magnesium?

    a. It should be routinely administered owing to its significant survival benefit.
    b. It should be administered as an adjunct to primary PCI.
    c. It does not have a clear benefit in patients undergoing reperfusion therapy.
    d. It has a significant additive effect when used with fibrinolytics.

46. Warfarin is strongly indicated in patients with acute MI who have which of the following conditions?

    a. AFib
    b. symptomatic LV dysfunction
    c. asymptomatic LV dysfunction
    d. all of the above
    e. none of the above

47. Which of the following statements is *true* regarding MI owing to cocaine abuse?

    a. Cocaine promotes coagulation.
    b. Cocaine accelerates atherosclerosis.
    c. Cocaine can trigger coronary spasm.
    d. Cocaine can raise BP.
    e. All of the above are true.
    f. None of the above is true.

48. A 64-year-old man presents with chest pain and is noted to have ST elevation in his inferior leads. His BP is 80/40, and his pulse is 130 bpm. The heart sounds are distant, and the neck veins are elevated. Which of the following would be the best next step?

    a. fibrinolysis
    b. coronary angiography
    c. TTE
    d. heparinization
    e. all of the above

49. A quick bedside TTE is performed and shows a large pericardial effusion. Which of the following would be the best next step?

    a. fibrinolysis
    b. IABP placement
    c. pericardiocentesis
    d. all of the above
    e. none of the above

50. Which of the following is approximately the 30-day mortality in the GUSTO-I trial in patients aged 75 years or older?

a. 1%
b. 5%
c. 20%
d. 50%
e. 90%

**51.** In the GUSTO-I trial, the benefit of tPA over streptokinase was greatest in those patients who were treated

   a. within 2 hours after MI
   b. between 2 and 4 hours after MI
   c. between 4 and 6 hours after MI
   d. over 6 hours after MI
   e. there was no time dependency observed in this trial

**52.** Which of the following was a finding of the GUSTO-II angioplasty study?

   a. Primary percutaneous transluminal coronary angioplasty (PTCA) reduced 30-day mortality when compared with accelerated-dose tPA.
   b. Accelerated tPA reduced 30-day mortality when compared with primary PTCA.
   c. Accelerated tPA and primary PTCA produced almost identical outcomes at 30 days.
   d. Primary PTCA with abciximab was superior to accelerated-dose tPA.

**53.** Two weeks after a hospitalization for an anterior wall MI, a 58-year-old man returns with reports of fever and chest pain. Laboratory studies are significant for an elevated white blood cell count. An ECG reveals ST elevation in the anterior, lateral, and inferior leads. Which of the following is the correct diagnosis?

   a. recurrent MI
   b. aneurysm formation
   c. myocardial abscess
   d. Dressler's syndrome
   e. none of the above

**54.** Which of the following have been used as therapy for post-MI pericarditis?

   a. aspirin
   b. nonsteroidal antiinflammatory drugs
   c. steroids
   d. colchicine
   e. all of the above
   f. none of the above

**55.** Which of the following is *true* regarding pericarditis in acute MI?

   a. Fibrinolysis has no effect on the incidence of pericarditis in MI.
   b. Fibrinolysis reduces the incidence of pericarditis in MI.
   c. Fibrinolysis increases the incidence of pericarditis in MI.
   d. No data have examined this issue.

**56.** A 78-year-old woman with an inferior wall MI is receiving tPA. One hour later, she reports a headache and is subsequently noted to be lethargic and not able to raise her right arm or leg. Which of the following would be the best next step?

   a. getting a stat head CT
   b. getting a stat ECG; if ST elevation resolves, stopping tPA infusion
   c. stopping tPA
   d. giving platelets

**57.** Which of the following would be useful to reverse the action of tPA?

   a. protamine
   b. hirudin
   c. cryoprecipitate

**d.** epsilon aminocaproic acid

**e.** B and C

**f.** C and D

**58.** A 55-year-old man with a history of mild hypertension comes into the emergency department with severe chest pain. He reports exertional and nonexertional chest discomfort over the past several months. His internist performed a stress thallium 2 weeks ago. This was normal at 93% maximal predicted heart rate. He is given an aspirin and three sublingual nitroglycerin tablets, with partial relief of his chest discomfort. He is given a GI cocktail, with further improvement in his chest discomfort. His troponin and cardiac enzymes are negative. He is placed in the chest pain unit for further observation. What does his initial ECG show (Fig. 3–11)?

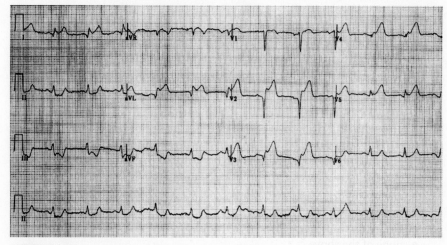

**FIGURE 3–11**

**a.** acute pericarditis

**b.** cardiac tamponade

**c.** ischemia

**d.** LV hypertrophy

**e.** AFib

**59.** Which of the following is *true* about ventricular septal rupture?

**a.** It is more common with inferior MI than with anterior MI.

**b.** It is less common with transmural MI than with nontransmural MI.

**c.** It is more common with a first MI.

**d.** All of the above are true.

**e.** None of the above is true.

**60.** Which of the following is *true* about acute MR in the setting of acute MI?

**a.** It is more common in women than in men.

**b.** It is more common in older patients than in younger patients.

**c.** It is more common in patients with a prior MI.

**d.** All of the above are true.

**e.** None of the above is true.

**61.** Regarding acute MR owing to MI, which of the following statements is *false*?

**a.** The posteromedial papillary muscle is supplied by the posterior descending artery.

**b.** The anterolateral papillary muscle is supplied by the LAD.

**c.** The anterolateral papillary muscle is supplied by the LCx.

**d.** Medical therapy is preferred over surgical therapy for definitive management.

**e.** All of the above are true.

**f.** All of the above are false.

**62.** The patient's second set of cardiac enzymes comes back elevated, and he is admitted to the cardiac care unit. An angiogram is performed. What is the infarct-related lesion on this angiogram (Fig. 3–12)?

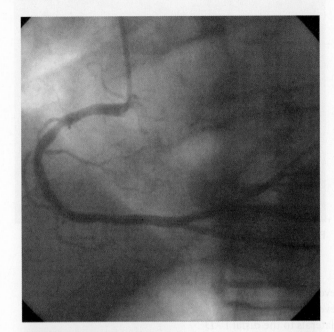

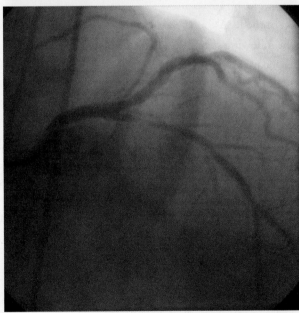

**FIGURE 3–12**

**a.** RCA stenosis

**b.** LCx stenosis

**c.** LAD stenosis

**d.** left main stenosis

**e.** no significant lesion

**63.** This patient is taken to the catheterization suite for an angiogram. What do you see in Figure 3–13?

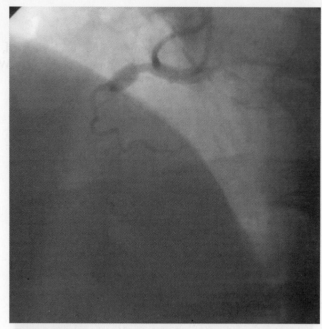

**FIGURE 3–13**

    **a.** a severe diagonal lesion
    **b.** a severe lateral circumflex lesion
    **c.** collaterals to the distal LAD
    **d.** collaterals to the RCA
    **e.** occlusion of the RCA

**64.** Which of the following statements about the use of IABPs is *false*?

    **a.** They may be useful in aortic stenosis.
    **b.** They may be useful in aortic regurgitation.
    **c.** They may be useful in MR.
    **d.** They may be useful in ventricular septal rupture.
    **e.** They may be useful in RV infarction.

**65.** A 68-year-old man presents with an anterior wall MI. His symptoms started 3 hours before. He has a history of hypertension and smoking. His heart rate is 90 bpm, and his BP is 240/120. He has an $S_3$ on examination. His lungs have rales at the bases. Which of the following is true?

    **a.** With his BP, fibrinolysis would be safer than primary angioplasty.
    **b.** His risk of intracranial hemorrhage is increased with tPA.
    **c.** Placement of an IABP is strongly indicated.
    **d.** A TEE should be the next step.
    **e.** None of the above is true.

**66.** A 72-year-old man has sustained an inferior wall MI. His BP is 200/100. Appropriate therapies may include all of the following *except*

    **a.** sublingual nifedipine
    **b.** IV metoprolol
    **c.** PO captopril
    **d.** IV nitroglycerin
    **e.** sublingual nitroglycerin

**67.** The patient remains hypotensive as these angiograms (Fig. 3–14) are performed. Now what do you think is the likely etiology of the hypotension?

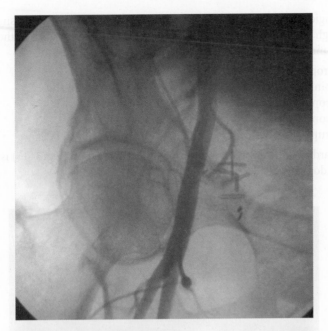

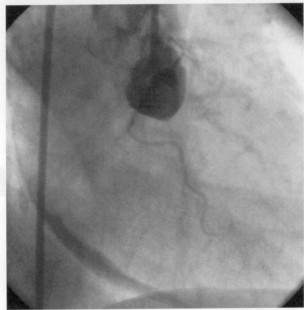

**FIGURE 3–14**

   **a.** retroperitoneal bleed
   **b.** groin hematoma
   **c.** coronary perforation
   **d.** coronary dissection
   **e.** abrupt vessel occlusion

**68.** An 84-year-old woman presents with an acute inferior MI. She is treated conservatively with aspirin, heparin, and nitroglycerin. You are asked to evaluate her 3 days after her infarction. She has been pain free since the day of her presentation, with no angina, CHF, or arrhythmia. Which of the following would be the best next step?

   **a.** diagnostic angiography only
   **b.** diagnostic angiography with ad hoc PCI if the anatomy is suitable
   **c.** symptom-limited treadmill exercise stress test before discharge
   **d.** discharge with no further evaluation

**NOTES**

**69.** An angioplasty is attempted, but difficulty is encountered in passing the wire through the lesion. The patient starts to get hypotensive. Which of the following is the most likely possibility to explain the hypotension?

**a.** retroperitoneal bleed
**b.** groin hematoma
**c.** coronary perforation
**d.** coronary dissection
**e.** abrupt vessel occlusion

**70.** The cardiac catheterization is performed. The angiogram (Fig. 3–15) is as follows. What do you see?

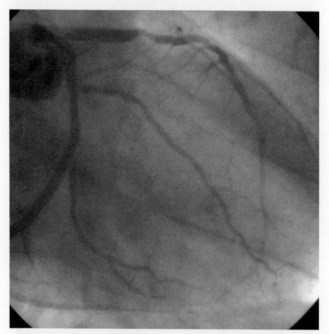

**FIGURE 3–15**

**a.** totally occluded LAD
**b.** collaterals to the LAD
**c.** severe lesion in the diagonal branch
**d.** severe lesion in the LCx
**e.** none of the above

**71.** A 68-year-old man is brought to the emergency department reporting chest pain for the past 2 hours. The bedside troponin is positive, and the initial ECG shows ST segment depression in the anterior leads. Appropriate next steps include any of the following *except*

**a.** aspirin
**b.** clopidogrel
**c.** tirofiban
**d.** eptifibatide
**e.** abciximab

**72.** The patient is given aspirin, heparin, nitroglycerin, metoprolol, and tirofiban, and his pain and ECG changes resolve. Which of the following would be the best next step?

**a.** exercise treadmill stress test
**b.** cardiac catheterization
**c.** TTE

**d.** positron emission tomography
**e.** IABP placement

**73.** What does this angiogram (Fig. 3–16) show?

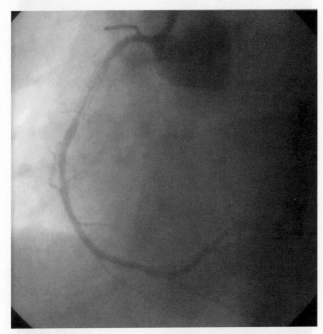

**FIGURE 3–16**

**a.** severe restenosis of the RCA
**b.** an intraluminal filling defect consistent with thrombus
**c.** stent edge dissection
**d.** extrinsic stent compression

**74.** A 47-year-old woman with a history of hypertension presents to your emergency department reporting chest pain. She tells you she had a stent placed in her RCA 4 months ago. Her ECG shows ST elevation in the inferior leads. Which of the following is a possible explanation of her chest pain?

**a.** stent thrombosis
**b.** stent restenosis
**c.** plaque rupture at a site elsewhere in her RCA
**d.** all of the above
**e.** none of the above

**75.** A 65-year-old woman sustains a non–ST segment elevation MI from which she recovers uneventfully. She had been taking aspirin, 325 mg per day. Appropriate steps on discharge may include all of the following *except*

**a.** increasing the dose of aspirin to 650 mg per day
**b.** starting clopidogrel, 75 mg per day
**c.** continuing aspirin at a dose of 81 mg per day
**d.** continuing aspirin at a dose of 162 mg per day

**76.** Which of the following is *true* regarding the placement of stents during acute MI angioplasty?

**a.** It decreases mortality.
**b.** It decreases TVR.
**c.** It leads to large improvements in rates of TIMI-3 flow.
**d.** It increases the risk of arrhythmia.
**e.** It decreases the rate of CHF.

**77.** An 83-year-old man presents to the catheterization suite with a chest pain syndrome. What does the LV angiogram show (Fig. 3–17)?

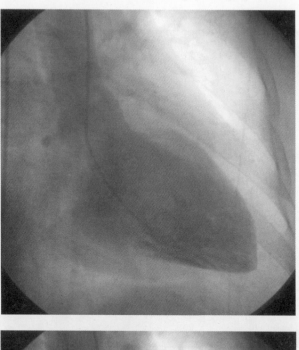

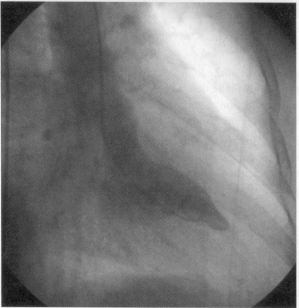

**FIGURE 3–17**

a. akinetic anterior wall
b. normal LV function
c. ventricular aneurysm
d. ventricular pseudoaneurysm
e. MR

**78.** Which of the following are indicators of successful reperfusion for acute MI?

a. resolution of chest pain
b. TIMI-3 flow on angiography
c. resolution of ST segment elevation

**d.** all of the above
**e.** none of the above

**79.** Which of the following is the most likely explanation for the patient's MI (Fig. 3–18)?

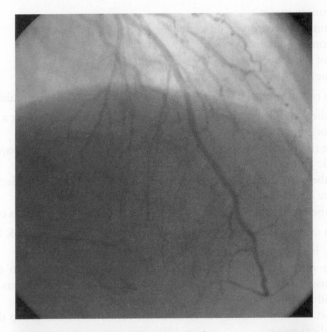

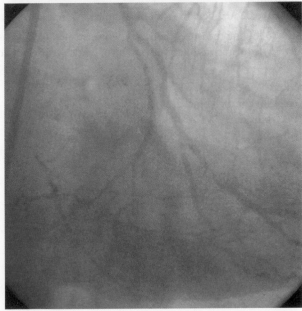

**FIGURE 3–18**

**a.** RCA occlusion
**b.** LAD occlusion
**c.** LCx occlusion
**d.** coronary dissection

**80.** Which of the following statements is *true* regarding the effect of gender on outcome after acute MI?

**a.** Female gender doubles the risk of mortality from MI.
**b.** Female gender triples the risk of mortality from MI.

**NOTES**

**c.** There is no large difference in outcome based on gender when age and other comorbidities are considered.

**d.** Women have one fourth the risk of death that men do.

**81.** Other than atherosclerosis, which of the following causes acute MI?

**a.** coronary spasm

**b.** spontaneous coronary dissection

**c.** coronary embolization

**d.** all of the above

**e.** none of the above

**82.** Which of the following statements is *true* regarding diabetes mellitus?

**a.** Diabetes raises the risk of MI the same amount as does having a history of prior MI.

**b.** The risk of MI owing to diabetes is entirely confined to insulin-requiring diabetic patients.

**c.** Diabetes increases the risk of MI but does not significantly affect outcome once an MI has occurred.

**d.** Diabetes has minimal impact on the risk of MI once patient age is considered.

**83.** Which of the following statements is *not* true regarding the SHOCK trial?

**a.** The majority of infarctions were anterior.

**b.** The difference in mortality between patients randomized to emergency revascularization versus initial medical stabilization at 30 days was not statistically significant.

**c.** Mortality at 6 months was lower in the revascularization group than in the medical group.

**d.** Patients derived equal benefit from revascularization, regardless of age.

**84.** Which of the following measures has been demonstrated to decrease the risk of perioperative MI during vascular surgery in patients with evidence of cardiac ischemia?

**a.** routine PA catheterization

**b.** use of calcium channel blockers

**c.** use of beta-blockers

**d.** use of nitrates

# Answers

1. **a.** Give aspirin. All the answers may be appropriate, but the question asked for the next step. This sort of question is common: Several correct answers are given, but you need to pick the most important one to do first.

2. **d.** Esophageal spasm. If anything, nitroglycerin would be expected to improve esophageal spasm. Not all nitrate-responsive pain is cardiac in etiology. Be aware of preload-dependent states, such as aortic stenosis, dehydration, cardiac tamponade, and RV infarction, in which nitroglycerin may cause hypotension.

3. **e.** Ticlopidine is the least appropriate treatment in this case. Clopidogrel in Unstable Angina to Prevent Recurrent Ischemic Events (CURE) data on clopidogrel are important but unlikely to be on the board examination (too recent). On the other hand, the LMWH and GP IIb/IIIa inhibitor data are old enough that you should know these agents have a role in ACS.

4. **e.** Angioplasty and stenting. Given the data from FRISC II (with LMWH) and TACTICS (Treat Angina with Aggrastat and Determine Costs of Therapy with Invasive or Conservative Strategies), TIMI-18 (with tirofiban), an invasive approach, is preferred to a conservative approach in patients presenting with ACSs. This is particularly true in patients with elevated troponin or ST depression. Even with a conservative approach, a patient with refractory ischemia on medical therapy would be a candidate for early revascularization.

5. **b.** Hypertrophic cardiomyopathy. There is no significant disease in the LAD, just prominent septal perforators. The comment about the normal RCA, while showing you the LAD, is a trick the board examinations like to play. The real abnormality is in the ventriculography. If systolic and diastolic frames are shown, wall motion abnormalities and hypertrophic obstructive cardiomyopathy should both be considered; for coronaries, myocardial bridging should be considered.

6. **c.** MR. MR is often caused by systolic anterior motion of the mitral valve. However, there can also be intrinsic mitral valvular abnormalities. Part of knowing the answer to questions regarding still-frame images, often of poor quality, is to know what you are looking for. The key point from this case is that you must remember that all chest pain is not caused by coronary ischemia.

7. **e.** Diuresis is not appropriate to treat RV infarction. Aggressive volume repletion is often necessary in RV infarction. Several liters of fluid may be necessary to maintain the preload. Diuresis can dramatically worsen the hypotension of RV infarction. Sequential AV pacing can be extremely useful in cases of heart block. An IABP can be used in cardiogenic shock, especially when there is concomitant LV dysfunction or ischemia. Reperfusion therapy is obviously indicated.

8. **e.** All of the above. All of the listed factors have been shown to be potential triggers for acute MI.

9. **c.** Adenosine diphosphate blockade. Clopidogrel blocks the adenosine diphosphate receptor and ultimately prevents GP IIb/IIIa receptor–mediated platelet aggregation. The board examination stresses knowledge of the basic pharmacology of the drugs used in cardiology.

10. **a.** Give aspirin. The initial ECG is rather unremarkable, although there may be slight ST elevation noted in some of the inferior leads. A middle-aged or older patient coming into the emergency department reporting chest pain deserves an aspirin while serial troponins, creatine kinases, and ECGs are being obtained (while the patient remains on telemetry). Early fibrinolytic therapy is important, but there is no clear-cut ST elevation or LBBB. Response to nitroglycerin, as was discussed earlier, does not necessarily indicate cardiac origin of pain.

11. **d.** Occluded LCx. An LCx infarction may be electrocardiographically silent, as in this patient's case. The angiogram reveals that the LCx is occluded.

12. **c.** Simvastatin. All of the statins appear to have an effect on lowering CRP.

13. **d.** Severe stenosis with thrombus. This patient's ACS is caused by a severe underlying stenosis with superimposed thrombus seen on angiography. Even when the thrombus is not angiographically apparent, ACS lesions are rich in platelet thrombus. Thus, antiplatelet agents, such as aspirin, clopidogrel, and IV GP IIb/IIIa inhibitors, are useful.

14. **a.** Aspirin, heparin, and full-dose tPA. The patient has an ST elevation MI. Anterior MI in particular is associated with increased mortality, and prompt reperfusion is indicated. Don't be confused by recent trial data—recent data will not be on the test. *Rural* is often a key word: If the time to primary PCI is longer than 90 to 120 minutes, fibrinolysis is probably preferred.

15. **b.** Bupropion. Bupropion has been shown in randomized studies to be associated with a modest increase in the rate of smoking cessation.

16. **a.** Seizures. Bupropion can rarely cause seizures and is generally best avoided in patients with a history of seizures. It is also contraindicated in patients with a history of bulimia and anorexia nervosa. It can be used safely in patients with recent MI.

17. **c.** Streptokinase and aspirin each have a similar effect on outcome. The ISIS-2 trial demonstrated that both aspirin and streptokinase had similar effects on mortality, with additive benefits.

18. **c.** The COMMIT trial (also referred to as CCS-2) randomized patients to clopidogrel or placebo, with patients receiving aspirin in both arms. There was a significant reduction in mortality in patients receiving clopidogrel. More recently, in patients with ACS undergoing PCI, including STEMI patients, prasugrel was found to be superior to clopidogrel, though with an increased risk of bleeding. In the future it may be an approved option.

19. **e.** Presence or absence of diabetes is least predictive of mortality. Based on the GUSTO model of mortality after acute MI, the other factors listed are major determinants of outcome. Although diabetes also increases the risk of adverse outcomes, it is not as potent as the other listed factors.

20. **b.** LAD occlusion. Always look for the LAD with its septal perforators. Although it is not uncommon to find a moderate stenosis with superimposed thrombus after fibrinolysis, this patient has not reperfused after lytics. This rather proximal infarction is likely to be associated with significant LV dysfunction and arrhythmic risk.

21. **b.** RV infarction. The coronary angiogram shows an almost occluded RCA. RV infarction may complicate an RCA infarct, leading to marked hypotension.

22. **d.** All of the above. Although much of the data regarding the benefits of beta-blockade were obtained before the fibrinolytic era, these agents appear to decrease the rate of intracranial hemorrhage in patients receiving lytics. Older data have shown their value in preventing VF. Intravenous beta blockers should be avoided, especially in patients with low blood pressure or impending shock.

23. **a.** Decrease subsequent repeat TVR. Stents have clearly been shown to decrease TVR in the setting of primary angioplasty.

24. **e.** All of the above. High-sensitivity CRP is a potent predictor of risk in a variety of populations with atherosclerotic disease. An elevated CRP is an independent risk factor for MI and stroke.

25. **d.** All of the above. All the listed factors are believed to be important in initiating plaque rupture.

26. **d.** Patent vessel with TIMI-3 flow. The vessel is patent, with excellent angiographic result. It is not really possible to comment on TIMI flow on a still-frame

image, but contrast dye is present distally in both the LAD and LCx, which implies that there is now TIMI-3 flow in the LCx.

27. **b.** Systolic and diastolic murmur. The angiograms demonstrate a VSD. Mechanical complications from an acute MI are favorite topics for board examinations.

28. **c.** 1%. The rate of stroke in most contemporary trials of fibrinolysis is approximately 1%.

29. **d.** It had similar rates of mortality to alteplase. The rates of mortality and stroke were similar for reteplase and alteplase. The major advantage of reteplase was that it could be given as two boluses rather than as an infusion.

30. **a.** The GISSI (Gruppo Italiano Per lo Studio Della Streptokinase Nell'Infarto Miocardio)–Prevenzione trial did not find a benefit of vitamin E in acute MI. Fibrinolysis for acute MI does lead to platelet activation. Non–ST-elevation ACS is more common than ST-elevation MI. Interestingly, troponin elevation at baseline does help predict risk even in acute MI, just as it does in ACS.

31. **a.** They benefit from an ICD more than antiarrhythmic therapy. Patients with VF or high-risk VT who were randomized to ICD versus empiric use of a type III antiarrhythmic (predominantly amiodarone) had significantly lower rates of all-cause mortality. The strategy was not guided by EP testing.

32. **c.** It decreased the need for subsequent CHF-related hospitalization. In the Survival and Ventricular Enlargement trial, the ACE inhibitor captopril was demonstrated to decrease all-cause mortality in patients with *asymptomatic* LV dysfunction (EF ≤40%) after acute MI. The benefits were present even in patients receiving aspirin, fibrinolysis, or beta-blockade. There were also significant decreases in subsequent severe CHF, hospitalization for CHF, and recurrent MI.

33. **c.** Nitrates. Doctors need to be aware of the potential for marked hypotension when nitrates are administered to a patient who has taken sildenafil acetate recently.

34. **d.** All of the above are true. The GUSTO-I trial showed that accelerated tPA reduced mortality when compared with streptokinase (either with SC heparin or IV heparin). There was an increase in the rate of hemorrhagic stroke, but this was outweighed by the reduction in overall mortality.

35. **e.** None of the above is true. The SHOCK trial found a significant reduction in mortality at 6 months in those patients who were randomized to emergency revascularization as opposed to initial medical therapy (50.3% vs. 63.1%; $p = 0.027$). This benefit was present at 30 days but was not statistically significant at that time (46.7% vs. 56.0%; $p = 0.11$). Despite early revascularization, the rate of mortality in patients with acute MI and cardiogenic shock is quite high, at least 50%.

36. **b.** VF in the first 48 hours is associated with a worse prognosis. In one study, the overall incidence of primary VF was 2.8%; in-hospital mortality nearly doubled for these patients, from 5.9% to 10.8%. In this same study, IV streptokinase did not reduce the incidence of primary VF. However, fibrinolytics do appear to reduce the incidence of secondary VF, probably by limiting infarct size. Other studies have corroborated the relationship between primary VF and worse outcome. VF after 2 days also correlates with worse outcome.

37. **e.** None of the above. The CAST-I and CAST-II studies found that there was no benefit, and that there was in fact detriment, in trying to suppress asymptomatic or mildly symptomatic PVCs after acute MI. The BASIS study suggested that low-dose amiodarone may be useful in some patients with complex ventricular ectopy. The MUSTT study found that EP-guided therapy with ICDs reduced the risk of sudden death in high-risk patients.

38. **a.** ICD implantation decreased mortality in patients with an EF ≤35%. MADIT I showed that in patients with prior MI, LV dysfunction (EF ≤35%), asymptomatic nonsustained VT, and inducible, nonsuppressible VT on EP testing, there was a reduction in all-cause mortality in patients randomized to receive an ICD instead of conventional medical therapy.

**39. b.** TIMI-2 or -3 flow is associated with a patent artery. TIMI flow is a powerful determinant of mortality. TIMI-3 flow is associated with a lower rate of mortality than TIMI-2 flow, which is associated with a lower mortality than TIMI-0 or -1 flow. With TIMI-2 or -3 flow, the epicardial artery is patent, but with TIMI-2, the flow is sluggish, and studies have shown that this difference in angiographic flow translates into a difference in mortality.

**40. b.** Twice as high. The mortality of diabetic patients is approximately 1.5 to 2.0 times higher than for nondiabetic patients after an acute MI.

**41. d.** An elevated white blood cell count is associated with worse outcomes, including mortality, after acute MI. Converging lines of evidence support the role of inflammation in the pathogenesis of acute MI. Despite the data supporting their use, even in patients who do not have contraindications, aspirin, fibrinolysis, beta-blockers, statins, and ACE inhibitors are all underused. Passive smoking is a risk factor for heart disease. A history of CHF is no longer considered a contraindication for beta-blockade.

**42. b.** ACE inhibitors have been shown to reduce mortality. Despite the widespread use of nitrates and heparin for acute MI, the evidence basis for their use is not as robust as for ACE inhibitors.

**43. c.** It is effective for the treatment of AFib and flutter. The Danish Investigations of Arrhythmia and Mortality on Dofetilide (DIAMOND) study enrolled patients with a recent MI and an EF ≤35% and found no significant difference in mortality between dofetilide and placebo. It was significantly more effective in restoring NSR in the 8% of patients who had atrial flutter or fibrillation at study entry. However, it was associated with an increased risk of torsades de pointes.

**44. b.** It should not be used prophylactically. Prophylactic IV lidocaine appears to have at best a neutral effect on mortality. Therefore, routine use of prophylactic lidocaine is no longer recommended.

**45. c.** It does not have a clear benefit in patients undergoing reperfusion therapy. Although there were initially some data to suggest that magnesium may be useful in acute MI, the bulk of data does not show a significant benefit, particularly in the reperfusion era. However, further studies are ongoing in an attempt to determine if particular issues of timing and dose have affected the differing results of the magnesium trials.

**46. a.** AFib. The role of warfarin is clear in patients with AFib to decrease the risk of stroke. There is no clearly established role for warfarin in routine MI or even in patients with LV dysfunction without LV aneurysm or thrombus.

**47. e.** All of the above are true. Cocaine has a number of adverse effects on the cardiovascular system.

**48. c.** TTE.

**49. e.** None of the above. Possible explanations for this patient's presentation include inferior MI with RV involvement. This could explain the inferior ST elevation and the hypotension. Other possibilities to consider include contained cardiac rupture or aortic dissection (which was the diagnosis in this case, along with compromise of the RCA ostium). When a pericardial effusion is caused by aortic dissection, pericardiocentesis can precipitate hemodynamic deterioration, and unless patient death is imminent, the patient should be transferred to the operative suite for further management.

**50. c.** 20%. The 30-day mortality in the subgroup of patients 75 years of age or older in the streptokinase arm was 20.4%, and in the tPA arm it was 19.1%. These results emphasize the high risk of death for elderly patients presenting with MI.

**51. a.** Within 2 hours after MI. The benefit of tPA over streptokinase was amplified in the earlier patients who were treated after the onset of their infarctions.

52. **a.** Primary PTCA reduced 30-day mortality when compared with accelerated-dose tPA. The GUSTO-IIb study found that primary PTCA was superior to accelerated-dose tPA.

53. **d.** Dressler's syndrome. Dressler's syndrome refers to pericarditis that occurs after MI. It can occur days to months after the MI. It is associated with chest pain, fever, and elevations of the white blood cell count and erythrocyte sedimentation rate. Cardiac or pulmonary effusions may be present. Rarely, it can lead to cardiac tamponade or constrictive pericarditis. Generally, however, it follows a more benign course.

54. **e.** All of the above. Aspirin, ibuprofen, and indomethacin have typically been used as first-line agents for post-MI pericarditis. Steroids or colchicine have been used in more refractory cases.

55. **b.** Fibrinolysis reduces the incidence of pericarditis in MI. Several studies, including GISSI 1, have examined this issue and found that fibrinolysis reduces the incidence of pericarditis in the setting of acute MI. Indeed, in the era of reperfusion therapy, the rate of both early and late pericarditis has decreased. Probably, by reducing infarct size, reperfusion decreases the incidence of pericarditis, which is more common with large MIs.

56. **c.** Stopping tPA. With a strong suspicion of intracranial hemorrhage, the tPA should be stopped, regardless of the cardiac situation. A head CT would be useful, but only after initial medical stabilization.

57. **f.** C and D. Protamine would be useful to reverse the action of heparin. However, to reverse the action of fibrinolytics, cryoprecipitate and epsilon aminocaproic acid would be necessary. Prompt neurosurgical consultation would also be indicated.

58. **c.** Ischemia. The patient has clear anterior ST segment elevation (as well as ST elevation in the high lateral leads) and ST segment depression inferiorly. This is indicative of ischemia. This sort of patient should be admitted to the hospital, not observed in a chest pain center.

59. **c.** It is more common with a first MI. Ventricular septal rupture is more common with a first MI that is transmural. Anterior MI is a somewhat more common cause than inferior MI, although ventricular septal rupture with inferior MI generally has a worse outcome.

60. **d.** All of the above are true. Patients with acute MR are more likely to be older, female, and have a history of prior MI.

61. **d.** The posteromedial papillary muscle is supplied by the posterior descending artery, typically from the RCA. This is why inferior infarcts are more often associated with acute MR. The anterolateral papillary muscle is supplied by both the LAD and the LCx. Surgical therapy is usually warranted.

62. **c.** LAD stenosis. The patient has a lesion of his proximal LAD.

63. **e.** Occlusion of the RCA. The RCA is occluded proximally.

64. **b.** IABPs are contraindicated in the presence of moderate or severe aortic insufficiency, as the degree of regurgitation can significantly worsen.

65. **b.** His risk of intracranial hemorrhage is increased with tPA. This level of hypertension greatly increases this patient's risk of intracranial hemorrhage. Control of his BP is clearly indicated. However, this will not entirely remove the associated risk of intracranial hemorrhage. If it is an option, primary angioplasty would be preferable.

66. **a.** Sublingual nifedipine is not an appropriate therapy. Although a few years ago sublingual nifedipine was often the treatment of choice for rapid lowering of BP, reports of MIs and strokes with this therapy, in particular associated with the practice of poking a hole in the capsule and placing it under the tongue, have led to its falling out of favor. The other listed choices are all appropriate means to lower BP.

**67. c.** Coronary perforation. There is contrast-dye layering in the pericardium. The femoral artery bifurcation is unremarkable.

**68. c.** Symptom-limited treadmill exercise stress test before discharge. Of the choices listed, the treadmill exercise stress test is best, because the evidence supports a noninvasive evaluation of ischemia before discharge. Historically, this has been the submaximal exercise stress test, with a maximal stress test at a later point after discharge. Some doctors prefer to get a dipyridamole thallium scan while the patient is hospitalized to avoid the need for a subsequent imaging study.

**69. c.** Coronary perforation. Bleeding in the groin or retroperitoneum should always be suspected in a patient with hypotension. Coronary dissection or abrupt vessel occlusion is less likely a cause in this patient, in whom the vessel was initially occluded. The temporal relationship with wire passage and hypotension makes coronary perforation highest on the list of immediate concerns.

**70. e.** None of the above. There is a severe lesion in the LAD itself, which is most likely the culprit.

**71. e.** The GUSTO-IV trial did not find a benefit to giving abciximab as empiric therapy for non–ST segment elevation ACSs. However, abciximab is of proven benefit during PCI in ACS patients.

**72. b.** Cardiac catheterization. The TACTICS–TIMI-18 trial demonstrated that high-risk patients, such as those with ST segment changes or elevated troponin, benefit from an invasive evaluation and subsequent revascularization, as opposed to a conservative strategy of initial medical stabilization followed by noninvasive risk stratification.

**73. a.** Severe restenosis of the RCA. There is severe in-stent restenosis. There is likely also thrombus present, but this is not evident angiographically.

**74. d.** All of the above. Stent thrombosis is more common in the first 2 weeks after stent placement, in particular if the patient is not on appropriate antiplatelet therapy, namely, aspirin and clopidogrel. However, it can occur later and is a possibility in this patient with an acute MI. Restenosis is often thought of as a benign process but can present in an acute fashion. Patients with CAD in one location are at risk for plaque rupture at sites other than those with severe angiographic lesions; thus, this patient could have a lesion somewhere other than the stented segment of the RCA.

**75. a.** The practice of increasing aspirin doses to this range has been out of favor in cardiology for a while and has fallen out of favor in neurology circles as well. In fact, for chronic therapy, there is no good evidence that more than 162 mg/day is of any added benefit, although the risks of gastric intolerance and perhaps bleeding appear to rise with higher aspirin doses.

**76. b.** It decreases TVR. Stents decrease the rate of subsequent TVR compared to balloon angioplasty alone, although there is no appreciable benefit for TIMI-3 flow or mortality. Whether drug eluting stents are better than bare metal stents in STEMI is the topic of ongoing study.

**77. b.** Normal LV function. Make sure you get some practice looking at still frames in systole and diastole. Don't be fooled into over-interpreting random shadows that you might notice on the reproductions of the still frames.

**78. d.** All of the above. Resolution of chest pain is a common method to indicate successful reperfusion. Resolution of ST-segment elevation is a more sensitive method to detect reperfusion. TIMI-3 flow on angiography suggests epicardial reperfusion, although not necessarily reperfusion at a microvascular level.

**79. a.** RCA occlusion. This patient likely has an occluded or severely stenotic RCA with collaterals from the LAD. When more distal portions of vessels are shown, think of collaterals.

**80. c.** There is no large difference in outcome based on gender when age and other comorbidities are considered. Although conclusions from various studies have differed regarding the impact of gender on outcome after acute MI, when age and associated comorbidities, such as diabetes, are factored in, women do not appear to have a significantly worse outcome than men. However, board examinations tend to steer away from such potentially controversial areas.

**81. d.** All of the above. Although the predominant causes of acute MI are atherosclerotic plaque rupture and subsequent thrombosis, other rarer causes remain in the differential.

**82. a.** Diabetes raises the risk of MI the same amount as does having a history of prior MI. The risk of an MI is similar for diabetic patients without a history of MI and nondiabetic patients who have already had an MI.

**83. d.** Unlike younger patients, patients over the age of 75 did not appear to derive substantial benefit from early revascularization. Although care must be used in interpreting a subgroup from a trial, elderly patients with cardiogenic shock often have multiple comorbidities; individualized decisions should be made about the appropriateness of emergency revascularization in the elderly.

**84. c.** Use of beta-blockers. Use of perioperative beta-blockers appears to reduce the rate of MI and cardiac death in high-risk patients with evidence of ischemia undergoing vascular surgery, at least in small studies.

## Suggested Reading

Alexander JH, Granger CB, Sadowski Z, et al. Prophylactic lidocaine use in acute myocardial infarction: incidence and outcomes from two international trials. The GUSTO-I and GUSTO-IIb Investigators. *Am Heart J.* 1999;137:799–805.

Anderson JL, Karagounis LA, Califf RM. Metaanalysis of five reported studies on the relation of early coronary patency grades with mortality and outcomes after acute myocardial infarction. *Am J Cardiol.* 1996;78:1–8.

Antman EM, Berlin JA. Declining incidence of ventricular fibrillation in myocardial infarction. Implications for the prophylactic use of lidocaine. *Circulation.* 1992;86:764–773.

Aronson D, Rayfield EJ, Chesebro JH. Mechanisms determining course and outcome of diabetic patients who have had acute myocardial infarction. *Ann Intern Med.* 1997;126:296–306.

Barron HV, Cannon CP, Murphy SA, et al. Association between white blood cell count, epicardial blood flow, myocardial perfusion, and clinical outcomes in the setting of acute myocardial infarction: a Thrombolysis in Myocardial Infarction 10 substudy. *Circulation.* 2000;102:2329–2334.

Barron HV, Michaels AD, Maynard C, et al. Use of angiotensin-converting enzyme inhibitors at discharge in patients with acute myocardial infarction in the United States: data from the National Registry of Myocardial Infarction 2. *J Am Coll Cardiol.* 1998;32:360–367.

Barron HV, Rundle AC, Gore JM, et al. Intracranial hemorrhage rates and effect of immediate beta-blocker use in patients with acute myocardial infarction treated with tissue plasminogen activator. Participants in the National Registry of Myocardial Infarction-2. *Am J Cardiol.* 2000;85:294–298.

Buxton AE, Lee KL, Fisher JD, et al. A randomized study of the prevention of sudden death in patients with coronary artery disease. Multicenter Unsustained Tachycardia Trial Investigators. *N Engl J Med.* 1999;341:1882–1890.

Cannon CP, McCabe CH, Wilcox RG, et al. Association of white blood cell count with increased mortality in acute myocardial infarction and unstable angina pectoris. OPUS–TIMI-16 Investigators. *Am J Cardiol.* 2001;87:636–639, A10.

The Cardiac Arrhythmia Suppression Trial (CAST) Investigators. Preliminary report: effect of encainide and flecainide on mortality in a randomized trial of arrhythmia suppression after myocardial infarction. *N Engl J Med.* 1989;321:406–412.

The Cardiac Arrhythmia Suppression Trial II Investigators. Effect of the antiarrhythmic agent moricizine on survival after myocardial infarction. *N Engl J Med.* 1992;327:227–233.

Chen J, Radford MJ, Wang Y, et al. Do "America's Best Hospitals" perform better for acute myocardial infarction? *N Engl J Med.* 1999;340:286–292.

**NOTES**

**NOTES**

Chen ZM, Jiang LX, Chen YP, et al. Addition of clopidogrel to aspirin in 45,852 patients with acute myocardial infarction: randomised placebo-controlled trial. *Lancet.* 2005;366(9497): 1607–1621.

de Lemos JA, Braunwald E. ST segment resolution as a tool for assessing the efficacy of reperfusion therapy. *J Am Coll Cardiol.* 2001;38:1283–1294.

Ellerbeck EF, Jencks SF, Radford MJ, et al. Quality of care for Medicare patients with acute myocardial infarction. A four-state pilot study from the Cooperative Cardiovascular Project. *JAMA.* 1995;273:1509–1514.

Glantz SA, Parmley WW. Passive smoking and heart disease. Epidemiology, physiology, and biochemistry. *Circulation.* 1991;83:1–12.

Gottlieb SS, McCarter RJ, Vogel RA. Effect of beta-blockade on mortality among high-risk and low-risk patients after myocardial infarction. *N Engl J Med.* 1998;339:489–497.

Haffner SM, Lehto S, Ronnemaa T, et al. Mortality from coronary heart disease in subjects with type 2 diabetes and in nondiabetic subjects with and without prior myocardial infarction. *N Engl J Med.* 1998;339:229–234.

Hine LK, Laird N, Hewitt P, et al. Meta-analytic evidence against prophylactic use of lidocaine in acute myocardial infarction. *Arch Intern Med.* 1989;149:2694–2698.

Hochman JS, Sleeper LA, Webb JG, et al. Early revascularization in acute myocardial infarction complicated by cardiogenic shock. SHOCK Investigators. Should We Emergently Revascularize Occluded Coronaries for Cardiogenic Shock. *N Engl J Med.* 1999;341:625–634.

ISIS-4: a randomised factorial trial assessing early oral captopril, oral mononitrate, and intravenous magnesium sulphate in 58,050 patients with suspected acute myocardial infarction. ISIS-4 (Fourth International Study of Infarct Survival) Collaborative Group. *Lancet.* 1995;345:669–685.

Kober L, Bloch Thomsen PE, Moller M, et al. Effect of dofetilide in patients with recent myocardial infarction and left-ventricular dysfunction: a randomised trial. Danish Investigations of Arrhythmia and Mortality on Dofetilide (DIAMOND) Study Group. *Lancet.* 2000;356:2052–2058.

MacIntyre K, Stewart S, Capewell S, et al. Gender and survival: a population-based study of 201,114 men and women following a first acute myocardial infarction. *J Am Coll Cardiol.* 2001;38:729–735.

MacMahon S, Collins R, Peto R, et al. Effects of prophylactic lidocaine in suspected acute myocardial infarction. An overview of results from the randomized, controlled trials. *JAMA.* 1988;260:1910–1916.

Moss AJ, Hall WJ, Cannom DS, et al. Improved survival with an implanted defibrillator in patients with coronary disease at high risk for ventricular arrhythmia. Multicenter Automatic Defibrillator Implantation Trial Investigators. *N Engl J Med.* 1996;335:1933–1940.

Mukamal KJ, Nesto RW, Cohen MC, et al. Impact of diabetes on long-term survival after acute myocardial infarction: comparability of risk with prior myocardial infarction. *Diabetes Care.* 2001;24:1422–1427.

Newby KH, Thompson T, Stebbins A, et al. Sustained ventricular arrhythmias in patients receiving thrombolytic therapy: incidence and outcomes. The GUSTO Investigators. *Circulation.* 1998;98:2567–2573.

Pfisterer ME, Kiowski W, Brunner H, et al. Long-term benefit of 1-year amiodarone treatment for persistent complex ventricular arrhythmias after myocardial infarction. *Circulation.* 1993;87:309–311.

Poldermans D, Boersma E, Bax JJ, et al. Bisoprolol reduces cardiac death and myocardial infarction in high-risk patients as long as 2 years after successful major vascular surgery. *Eur Heart J.* 2001;22:1353–1358.

Ryden L, Ariniego R, Arnman K, et al. A double-blind trial of metoprolol in acute myocardial infarction. Effects on ventricular tachyarrhythmias. *N Engl J Med.* 1983;308:614–618.

Sadowski ZP, Alexander JH, Skrabucha B, et al. Multicenter randomized trial and a systematic overview of lidocaine in acute myocardial infarction. *Am Heart J.* 1999; 137:792–798.

Santoro GM, Antoniucci D, Bolognese L, et al. A randomized study of intravenous magnesium in acute myocardial infarction treated with direct coronary angioplasty. *Am Heart J.* 2000;140:891–897.

Second Chinese Cardiac Study (CCS-2) Collaborative Group. Rationale, design and organization of the Second Chinese Cardiac Study (CCS-2): a randomized trial of clopidogrel plus aspirin, and of metoprolol, among patients with suspected acute myocardial infarction. *J Cardiovasc Risk.* 2000;7:435–441.

Volpi A, Cavalli A, Santoro E, et al. Incidence and prognosis of secondary ventricular fibrillation in acute myocardial infarction. Evidence for a protective effect of thrombolytic therapy. GISSI Investigators. *Circulation.* 1990;82:1279–1288.

Volpi A, Maggioni A, Franzosi MG, et al. In-hospital prognosis of patients with acute myocardial infarction complicated by primary ventricular fibrillation. *N Engl J Med.* 1987;317:257–261.

Woods KL, Fletcher S. Long-term outcome after intravenous magnesium sulphate in suspected acute myocardial infarction: the second Leicester Intravenous Magnesium Intervention Trial (LIMIT-2). *Lancet.* 1994;343:816–819.

Woods KL, Fletcher S, Roffe C, et al. Intravenous magnesium sulphate in suspected acute myocardial infarction: results of the second Leicester Intravenous Magnesium Intervention Trial (LIMIT-2). *Lancet.* 1992;339:1553–1558.

Ziegelstein RC, Hilbe JM, French WJ, et al. Magnesium use in the treatment of acute myocardial infarction in the United States (observations from the Second National Registry of Myocardial Infarction). *Am J Cardiol.* 2001;87:7–10.

**NOTES**

# chapter 4

# Coronary Artery Disease

DEBABRATA MUKHERJEE • MARCO ROFFI

## QUESTIONS

1. A 67-year-old male presents to the emergency room with increasing frequency of chest pain on exertion and one episode of rest pain lasting 5 minutes. Other than for hypertension and hyperlipidemia his medical history is unremarkable. He quit smoking (1 pack a year for 20 years) 11 years ago. On physical exam he is afebrile, his pulse is 78, and his blood pressure is 138/76. Chest auscultation reveals an $S_3$ gallop in the absence of basilar crackles. His current medications include aspirin, metoprolol, ramipril, and atorvastatin. His presenting ECG reveals sinus rhythm and ST-segment depression in I, aVL, $V_5$ to $V_6$. You admit him to the hospital and start intravenous heparin, nitroglycerin, and tirofiban. His initial troponin I level is 1.4 µg/L. The next step in his management would be

   a. low-level stress test next morning
   b. continue intravenous heparin, nitroglycerin, and tirofiban until completely free of chest pain for 24 hours, then discharge home
   c. coronary angiography within 48 hours followed by percutaneous intervention/surgical revascularization if indicated
   d. dobutamine echocardiogram after 48 hours

2. The effects of exercise training in patients who received percutaneous transluminal coronary angioplasty or coronary stenting include

   a. reduced restenosis
   b. lower rate of hospital readmission
   c. reduction in $\dot{V}o_2$
   d. higher event rate related to exercise

3. Which of the following parameters predicts future risk of coronary heart disease in initially healthy middle-aged men?

   a. Erythrocyte sedimentation rate (ESR)
   b. High sensitivity C-reactive protein (hsCRP)
   c. immunoglobulin G (IgG)
   d. immunoglobulin E (IgE)

4. A 58-year-old male with coronary artery disease had stenting of the mid LAD 10 months ago with a bare metal stent. He presents now with recurrent angina, and angiography reveals a severe and diffuse in-stent restenosis (ISR). A reasonable next therapeutic option would be

   a. plain balloon angioplasty
   b. repeat stenting with a bare metal stent
   c. drug-eluting stent implantation (stent-in-stent)

    **d.** medical therapy

    **e.** brachytherapy

**5.** The HOPE trial demonstrated that treatment with ramipril reduces all of the following *except*

    **a.** death from cardiovascular causes

    **b.** myocardial infarction

    **c.** stroke

    **d.** hospitalization for unstable angina

    **e.** complications related to diabetes

**6.** Which type of atherosclerotic lesion (Stary type) is most likely to disrupt, thrombose, and lead to myocardial infarction?

    **a.** I–III

    **b.** IV–Va

    **c.** Vb–Vc

    **d.** VI

**7.** The determinants of myocardial oxygen demand include all of the following *except*

    **a.** heart rate

    **b.** contractility

    **c.** myocardial wall tension

    **d.** *oxygen-carrying* capacity of the blood

**8.** Which area of the myocardium is more vulnerable to ischemic damage?

    **a.** subepicardium

    **b.** midmyocardium

    **c.** subendocardium

    **d.** pericardium

**9.** A 73-year-old male presents to the emergency room with severe mid-sternal chest discomfort. He appears anxious and in distress. His heart rate is 66, blood pressure is 92/68 mm Hg, and respiratory rate is 14. There is marked jugular venous distention. On auscultation an $S_4$ gallop sound is audible and the lung fields are clear. ECG reveals 2-mm ST-segment elevation in leads II, III, and aVF. The most likely diagnosis is

    **a.** acute pericarditis

    **b.** aortic dissection

    **c.** right ventricular infarction

    **d.** inferior wall myocardial infarction with right ventricular infarction

    **e.** pneumonia

**10.** A fourth heart sound ($S_4$) in patients with acute myocardial infarction is related to

    **a.** reduction in left ventricular compliance

    **b.** rapid deceleration of transmitral flow during protodiastolic filling of the left ventricle

    **c.** increased inflow into the left ventricle

    **d.** reduced left ventricular systolic function

**11.** The GUSTO-I trial demonstrated

    **a.** decreased stroke risk with tPA

    **b.** survival benefit of tPA over streptokinase

    **c.** equivalence of tPA and streptokinase

    **d.** decreased reocclusion with tPA

**12.** Of the following cardiac markers of necrosis, the earliest initial rise is seen with

    **a.** troponin I

    **b.** troponin T

    **c.** myoglobin

**d.** creatine kinase myocardial band (CK-MB)

**e.** lactate dehydrogenase (LDH)

**13.** Among the four listed predictors of 30-day mortality identified in acute myocardial infarction patients treated with thrombolytic therapy within the GUSTO-I trial, which one was the least contributive?

**a.** systolic blood pressure

**b.** age

**c.** heart rate

**d.** choice of thrombolytic agent

**14.** High-risk exercise ECG criteria on stress testing include

**a.** achievement of a workload of less than 7 METS

**b.** ST-segment depression for greater than 2 minutes during the recovery period

**c.** ≥1 mm ST-segment depression in stage I

**d.** increase in heart rate

**15.** The 10-year follow-up of the Coronary Artery Surgery Study (CASS) study demonstrated which of the following?

**a.** Patients with left ventricular dysfunction exhibit long-term benefit from an initial strategy of surgical treatment.

**b.** At 10 years, there was significant improvement in cumulative survival and difference in percentage free of death and nonfatal myocardial infarction with surgery compared to medical therapy.

**c.** Patients with an ejection fraction ≥0.50 exhibited a higher proportion free of death and myocardial infarction with initial surgical therapy.

**d.** Patients with mild stable angina and normal left ventricular function randomized to initial surgical treatment have improved survival compared to medical therapy.

**16.** The Asymptomatic Cardiac Ischemia Pilot (ACIP) study demonstrated at 1 year

**a.** significant mortality benefit with revascularization compared to angina-guided medical therapy

**b.** equivalent clinical outcomes with angina-guided, ischemia-guided, and revascularization strategies

**c.** improved clinical outcome with angina-guided therapy compared to revascularization

**d.** improved clinical outcome with ischemia-guided therapy compared to revascularization

**17.** Class I ACC/AHA guidelines regarding early risk stratification for the management of patients with unstable angina and non–ST-segment elevation myocardial infarction include all of the following *except*

**a.** A rapid clinical determination of the likelihood risk of obstructive CAD (i.e., high, intermediate, or low) should be made in all patients with chest discomfort or other symptoms suggestive of an ACS and considered in patient management.

**b.** Patients who present with chest discomfort or other ischemic symptoms should undergo early risk stratification for the risk of cardiovascular events (e.g., death or [re]MI) that focuses on history, including anginal symptoms, physical findings, ECG findings, and biomarkers of cardiac injury, and results should be considered in patient management.

**c.** A 12-lead ECG should be performed and shown to an experienced emergency physician after emergency department arrival, with a goal of within 30 minutes of emergency department arrival for all patients with chest discomfort (or anginal equivalent) or other symptoms suggestive of ACS.

**d.** Cardiac biomarkers should be measured in all patients who present with chest discomfort consistent with ACS.

**18.** Class I ACC/AHA guidelines regarding immediate management of patients with unstable angina and non–ST-segment elevation myocardial infarction include all of the following *except*

  **a.** The history, physical examination, 12-lead ECG, and initial cardiac biomarker tests should be integrated to assign patients with chest pain into one of four categories: a noncardiac diagnosis, chronic stable angina, possible ACS, and definite ACS.

  **b.** Patients with probable or possible ACS but whose initial 12-lead ECG and cardiac biomarker levels are normal should be observed in a facility with cardiac monitoring (e.g., chest pain unit or hospital telemetry ward), and repeat ECG (or continuous 12-lead ECG monitoring) and repeat cardiac biomarker measurement(s) should be obtained at predetermined, specified time intervals.

  **c.** In patients with suspected ACS in whom ischemic heart disease is present or suspected, if the follow-up 12-lead ECG and cardiac biomarkers measurements are normal, a stress test (exercise or pharmacological) to provoke ischemia should be performed in the emergency department, in a chest pain unit, or on an outpatient basis in a timely fashion (within 72 hours) as an alternative to inpatient admission. Low-risk patients with a negative diagnostic test can be managed as outpatients.

  **d.** In low-risk patients who are referred for outpatient stress testing (see above), precautionary appropriate pharmacotherapy (e.g., ASA, sublingual NTG, and/or beta-blockers) should be given while awaiting results of the stress test.

  **e.** Patients with possible ACS and negative cardiac markers who are unable to exercise or who have an abnormal resting ECG should have a coronary angiogram.

  **f.** Patients with definite ACS and ST-segment elevation in leads $V_7$ to $V_9$ caused by left circumflex occlusion should be evaluated for immediate reperfusion therapy.

**19.** Class I ACC/AHA guidelines regarding anti-ischemic therapy for patients with unstable angina and non–ST-segment elevation myocardial infarction include all of the following *except*

  **a.** Bed/chair rest with continuous ECG monitoring is recommended for all UA/NSTEMI patients during the early hospital phase.

  **b.** Supplemental oxygen should be administered to patients with UA/NSTEMI with an arterial saturation less than 90%, respiratory distress, or other high-risk features for hypoxemia.

  **c.** Patients with UA/NSTEMI with ongoing ischemic discomfort should receive sublingual NTG (0.4 mg) every 5 minutes for a total of three doses, after which assessment should be made about the need for intravenous NTG, if not contraindicated.

  **d.** Intravenous NTG is indicated in the first 48 hours after UA/NSTEMI for treatment of persistent ischemia, heart failure (HF), or hypertension. The decision to administer intravenous NTG and the dose used should not preclude therapy with other proven mortality-reducing interventions such as beta-blockers or ACE inhibitors.

  **e.** Oral beta-blocker therapy should be initiated within the first 24 hours for patients who do not have one or more of the following: (a) signs of HF, (b) evidence of a low-output state, (c) increased risk for cardiogenic shock, or (d) other relative contraindications to beta-blockade (PR interval greater than 0.24 seconds, second- or third-degree heart block, active asthma, or reactive airway disease).

  **f.** A nondihydropyridine calcium antagonist (e.g., verapamil or diltiazem), followed by oral therapy, as initial therapy.

  **g.** An ACE inhibitor should be administered orally within the first 24 hours to UA/NSTEMI patients with pulmonary congestion or LV ejection fraction

(LVEF) ≤0.40, in the absence of hypotension (systolic blood pressure <100 mm Hg or <30 mm Hg below baseline) or known contraindications to that class of medications.

**h.** An angiotensin receptor blocker should be administered to UA/NSTEMI patients who are intolerant of ACE inhibitors and have either clinical or radiological signs of HF or LVEF ≤0.40. (Level of evidence: A)

**i.** Because of the increased risks of mortality, reinfarction, hypertension, HF, and myocardial rupture associated with their use, nonsteroidal anti-inflammatory drugs (NSAIDs), except for ASA, whether nonselective or cyclo-oxygenase (COX)-2–selective agents, should be discontinued at the time a patient presents with UA/NSTEMI.

**20.** Class I ACC/AHA guidelines regarding antiplatelet and anticoagulant therapy for patients with unstable angina and non–ST-segment elevation myocardial infarction include all of the following *except*

**a.** Aspirin should be administered to UA/NSTEMI patients as soon as possible after hospital presentation and continued indefinitely in patients not known to be intolerant of that medication.

**b.** Clopidogrel (loading dose followed by daily maintenance dose) should be administered to UA/NSTEMI patients who are unable to take ASA because of hypersensitivity or major gastrointestinal intolerance.

**c.** In UA/NSTEMI patients with a history of gastrointestinal bleeding, when ASA and clopidogrel are administered alone or in combination, drugs to minimize the risk of recurrent gastrointestinal bleeding (e.g., proton-pump inhibitors) should be prescribed concomitantly.

**d.** For UA/NSTEMI patients in whom an initial invasive strategy is selected, antiplatelet therapy in addition to aspirin should be initiated before diagnostic angiography (upstream) with either clopidogrel (loading dose followed by daily maintenance dose) or an intravenous GP IIb/IIIa inhibitor. Abciximab as the choice for upstream GP IIb/IIIa therapy is indicated only if there is no appreciable delay to angiography and PCI is likely to be performed; otherwise, IV eptifibatide or tirofiban is the preferred choice of GP IIb/IIIa inhibitor.

**e.** For UA/NSTEMI patients in whom an initial conservative (i.e., noninvasive) strategy is selected clopidogrel (loading dose followed by daily maintenance dose) should be added to ASA and anticoagulant therapy as soon as possible after admission and administered for at least 1 month and ideally up to 1 year.

**f.** A platelet GP IIb/IIIa receptor antagonist should be administered to all patients.

**21.** Class I recommendations for revascularization with PCI and CABG in patients with acute coronary syndrome include all of the following *except*

**a.** An early invasive PCI strategy is indicated for patients with UA/NSTEMI who have no serious comorbidity and who have coronary lesions amenable to PCI and any of the high-risk features listed in Table 1–1.

**b.** Percutaneous coronary intervention (or CABG) is recommended for UA/NSTEMI patients with one- or two-vessel CAD with or without significant proximal left anterior descending CAD.

**c.** Percutaneous coronary intervention (or CABG) is recommended for UA/NSTEMI patients with multivessel coronary disease with suitable coronary anatomy and normal LV function, and without diabetes mellitus.

**d.** An intravenous platelet GP IIb/IIIa inhibitor is generally recommended in UA/NSTEMI patients undergoing PCI.

**22.** Class I recommendations regarding post-discharge care of patients with unstable angina/non-Q MI include all of the following *except*

**a.** Medications required in the hospital to control ischemia should be discontinued after hospital discharge in patients with UA/NSTEMI who do not

**TABLE 4–1   Selection of Initial Treatment Strategy: Invasive Versus Conservative Strategy**

| Preferred Strategy | Patient Characteristics |
|---|---|
| Invasive | Recurrent angina or ischemia at rest or with low-level activities despite intensive medical therapy |
| | Elevated cardiac biomarkers (TnT or TnI) |
| | New or presumably new ST-segment depression |
| | Signs or symptoms of HF or new or worsening mitral regurgitation |
| | High-risk findings from noninvasive testing |
| | Hemodynamic instability |
| | Sustained ventricular tachycardia |
| | PCI within 6 mo |
| | Prior CABG |
| | High risk score (e.g., TIMI, GRACE) |
| | Reduced left ventricular function (LVEF <40%) |
| Conservative | Low risk score (e.g., TIMI, GRACE) |
| | Patient or physician preference in the absence of high-risk features |

Adapted from Anderson JL, Adams CD, Antman EM, et al. ACC/AHA 2007 guidelines for the management of patients with unstable angina/non-ST-Elevation myocardial infarction: a report of the American College of Cardiology/American Heart Association Task Force on Practice Guidelines (Writing Committee to Revise the 2002 Guidelines for the Management of Patients with Unstable Angina/Non-ST-Elevation Myocardial Infarction) developed in collaboration with the American College of Emergency Physicians, the Society for Cardiovascular Angiography and Interventions, and the Society of Thoracic Surgeons endorsed by the American Association of Cardiovascular and Pulmonary Rehabilitation and the Society for Academic Emergency Medicine. *J Am Coll Cardiol.* 2007;50:e1–e157, with permission.

undergo coronary revascularization, patients with unsuccessful revascularization, and patients with recurrent symptoms after revascularization.

**b.** All post-UA/NSTEMI patients should be given sublingual or spray NTG and instructed in its use.

**c.** Before hospital discharge, patients with UA/NSTEMI should be informed about symptoms of worsening myocardial ischemia and MI and should be instructed in how and when to seek emergency care and assistance if such symptoms occur.

**d.** Before hospital discharge, post-UA/NSTEMI patients and/or designated responsible caregivers should be provided with supportable, easily understood, and culturally sensitive instructions with respect to medication type, purpose, dose, frequency, and pertinent side effects.

**e.** In post-UA/NSTEMI patients, anginal discomfort lasting more than 2 or 3 minutes should prompt the patient to discontinue physical activity or remove himself or herself from any stressful event. If pain does not subside immediately, the patient should be instructed to take one dose of NTG sublingually. If the chest discomfort/pain is unimproved or worsening 5 minutes after one NTG dose has been taken, it is recommended that the patient or a family member or friend call 9-1-1 immediately to access EMS. While activating EMS access, additional NTG (at 5-minute intervals two times) may be taken while lying down or sitting.

**f.** If the pattern or severity of anginal symptoms changes, which suggests worsening myocardial ischemia (e.g., pain is more frequent or severe or is precipitated by less effort or now occurs at rest), the patient should contact his or her physician without delay to assess the need for additional treatment or testing.

**23.** Class I recommendations regarding management of patients with diabetes mellitus presenting with unstable angina/non-Q MI include all of the following *except*

**a.** Medical treatment in the acute phase of UA/NSTEMI and decisions on whether to perform stress testing, angiography, and revascularization should be geared toward more aggressive strategy in diabetic compared to nondiabetic patients.

**b.** In all patients with diabetes mellitus and UA/NSTEMI, attention should be directed toward aggressive glycemic management in accordance with current standards of diabetes care endorsed by the American Diabetes Association and the American College of Endocrinology. Goals of therapy should include a preprandial glucose target of less than 110 mg/dL and a maximum daily target of less than 180 mg/dL. The post-discharge goal of therapy should be HbA1C less than 7%, which should be addressed by primary care and cardiac caregivers at every visit.

**c.** An intravenous platelet GP IIb/IIIa inhibitor should be administered for patients with diabetes mellitus as recommended for all UA/NSTEMI patients. The benefit may be enhanced in patients with diabetes mellitus.

**24.** Regarding women and acute coronary syndromes, all of the following statements are true *except*

**a.** Women with UA/NSTEMI should be managed with the same pharmacological therapy as men both in the hospital and for secondary prevention, with attention to antiplatelet and anticoagulant doses based on weight and renal function; doses of renally cleared medications should be based on estimated creatinine clearance.

**b.** Recommended indications for noninvasive testing in women with UA/NSTEMI are similar to those for men.

**c.** Women benefit less with invasive therapy compared to men, and women with high-risk features should be treated primarily noninvasively.

**d.** In women with low-risk features, a conservative strategy is recommended.

**25.** Class I indications for coronary angiography for risk stratification in patients with chronic stable angina include all of the following except

**a.** Patients with disabling (Canadian Cardiovascular Society [CCS] classes III and IV) chronic stable angina not on medical therapy.

**b.** Patients with high-risk criteria on noninvasive testing regardless of anginal severity.

**c.** Patients with angina who have survived sudden cardiac death or serious ventricular arrhythmia.

**d.** Patients with angina and symptoms and signs of congestive heart failure.

**e.** Patients with clinical characteristics that indicate a high likelihood of severe CAD.

**26.** Class I Indications for CABG in asymptomatic patients include all of the following *except*

**a.** significant left main coronary artery stenosis

**b.** proximal LAD stenosis with single vessel disease

**c.** three-vessel disease (survival benefit is greater in patients with abnormal LV function, e.g., with an EF <0.50)

**c.** coronary artery bypass grafting for patients with two-vessel disease with significant proximal LAD CAD and either abnormal LV function (ejection fraction <50%) or demonstrable ischemia on noninvasive testing

**27.** Class I recommendations for cardiac stress imaging as the initial test for diagnosis in patients with chronic stable angina who are able to exercise include all of the following *except*

**a.** exercise myocardial perfusion imaging or exercise echocardiography in patients with an intermediate pretest probability of CAD who have one of the following baseline ECG abnormalities: (i) pre-excitation (Wolff-Parkinson-White) syndrome, or (ii) more than 1 mm of ST depression at rest

**b.** exercise myocardial perfusion imaging or exercise echocardiography in patients with prior revascularization (either PCI or CABG)

**c.** adenosine or dipyridamole myocardial perfusion imaging in patients with an intermediate pretest probability of CAD and one of the following baseline ECG abnormalities: (i) electronically paced ventricular rhythm, or (ii) left bundle-branch block

**d.** exercise myocardial perfusion imaging, exercise echocardiography, adenosine or dipyridamole myocardial perfusion imaging, or dobutamine echocardiography as the initial stress test in a patient with a normal rest ECG who is not taking digoxin

**28.** The following variables are multivariate predictors of stent thrombosis after drug eluting stents *except*

**a.** renal failure
**b.** bifurcation stensosis
**c.** in-stent restenotic lesion
**d.** reference diameter or vessel size
**e.** lack of clopidogrel therapy or clopidogrel withdrawal

**29.** The Prospective Pravastatin Pooling (PPP) project demonstrated an approximate stroke reduction (relative reduction) of

**a.** 10%
**b.** 20%
**c.** 40%
**d.** 45%

**30.** Prognostic factors for atherosclerosis progression in saphenous vein grafts (SVGs) include all of the following *except*

**a.** maximum stenosis of the graft at baseline angiography
**b.** years post-SVG placement
**c.** warfarin therapy
**d.** female gender
**e.** high triglyceride level

**31.** The AVERT trial demonstrated that in patients with ischemic heart disease and stable angina pectoris

**a.** Percutaneous coronary revascularization is more effective than aggressive lipid lowering therapy.
**b.** Aggressive lipid lowering therapy is more effective than percutaneous coronary revascularization.
**c.** Aggressive lipid lowering therapy is as effective as percutaneous coronary revascularization.

**32.** The relative risk of death in the simvastatin group in the Scandinavian Simvastatin Survival Study (4S) was

**a.** 0.50
**b.** 0.60
**c.** 0.70
**d.** 0.80
**e.** 0.85

**33.** The main outcome measure of the primary prevention of acute coronary events with lovastatin in men and women with average cholesterol levels in the Air Force/Texas Coronary Atherosclerosis Prevention Study (AFCAPS/TexCAPS) was

**a.** cardiovascular mortality
**b.** first acute major coronary event defined as fatal or nonfatal myocardial infarction, unstable angina, or sudden cardiac death
**c.** total mortality
**d.** stroke

**34.** The West of Scotland Coronary Prevention Study (WOSCOPS) trial demonstrated that a fall in what percentage point in LDL is sufficient to produce the full benefit in patients taking 40-mg dose of pravastatin?

**a.** 12%
**b.** 24%

**c.** 30%

**d.** 36%

**35.** The Bypass Angioplasty Revascularization Investigation (BARI) randomized trial and registry both demonstrated

    **a.** CABG is associated with equivalent survival to PTCA in treated diabetic patients with multivessel coronary disease suitable for either surgical or catheter-based revascularization.

    **b.** CABG is associated with better long-term survival than PTCA in treated diabetic patients with multivessel coronary disease suitable for either surgical or catheter-based revascularization.

    **c.** PTCA is associated with better long-term survival than CABG in treated diabetic patients with multivessel coronary disease suitable for either surgical or catheter-based revascularization.

**36.** The effect of cigarette smoking on the activity of ischemic heart disease is

    **a.** increased frequency of episodes of angina and no effect on the duration of ischemia

    **b.** increased frequency of episodes of angina and increased duration of ischemia

    **c.** increased duration of ischemia but no effect on frequency of angina

    **d.** no significant effect on either duration or frequency of angina

**37.** The primary end point of the Should We Emergently Revascularize Occluded Coronaries for Cardiogenic Shock (SHOCK) trial revealed

    **a.** significant benefit with early revascularization compared to intensive medical therapy at 30 days

    **b.** no significant difference with early revascularization compared to intensive medical therapy at 30 days

    **c.** significant benefit with intensive medical therapy compared to early revascularization at 30 days

    **d.** significant benefit with combination of thrombolysis and IABP compared to early revascularization at 30 days

**38.** A 66-year-old female presents to your outpatient department with stable angina. You order a perfusion stress study, which reveals inferior and inferoseptal ischemia. Coronary angiogram reveals an 80% calcified lesion in the midportion of the right coronary artery. The left anterior descending artery and the left circumflex artery have mild luminal irregularities. Based on the available literature you quote her a survival of

    **a.** >90% at 5 years

    **b.** 80% at 5 years

    **c.** 70% at 5 years

    **d.** 60% at 5 years

    **e.** 50% at 5 years

**39.** All of the following were multivariate predictors in identifying high-risk patients with left main and three-vessel coronary artery disease by adenosine single photon emission computed tomographic (SPECT) thallium imaging *except*

    **a.** multivessel thallium abnormality

    **b.** increased lung thallium uptake

    **c.** extent of thallium abnormality

    **d.** ST depression on resting ECG

**40.** The following statement is correct regarding risk of stroke associated with abciximab among patients undergoing percutaneous coronary intervention.

    **a.** Abciximab in addition to aspirin and heparin does not increase the risk of stroke in patients undergoing PCI.

**b.** Abciximab in addition to aspirin and heparin increases the risk of stroke in patients undergoing PCI.

**c.** Abciximab in addition to aspirin and heparin decreases the risk of stroke in patients undergoing PCI.

**41.** Clinical factors predictive of global and regional ventricular function among patients undergoing reperfusion therapy for acute myocardial infarction as well as of improvement in function between 90 minutes and 5 to 7 days include all of the following *except*

    **a.** time to treatment

    **b.** early infarct-related artery flow grade

    **c.** age

    **d.** body mass index

**42.** Factors associated with failure of medical therapy in patients with unstable angina and non-Q wave myocardial infarction include all of the following *except*

    **a.** ST-segment depression on the qualifying ECG

    **b.** history of prior angina

    **c.** family history of premature coronary disease (i.e., onset <55 years of age)

    **d.** prior use of heparin or aspirin

    **e.** female gender

    **f.** increasing age

**43.** Based on the National Cholesterol Education Program (NCEP) Expert Panel on Detection, Evaluation, and Treatment of High Blood Cholesterol in Adults (Adult Treatment Panel III), the LDL level at which to consider drug therapy for patients with coronary artery disease is

    **a.** 190 mg/dL

    **b.** 160 mg/dL

    **c.** 130 mg/dL

    **d.** 100 mg/dL

**44.** The TIMI 11B–ESSENCE meta-analysis demonstrated what in regard to the use of low-molecular-weight heparin (LMWH) compared to unfractionated heparin (UFH) in patients with acute coronary syndromes?

    **a.** Use of LMWH compared to UFH resulted in no significant difference in outcomes.

    **b.** Use of UFH was associated with a 20% reduction in death and serious cardiac ischemic events that appeared within the first few days of treatment, and this benefit was sustained through 43 days.

    **c.** Use of LMWH was associated with a 20% reduction in death and serious cardiac ischemic events that appeared within the first few days of treatment, and this benefit was sustained through 43 days.

**45.** The incidence of nonsignificant coronary artery disease on angiography in patients presenting with acute coronary syndromes is

    **a.** 3%

    **b.** 6%

    **c.** 12%

    **d.** 20%

    **e.** 24%

**46.** A bleeding episode in a patient treated with hirudin can be effectively reversed with

    **a.** fresh frozen plasma

    **b.** prothrombin complex

    **c.** epsilon aminocaproic acid

    **d.** bivalirudin

**47.** The overall, 30-day mortality in patients with prior bypass who present with acute myocardial infarction is

**a.** 3%
**b.** 6%
**c.** 11%
**d.** 16%

**48.** Thrombolysis in Myocardial Infarction (TIMI) trial flow grade 3 is achieved in what percentage of patients with acute myocardial infarction and prior CABG following primary angioplasty?

**a.** 50%
**b.** 70%
**c.** 90%
**d.** 95%

**49.** A 76-year-old male presents to the emergency department with substernal chest pressure for 40 minutes. Physical examination reveals a diaphoretic male, with heart rate of 82 and a blood pressure of 76/42. He has a jugular venous pressure of 12 cms of $H_2O$. On auscultation he has an $S_3$ gallop and clear lung fields. ECG reveals ST-segment elevation in leads II, III, and aVF. The diagnosis is

**a.** severe left ventricular failure with cardiogenic shock
**b.** ventricular septal defect
**c.** acute mitral regurgitation
**d.** right ventricular infarction
**e.** cardiac rupture

**50.** In patients presenting with right ventricular infarction, which of the following has been shown to have survival advantage?

**a.** fluid loading
**b.** nitroglycerin
**c.** pulmonary artery catheter placement
**d.** primary angioplasty

**51.** The potential causes of a new systolic murmur after an acute myocardial infarction include all of the following *except*

**a.** mitral regurgitation
**b.** ventricular septal defect
**c.** aortic stenosis
**d.** dynamic left ventricular outflow tract obstruction

**52.** In patients with coronary artery disease, use of oral glycoprotein IIb/IIIa receptor inhibitors results in

**a.** significant decrease in mortality
**b.** no effect on mortality
**c.** significant increase in mortality
**d.** mortality was not ascertained in these trials

**53.** The Clopidogrel versus Aspirin in Patients at Risk of Ischemic Events (CAPRIE) trial comparing aspirin and clopidogrel showed that

**a.** Long-term administration of clopidogrel to patients with atherosclerotic vascular disease is as effective as aspirin in reducing the combined risk of ischemic stroke, myocardial infarction, or vascular death.
**b.** Long-term administration of clopidogrel to patients with atherosclerotic vascular disease is more effective than aspirin in reducing the combined risk of ischemic stroke, myocardial infarction, or vascular death.
**c.** Long-term administration of clopidogrel to patients with atherosclerotic vascular disease is less effective than aspirin in reducing the combined risk of ischemic stroke, myocardial infarction, or vascular death.

**54.** Low, fixed-dose warfarin (1 mg or 3 mg) combined with low-dose aspirin (80 mg) in patients who have had myocardial infarction has what clinical effect in patients who have had myocardial infarction?

  **a.** It does not provide clinical benefit beyond that achievable with 160-mg aspirin monotherapy.

  **b.** It provides clinical benefit beyond that achievable with 160-mg aspirin monotherapy.

  **c.** It has worse clinical outcome compared to 160-mg aspirin monotherapy.

**55.** This figure (Fig. 4–1) shows the Brockenbrough response after a ventricular premature beat in a 57-year-old female with hypertrophic cardiomyopathy, which includes

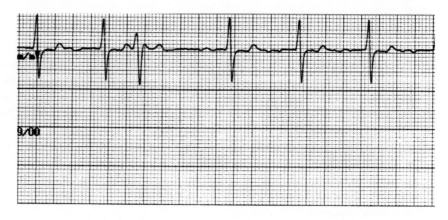

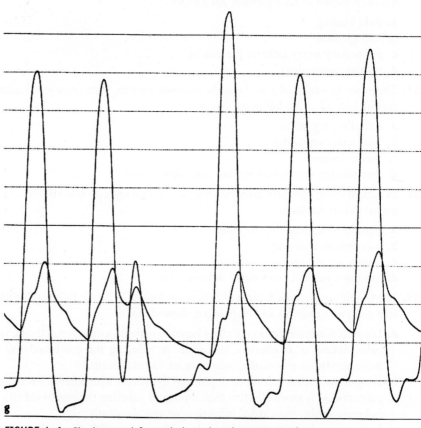

**FIGURE 4–1** Simultaneous left ventricular and aortic pressure tracing.

a. an increase in left ventricular systolic pressure, a decrease in aortic systolic pressure, an increase in left ventricular to aortic gradient, and diminished aortic pulse pressure

b. an increase in left ventricular systolic pressure, an increase in aortic systolic pressure, an increase in left ventricular to aortic gradient, and increased aortic pulse pressure

c. a decrease in left ventricular systolic pressure, a decrease in aortic systolic pressure, an increase in left ventricular to aortic gradient and diminished aortic pulse pressure

**56.** The angiogram in Fig. 4–2 shows the following:

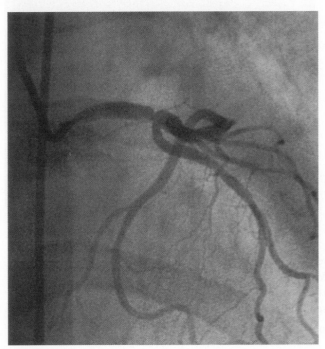

**FIGURE 4–2**

a. occluded left anterior descending artery
b. occluded left circumflex coronary artery
c. severe ostial and moderate distal left main trunk stenosis
d. normal coronary arteries

**57.** The Arterial Revascularization Therapies Study (ARTS) comparing bypass versus stenting in multivessel coronary disease demonstrated

a. At 1 year, there was no significant difference between the two groups in terms of the rates of death, stroke, or myocardial infarction.
b. At 1 year, bypass surgery had significantly better outcomes.
c. At 1 year, coronary stenting had significantly better outcomes.
d. The trial was aborted prior to 1 year.

**58.** The incidence of coronary artery aneurysms and/or ectasia in patients with Kawasaki disease is

a. 5% to 10%
b. 10% to 15%
c. 15% to 25%
d. 25% to 35%
e. ~ 40%

**59.** A 48-year-old female presents with congestive heart failure. The etiology of her heart failure based on the coronary angiogram in Fig. 4–3 is

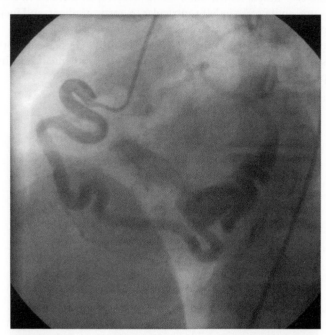

**FIGURE 4–3**

    **a.** severe coronary artery disease
    **b.** A-V fistula
    **c.** aortic regurgitation
    **d.** absent right coronary artery

**60.** The angiogram in Fig. 4–4 shows

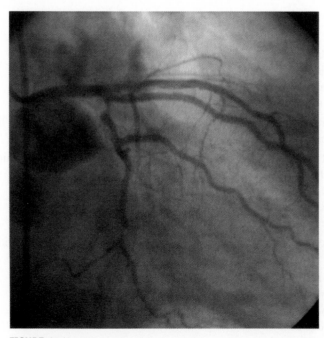

**FIGURE 4–4**

a. ostial left main trunk stenosis
b. ostial left anterior descending artery stenosis
c. ostial left circumflex artery stenosis
d. normal coronaries

**61.** The angiogram in Fig. 4–5 shows

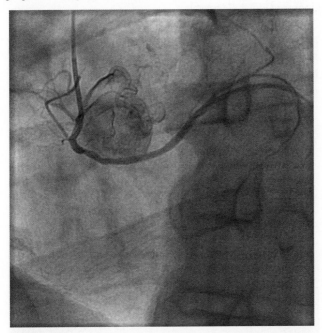

**FIGURE 4–5**

a. anomalous origin of the left main trunk
b. anomalous origin of the left anterior descending artery
c. anomalous origin of the left circumflex artery
d. normal coronaries

**62.** Coronary angiogram of a 59-year-old male with acute inferior myocardial infarction. The angiogram (Fig. 4–6) reveals

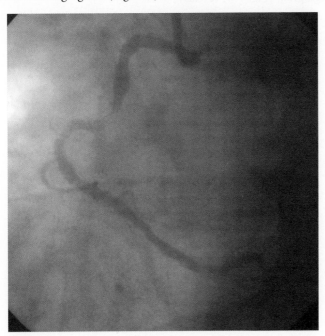

**FIGURE 4–6**

a. large angiographically visible thrombus in the mid portion of the right coronary artery distal to a severe stenosis
b. perforation of the mid portion of the right coronary artery
c. normal right coronary artery
d. absent right coronary artery

63. The angiogram (Fig. 4–7) reveals

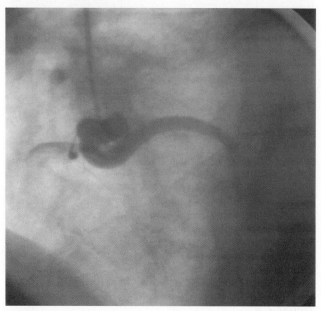

**FIGURE 4–7**

a. anomalous origin of the left main trunk
b. anomalous origin of the left anterior descending artery
c. anomalous origin of the left circumflex artery
d. anomalous origin of the right coronary artery

64. The angiogram (Fig. 4–8) reveals

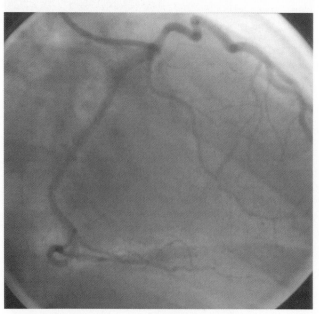

**FIGURE 4–8**

a. anomalous origin of the left main trunk
b. anomalous origin of the left anterior descending artery
c. anomalous origin of the left circumflex artery
d. anomalous origin of the left anterior descending artery and the right coronary artery

**65.** During coronary angioplasty of the right coronary artery, this 72-year-old patient developed sharp chest pain with rapid development of hypotension and tachycardia. The most likely etiology based on Fig. 4–9 is

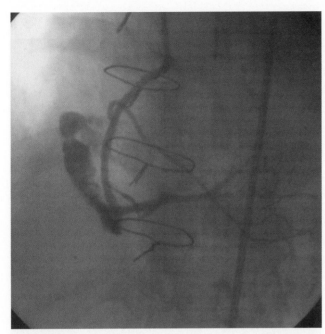

**FIGURE 4–9**

a. abrupt closure of the right coronary artery
b. dissection of the right coronary artery
c. perforation of the right coronary artery
d. allergic reaction

**66.** Patients with scleroderma have

a. increased coronary flow reserve
b. decreased coronary flow reserve
c. normal coronary flow reserve

**67.** The major difference in the morphology of coronary atherosclerotic lesion in patients with end-stage renal failure compared to nonuremic patients is

a. significantly more fibrous plaques of coronary arteries in patients with end-stage renal failure
b. significantly more calcified plaques of coronary arteries in patients with end-stage renal failure
c. significantly more cellular plaques of coronary arteries in patients with end-stage renal failure

**68.** Regarding homocysteine as a risk factor for coronary artery disease, which statement is most accurate?

a. In patients with angiographically defined coronary artery disease, homocysteine is a significant predictor of mortality, in conjunction with traditional risk factors, CRP, and methylenetetrahydrofolate reductase (MTHFR) genotype.

**b.** In patients with angiographically defined coronary artery disease, homocysteine is a significant predictor of mortality, independent of traditional risk factors, CRP, and methylenetetrahydrofolate reductase (MTHFR) genotype.

**c.** In patients with angiographically defined coronary artery disease, homocysteine is not a significant predictor of mortality, but CRP and methylenetetrahydrofolate reductase (MTHFR) genotype were predictors.

**69.** The angiogram (Fig. 4–10) in this 28-year-old male with hypercholesterolemia reveals

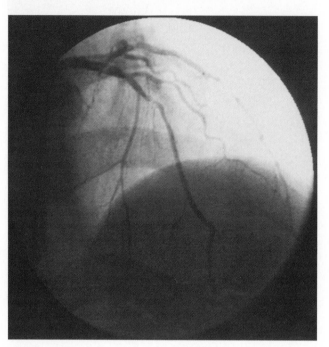

**FIGURE 4–10**

**a.** severe left circumflex artery stenosis
**b.** severe left main trunk stenosis
**c.** severe left anterior descending artery stenosis
**d.** severe right coronary artery stenosis

**70.** The Occluded Artery Trial (OAT), which tested a strategy of routine PCI for total occlusion of the infarct-related artery 3 to 28 days after acute myocardial infarction, demonstrated that

**a.** PCI reduced the occurrence of death, reinfarction, or heart failure, and there was a trend toward excess reinfarction during 4 years of follow-up in stable patients with occlusion of the infarct-related artery 3 to 28 days after myocardial infarction.

**b.** PCI did not reduce the occurrence of death, reinfarction, or heart failure, and there was a trend toward excess reinfarction during 4 years of follow-up in stable patients with occlusion of the infarct-related artery 3 to 28 days after myocardial infarction.

**c.** CABG did not reduce the occurrence of death, reinfarction, or heart failure, and there was a trend toward excess reinfarction during 4 years of follow-up in stable patients with occlusion of the infarct-related artery 3 to 28 days after myocardial infarction.

**71.** The Clopidogrel for High Atherothrombotic Risk and Ischemic Stabilization, Management, and Avoidance (CHARISMA) trial demonstrated that

a. Among patients with established atherothrombotic disease or at high risk for such disease, there was no significant benefit associated with clopidogrel plus aspirin as compared with placebo plus aspirin in reducing the incidence of the primary end point of myocardial infarction, stroke, or death from cardiovascular causes.

b. Among patients with established atherothrombotic disease or at high risk for such disease, there was a significant benefit associated with clopidogrel plus aspirin as compared with placebo plus aspirin in reducing the incidence of the primary end point of myocardial infarction, stroke, or death from cardiovascular causes.

c. The rate of severe or moderate bleeding was not significantly greater with clopidogrel than with placebo.

**72.** The angiogram (Fig. 4–11) in this 79-year-old female with inferolateral ischemia reveals

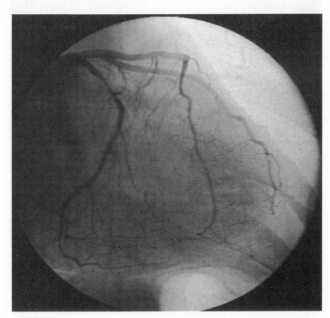

**FIGURE 4–11**

a. severe left circumflex artery stenosis
b. severe left main trunk stenosis
c. severe left anterior descending artery stenosis
d. severe right coronary artery stenosis

**73.** The use of combination evidence-based therapies (antiplatelet agents, statins, beta-blockers, angiotensin converting enzyme inhibitors) in patients with acute coronary syndrome is associated with

a. significant reduction in recurrent angina but no mortality benefit
b. significant survival advantage
c. no significant clinical benefits

**74.** The Clinical Outcomes Utilizing Revascularization and Aggressive Drug Evaluation (COURAGE) trial was designed to determine whether PCI coupled with optimal medical therapy reduces the risk of death and nonfatal myocardial infarction in patients with stable coronary artery disease, as compared with optimal medical therapy alone, and demonstrated that

a. PCI reduced the risk of death, myocardial infarction, or other major cardiovascular events when added to optimal medical therapy.

**b.** PCI did not reduce the risk of death, myocardial infarction, or other major cardiovascular events when added to optimal medical therapy.

**c.** PCI did not reduce the risk of death, myocardial infarction, the prevalence of angina or other cardiovascular events when added to optimal medical therapy.

**75.** The angiogram (Fig. 4–12) in this 67-year-old male with inferoposterior ischemia reveals

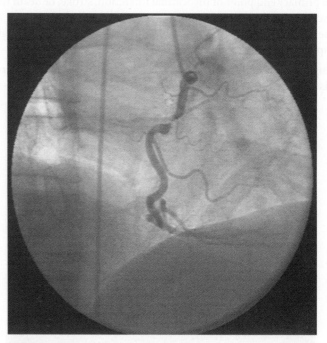

**FIGURE 4–12**

**a.** severe left circumflex artery stenosis

**b.** severe left main trunk stenosis

**c.** severe left anterior descending artery stenosis

**d.** severe right coronary artery stenosis

**76.** In the initial randomized trials of drug-eluting stents (DES), dual antiplatelet therapy with aspirin and clopidogrel was recommended for

**a.** 1 month for sirolimus-eluting and paclitaxel-eluting stents

**b.** 3 months for sirolimus-eluting and paclitaxel-eluting stents

**c.** 2 to 3 months for sirolimus-eluting and 6 months for paclitaxel-eluting stents

**d.** 6 months for sirolimus-eluting and paclitaxel-eluting stents

**e.** 12 months for sirolimus-eluting and paclitaxel-eluting stents

**77.** Your patient presented in an outside hospital with an acute coronary syndrome and underwent a drug-eluting stent (DES)-based percutaneous coronary intervention (PCI). Unfortunately, the patient has an absolute indication for oral anticoagulation because of a prosthetic mitral valve. Your best option at this moment is

**a.** Administer dual antiplatelet therapy for 3 months in addition to oral anticoagulation, and then continue with aspirin and oral anticoagulation indefinitely.

**b.** Administer dual antiplatelet therapy for 1 month in addition to oral anticoagulation, and then continue with aspirin and oral anticoagulation indefinitely.

**c.** Administer dual antiplatelet therapy for at least 6 months, if possible 12 months, in addition to oral anticoagulation, and then continue with aspirin and oral anticoagulation indefinitely.

**d.** Since the patient is anticoagulated, the combination with aspirin long-term is sufficient.

**e.** Since the patient is anticoagulated, the combination with clopidogrel long-term is sufficient.

**78.** The angiogram (Fig. 4–13) in this 54-year-old male with acute lateral wall myocardial infarction reveals

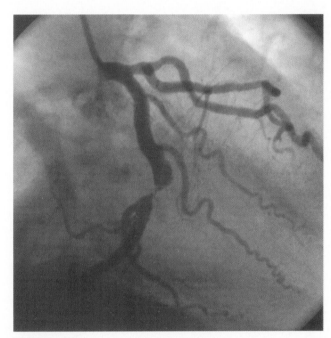

**FIGURE 4–13**

**a.** severe left circumflex artery stenosis

**b.** severe left main trunk stenosis

**c.** severe left anterior descending artery stenosis

**d.** severe right coronary artery stenosis

**79.** Which of the following statements regarding the implantation of coronary stents prior to noncardiac surgery is correct?

**a.** The implantation of drug-eluting stents (DESs) is not problematic as long as aspirin can be continued during surgery.

**b.** The implantation of DESs is not problematic as long as clopidogrel can be continued during surgery.

**c.** The implantation of DESs is not problematic as long as aspirin and clopidogrel can be continued during surgery.

**d.** The implantation of a bare-metal stent (BMS) is not problematic.

**e.** Stent thrombosis associated with noncardiac surgery may occur also with a BMS.

**80.** Which of the following statements on the use of long-term dual antiplatelet therapy post drug-eluting-stent (DES) implantation is correct?

**a.** Because of the possibility of DES late thrombosis, aspirin and clopidogrel are recommended indefinitely.

**b.** Based on the results of the CHARISMA trial, aspirin and clopidogrel should be administered for at least 3 years in patients with an acute coronary event, independently of the implantation of a DES.

**c.** At 1 year, clopidogrel can be discontinued but the aspirin dose should be increased to 325 mg/day.

**d.** In patients at particular high risk of stent thrombosis (e.g., patients who have already suffered a stent thrombosis) or patients in whom a stent thrombosis would be associated with catastrophic outcomes (e.g., patients with a left main trunk stent), dual antiplatelet therapy may be extended after 12 months, although currently there are no data to support this strategy.

**e.** Following DES implantation, aspirin should be discontinued at 12 months and clopidogrel administered indefinitely.

# ANSWERS

1. **c.** There is continued debate as to whether a routine, early invasive strategy is superior to a conservative strategy for the management of unstable angina and non–ST-segment elevation myocardial infarction (UA/NSTEMI). The TACTICS study enrolled 2,220 patients with UA/NSTEMI who had electrocardiographic evidence of changes in the ST segment or T wave, elevated levels of cardiac markers, a history of coronary artery disease, or all three findings. All patients were treated with aspirin, heparin, and the glycoprotein IIb/IIIa inhibitor tirofiban. They were randomly assigned to an early invasive strategy, which included routine catheterization within 4 to 48 hours and revascularization as appropriate, or to a more conservative (selectively invasive) strategy, in which catheterization was performed only if the patient had objective evidence of recurrent ischemia or an abnormal stress test. The primary end point was a composite of death, nonfatal myocardial infarction, and rehospitalization for an acute coronary syndrome at 6 months. At 6 months, the rate of the primary end point was 15.9% with use of the early invasive strategy and 19.4% with use of the conservative strategy (odds ratio [OR], 0.78; 95% confidence interval [CI], 0.62 to 0.97; $p = 0.025$). The rate of death or nonfatal myocardial infarction at 6 months was similarly reduced (7.3% vs. 9.5%; OR, 0.74; 95% CI, 0.54 to 1.00; $p < 0.05$). An early invasive strategy was particularly beneficial among patients—like the one just described—with elevated troponin at presentation. Accordingly. the incidence of the primary end point was 14.8% among troponin-positive patients undergoing early invasive strategy and 24.2% among those treated conservatively (OR, 0.55; 95% CI, 0.40 to 0.75; $p < 0.001$). The authors concluded that in patients with UA/NSTEMI who were treated with the glycoprotein IIb/IIIa inhibitor tirofiban, the use of an early invasive strategy significantly reduced the incidence of major cardiac events. These data support a policy involving broader use of the early inhibition of glycoprotein IIb/IIIa in combination with an early invasive strategy in this setting.[1] The ACC/AHA 2007 Guidelines for the Management of Patients with Unstable Angina/Non–ST-Elevation Myocardial Infarction recommends an early invasive strategy (i.e., diagnostic angiography with intent to perform revascularization) in patients who have refractory angina or hemodynamic or electrical instability, and in those initially stabilized who have an elevated risk for clinical events.[2] Table 4–1 (see question 21) lists patients at elevated risk and in whom invasive strategy is preferred based on the ACC/AHA 2007 guidelines. Our patient has several high-risk criteria including ST-segment depression and elevated troponin.

2. **b.** Belardinelli et al. addressed the effects of exercise training (ET) on functional capacity and quality of life (QOL) in patients who received percutaneous transluminal coronary angioplasty (PTCA) or coronary stenting (CS). The authors studied 118 consecutive patients with coronary artery disease (mean age 57 +/– 10 years) who underwent PTCA or CS on one (69%) or two (31%) native epicardial coronary arteries. Patients were randomized into two matched groups. Group T (n = 59) was exercised three times a week for 6 months at 60% of peak $\dot{V}o_2$. Group C (n = 59) was the control group. Only patients in the active group had significant improvements in peak $\dot{V}o_2$ (26%, $p < 0.001$) and quality of life (26.8%, $p = 0.001$ vs. C). The angiographic restenosis rate was unaffected by ET (T: 29%; C: 33%, $p =$ not significant). However, residual diameter stenosis was lower in trained patients ($-29.7\%$, $p = 0.045$). In patients with angiographic restenosis, thallium uptake improved only in group T (19%, $p < 0.001$). During the follow-up (33 +/– 7 months) trained patients had a significantly lower event rate than controls (11.9% vs. 32.2%; risk ratio [RR]: 0.71; 95% CI: 0.60 to 0.91; $p = 0.008$) and a lower rate of hospital readmission (18.6% vs. 46%; RR: 0.69; 95% CI: 0.55 to 0.93; $p < 0.001$).

Moderate ET improved functional capacity and QOL after PTCA or CS. During the follow-up, trained patients had fewer events and a lower hospital readmission rate than controls, despite an unchanged restenosis rate.[3]

3. **b.** Inflammatory reactions in coronary plaques play an important role in the pathogenesis of acute atherothrombotic events; inflammatory involvement of the peripheral arterial vasculature is also associated with both atherogenesis and its vascular events. Recent studies indicate that systemic markers of inflammation can identify subjects at high risk of coronary events. Koenig et al. used a sensitive immunoradiometric assay to examine the association of serum C-reactive protein (CRP), a sensitive systemic marker of inflammation, with the incidence of the first major coronary heart disease (CHD) event in 936 men 45 to 64 years of age. The subjects, who were sampled at random from the general population, participated in the first MONICA Augsburg survey (1984 to 1985) and were followed for 8 years. The study demonstrated a positive and statistically significant unadjusted relationship, which was linear on the log-hazards scale, between CRP values and the incidence of CHD events (n = 53). The hazard rate ratio (HRR) of CHD events associated with a 1-SD increase in log-CRP level was 1.67 (95% CI, 1.29 to 2.17). After adjustment for age, the HRR was 1.60 (95% CI, 1.23 to 2.08). Adjusting further for smoking behavior, the only variable selected from a variety of potential confounders by a forward-stepping process, with a 5% change in the relative risk of CRP as the selection criterion, yielded an HRR of 1.50 (95% CI, 1.14 to 1.97). These results demonstrate the prognostic relevance of CRP in terms of future cardiovascular event prediction in a large unselected cohort of healthy middle-aged men. These data support the concept that low-grade inflammation is involved in the pathogenesis of atherosclerosis and its thrombo-occlusive complications.[4] Similarly, within a prospective large cohort of apparently healthy men, baseline CRP level added to the predictive value of lipid parameters in determining risk of first MI.[5]

4. **c.** In the randomized trial TAXUS V ISR, the slow-release, polymer-based, paclitaxel-eluting stent was found to be not only noninferior to β source vascular brachytherapy, but also superior in terms of reducing clinical and angiographic restenosis at 9 months after treatment of bare-metal ISR lesions. Because of both greater acute gain and less late loss, luminal dimensions were significantly larger with paclitaxel-eluting stents compared with brachytherapy in the injury zone, at the distal edge, and over the entire analysis segment. Proximal edge luminal dimensions were also numerically larger with the paclitaxel-eluting stent.[6] Similarly, the Sirolimus-Eluting Stent with Vascular Brachytherapy for the Treatment of In-Stent Restenosis (SISR) trial demonstrated a marked reduction in target vessel failure with the sirolimus-eluting stent, driven predominantly by a reduction in the rate of target vessel revascularization.[7] Based on available data, drug-eluting stent implantation is the best option for patients with bare metal stent restenosis.[8] Brachytherapy is no longer available except in a few research centers.

5. **d.** Angiotensin-converting-enzyme inhibitors improve the outcome among patients with left ventricular dysfunction, whether or not they have overt heart failure. In the HOPE trial, a total of 9,297 high-risk patients (55 years of age or older, with evidence of vascular disease or diabetes plus one additional cardiovascular risk factor and/or low left ventricular ejection fraction or heart failure) were randomly assigned to receive ramipril (10 mg once per day orally) or matching placebo for a mean of 5 years. The primary outcome of the study was a composite of myocardial infarction, stroke, or cardiovascular death. A total of 651 patients allocated to ramipril (14.0%) reached the primary end point, as compared with 826 patients in the placebo group (17.8%) (RR 0.78; 95% CI 0.70 to 0.86; $p < 0.001$). Treatment with ramipril reduced the rates of death from cardiovascular causes (6.1%, as compared with 8.1% in the placebo group; RR 0.74; $p < 0.001$), myocardial infarction (9.9% vs. 12.3%; RR 0.80; $p < 0.001$), stroke

(3.4% vs. 4.9%; RR 0.68; *p* <0.001), death from any cause (10.4% vs. 12.2%; RR 0.84; *p* = 0.005), revascularization procedures (16.3% vs. 18.8%; RR 0.85; *p* <0.001), cardiac arrest (0.8% vs. 1.3%; RR 0.62; *p* = 0.02), heart failure (9.1% vs. 11.6%; RR 0.77; *p* <0.001), and complications related to diabetes (6.4% vs. 7.6%; RR 0.84; *p* = 0.03). In the study, ramipril also significantly reduced the rates of death, myocardial infarction, and stroke in patients without low ejection fraction or heart failure. However, treatment with ramipril had no effect on the likelihood of hospitalization for unstable angina.[9]

6. **d.** Myocardial infarction is the most frequent cause of mortality in the United States as well as in most western countries. Fuster and Lewis reviewed the processes leading to myocardial infarction based on studies of vascular biology. Five phases of the progression of coronary atherosclerosis (phases 1 to 5) and eight morphologically different lesions (Stary types I, II, III, IV, Va, Vb, Vc, and VI) in the various phases were defined. Type VI lesion is characterized by plaque rupture. This phenomenon is associated with local thrombus formation, vessel obstruction, and acute myocardial infarction.[10]

7. **d.** Oxygen-carrying capacity of the blood determines oxygen supply, not demand.

8. **c.** The subendocardium is most susceptible to ischemic damage. Although the mechanisms of subendocardial ischemia remain to be fully defined, they are clearly associated with the transmural distribution of intramyocardial systolic pressures. Even though almost all the myocardium is perfused in diastole, a reduction of diastolic perfusion pressure or duration will result in subendocardial ischemia.[11]

9. **d.** The association of inferior wall myocardial infarction on ECG and elevated jugular venous pressure with clear lungs is suggestive of additional right ventricular infarction. Tall *c–v* waves of tricuspid regurgitation may be evident in patients with necrosis or ischemia of the right ventricular papillary muscles.

10. **a.** An $S_4$ is frequently present in patients with acute myocardial infarction and is related to a reduction in left ventricular compliance. Rapid deceleration of transmitral flow during protodiastolic filling of the left ventricle and increased inflow into the left ventricle are responsible for the third heart sound ($S_3$).

11. **c.** The relative efficacy of streptokinase and tissue plasminogen activator and the roles of intravenous as compared with subcutaneous heparin as adjunctive therapy in acute myocardial infarction were studied in GUSTO-I. In 15 countries and 1,081 hospitals, 41,021 patients with evolving myocardial infarction were randomly assigned to four different thrombolytic strategies, consisting of the use of streptokinase and subcutaneous heparin, streptokinase and intravenous heparin, accelerated tissue plasminogen activator (tPA) and intravenous heparin, or a combination of streptokinase plus tPA with intravenous heparin. ("Accelerated" refers to the administration of tPA over a period of 1 1/2 hours, with two thirds of the dose given in the first 30 minutes, rather than the conventional period of 3 hours.) The primary end point was 30-day mortality. The mortality rates in the four treatment groups were as follows: streptokinase and subcutaneous heparin, 7.2%; streptokinase and intravenous heparin, 7.4%; accelerated tPA and intravenous heparin, 6.3%; and the combination of both thrombolytic agents with intravenous heparin, 7.0%. This represented a 14% (95% CI, 5.9% to 21.3%) in mortality for accelerated tPA as compared with the two streptokinase-only strategies (*p* = 0.001). The rates of hemorrhagic stroke were 0.49%, 0.54%, 0.72%, and 0.94% in the four groups, respectively, which represented a significant excess of hemorrhagic strokes for accelerated tPA (*p* = 0.03) and for the combination strategy (*p* < 0.001), as compared with streptokinase only. A combined end point of death or disabling stroke was significantly lower in the accelerated-tPA group than in the streptokinase-only groups (6.9% vs. 7.8%, *p* = 0.006). The authors concluded that accelerated tPA

**NOTES**

given with intravenous heparin provides a survival benefit over previous standard thrombolytic regimens. Reocclusion was infrequent and was similar in all four groups (range, 4.9% to 6.4%)[13,14]

**12. b.** The earliest rise is seen with myoglobin, followed by CK-MB, troponin, and then LDH[12] (Fig. 4–14). However, compared with troponins or CK-MB, the diagnostic value of myoglobin is limited by its lower specificity.

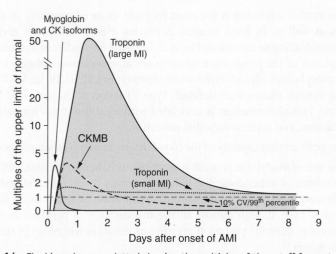

**FIGURE 4–14**   The biomarkers are plotted showing the multiples of the cutoff for acute myocardial infarction (AMI) over time. The dashed horizontal line shows the upper limit of normal (ULN; defined as the 99th percentile from a normal reference population without myocardial necrosis; the coefficient of variation of the assay should be 10% or less). The earliest rising biomarkers are myoglobin and CK isoforms *(leftmost curve)*. CK-MB *(dashed curve)* rises to a peak of 2 to 5 times the ULN and typically returns to the normal range within 2 to 3 days after AMI. The cardiac-specific troponins show small elevations above the ULN in small infarctions (e.g., as is often the case with NSTEMI) but rise to 20 to 50 times the ULN in the setting of large infarctions (e.g., as is typically the case in STEMI). The troponin levels may stay elevated above the ULN for 7 days or more after AMI. CK, creatine kinase; CK-MB, MB fraction of creatine kinase; CV, coefficient of variation; MI, myocardial infarction; NSTEMI, non–ST-elevation myocardial infarction; UA/NSTEMI, unstable angina/non–ST-elevation myocardial infarction. [Adapted from Anderson JL, Adams CD, Antman EM, et al. ACC/AHA 2007 guidelines for the management of patients with unstable angina/non-ST-Elevation myocardial infarction: a report of the American College of Cardiology/American Heart Association Task Force on Practice Guidelines (Writing Committee to Revise the 2002 Guidelines for the Management of Patients with Unstable Angina/Non-ST-Elevation Myocardial Infarction) developed in collaboration with the American College of Emergency Physicians, the Society for Cardiovascular Angiography and Interventions, and the Society of Thoracic Surgeons endorsed by the American Association of Cardiovascular and Pulmonary Rehabilitation and the Society for Academic Emergency Medicine. *J Am Coll Cardiol.* 2007;50:e1–e157, with permission.]

**13. d.** Individual patients reflect a combination of clinical features that influence prognosis, and these factors must be appropriately weighted to produce an accurate assessment of risk. Using the large population of the GUSTO-I trial, Lee et al. performed a comprehensive analysis of relations between baseline clinical data and 30-day mortality and developed a multivariable statistical model for risk assessment in candidates for thrombolytic therapy. For the 41,021 patients enrolled in GUSTO-I, a randomized trial of four thrombolytic strategies, relations between clinical descriptors routinely collected at initial presentation, and death within 30 days (which occurred in 7% of the population) were examined with both univariable and multivariable analyses. Variables studied included demographics, history and risk factors, presenting characteristics, and treatment assignment. Risk modeling was performed with logistic multiple regression and validated with bootstrapping techniques. Multivariable analysis identified age as the most significant factor influencing 30-day mortality, with rates of 1.1% in the youngest decile (<45 years) and 20.5% in patients >75 (adjusted chi 2 = 717, $p$ <.0001). Other factors most significantly associated with increased mortality were lower systolic blood pressure (chi 2 = 550, $p$ <.0001), higher Killip class (chi 2 = 350, $p$ <.0001), elevated heart rate (chi 2 = 275, $p$ <.0001), and anterior infarction (chi 2 = 143, $p$ <.0001). Together, these five characteristics contained 90% of the prognostic information in the baseline clinical data. Other significant though less important factors included previous myocardial infarction, height, time to treatment, diabetes, weight, smoking status, type of thrombolytic, previous bypass surgery, hypertension, and prior cerebrovascular disease. Choice of the thrombolytic agent contributed less than 1% to the proportional effect of mortality.[15]

**14. c.** High-risk exercise ECG variables include (a) ≥2.0 mm ST-segment depression, (b) ≥1 mm ST-segment depression in stage I, (c) ST-segment depression in multiple leads, (d) ST-segment depression > 1.0 for > 5 minutes during the recovery period, (e) achievement of a workload of less than 4 METS or a low maximal heart rate, (f) abnormal blood pressure response, and (g) ventricular arrhythmias.[16]

**15. a.** The CASS randomized 780 patients to an initial strategy of coronary surgery or medical therapy. Of medically randomized patients, 6% had surgery within 6 months and a total of 40% had surgery by 10 years. At 10 years, there was no difference in cumulative survival (medical, 79%, vs. surgical, 82%; NS) and no difference in percentage free of death and nonfatal myocardial infarction (medical, 69%, vs. surgical, 66%; NS). Patients with an ejection fraction of less than 0.50 exhibited a better survival with initial surgery treatment (medical, 61%, vs. surgical, 79%; $p$ = 0.01). Conversely, patients with an ejection fraction ≥0.50 exhibited a higher proportion free of death and myocardial infarction with initial medical therapy (medical, 75%, vs. surgical, 68%; $p$ = 0.04), although long-term survival remained unaffected (medical, 84%, vs. surgical, 83%; $p$ = 0.75). There were no significant differences either in survival and freedom from nonfatal myocardial infarction, whether stratified on presence of heart failure, age, hypertension, or number of vessels diseased. Thus, 10-year follow-up results confirm earlier reports from CASS that patients with left ventricular dysfunction exhibit long-term benefit from an initial strategy of surgical treatment. Patients with mild stable angina and normal left ventricular function randomized to initial medical treatment (with an option for later surgery if symptoms progress) have survival equivalent to those patients randomized to initial surgery.

**16 a.** The ACIP study assessed the ability of three treatment strategies to suppress ambulatory electrocardiographic ischemia to determine whether a large-scale trial studying the impact of these strategies on clinical outcomes was feasible. Five hundred fifty-eight patients with coronary anatomy amenable to revascularization, at least one episode of asymptomatic ischemia on the 48-hour ambulatory ECG, and ischemia on treadmill exercise testing were randomized to one of three treatment strategies: (a) medication to suppress angina (angina-guided strategy, n = 183); (b) medication to suppress both angina and ambulatory ECG ischemia (ischemia-guided strategy, n = 183); or (c) revascularization strategy (angioplasty or bypass surgery, n = 192). The revascularization group received less medication and had less ischemia on serial ambulatory ECG recordings and exercise testing than those assigned to the medical strategies. The ischemia-guided group received more medication but had suppression of ischemia similar to the angina-guided group. At 1 year, the mortality rate was 4.4% in the angina-guided group (8 of 183), 1.6% in the ischemia-guided group (3 of 183) and 0% in the revascularization group (overall, $p$ = 0.004; angina-guided vs. revascularization, $p$ = 0.003; other pair-wise comparisons, $p$ = NS). Frequency of myocardial infarction, unstable angina, stroke, and congestive heart failure was not significantly different among the three strategies. The revascularization group had significantly fewer hospital admissions and nonprotocol revascularizations at 1 year. The incidence of death, myocardial infarction, nonprotocol revascularization, or hospital admissions at 1 year was 32% with the angina-guided medical strategy, 31% with the ischemia-guided medical strategy, and 18% with the revascularization strategy ($p = 0.003$). After 1 year, revascularization was superior to both angina-guided and ischemia-guided medical strategies in suppressing asymptomatic ischemia, and was associated with better outcomes in terms of total mortality, death, or myocardial infarction, and death, myocardial infarction, or recurrent hospitalization for cardiac causes.[17,18]

17. **c.** A 12-lead ECG should be obtained immediately (within 10 minutes) in patients with ongoing chest discomfort and as rapidly as possible in patients who have a history of chest discomfort consistent with ACS but whose discomfort has resolved by the time of evaluation. The remainder are all class I recommendations.[2]

18. **e.** Patients with possible ACS and negative cardiac markers who are unable to exercise or who have an abnormal resting ECG should have a pharmacological stress test instead of proceeding to coronary angiograms directly.[2]

19. **f.** In patients with continuing or frequently recurring ischemia when beta-blockers are contraindicated, a nondihydropyridine calcium antagonist (e.g., verapamil or diltiazem), followed by oral therapy, is indicated as initial therapy in the absence of severe LV dysfunction or other contraindications.[2] Calcium antagonists are not considered for initial therapy unless beta-blockers are contraindicated. NSAIDs and COX-2 inhibitors should be discontinued in patients presenting with UA/NSTEMI based on potential prothrombotic effects.[19]

20. **f.** The cumulative event rates observed during the phase of medical management and at the time of PCI in the c7E3 Fab Antiplatelet Therapy in Unstable Refractory Angina (CAPTURE) (abciximab), Platelet Receptor Inhibition in Ischemic Syndrome Management in Patients Limited by Unstable Signs and Symptoms (PRISM-PLUS) (tirofiban), and Platelet Glycoprotein IIb/IIIa in Unstable Angina: Receptor Suppression Using Integrilin Therapy (PURSUIT) (eptifibatide) trials are shown in Fig. 4–15. Each trial has shown a statistically significant reduction in the rate of death or MI during the phase of medical management; the reduction in event rates was magnified at the time of the intervention.[20] Boersma et al. performed a meta-analysis of GP IIb/IIIa antagonists of six large, randomized, placebo-controlled trials involving 31,402 patients with UA/NSTEMI not routinely scheduled to undergo coronary revascularization.[21] In the overall population, the risk of death or myocardial infarction at 30 days was modestly reduced in the active treatment arms (11.8% vs. 10.8%, OR 0.91, 95% CI, 0.84 to 0.98, $p = 0.015$). Treatment effect appeared to be greater among higher-risk patients with troponin elevations or ECG ST-segment depressions. These data suggest troponin level to be a major factor in identifying patients likely to benefit from GP IIb/IIIa inhibitors. Major bleeding complications were increased in the GP IIb/IIIa antagonist-treated group compared with those who received placebo (2.4% vs. 1.4%, $p <0.0001$). It is difficult to extrapolate GP IIb/IIIa studies from the 1990s with more recent studies using clopidogrel loading, newer anticoagulants, and varying degrees of patient acuity and risk/benefit. The current evidence suggests that for UA/NSTEMI patients in whom an initial invasive strategy is selected, either an intravenous GP IIb/IIIa inhibitor or clopidogrel should be added to ASA and anticoagulant therapy before diagnostic angiography (upstream) for lower-risk, troponin-negative patients and that both (clopidogrel and GP IIb/IIIa) should be given before angiography for high-risk, troponin-positive patients (class I recommendations). For UA/NSTEMI patients in whom an initial noninvasive strategy is selected, the evidence for benefit of GP IIb/IIIa is less robust, but the addition of eptifibatide or tirofiban to

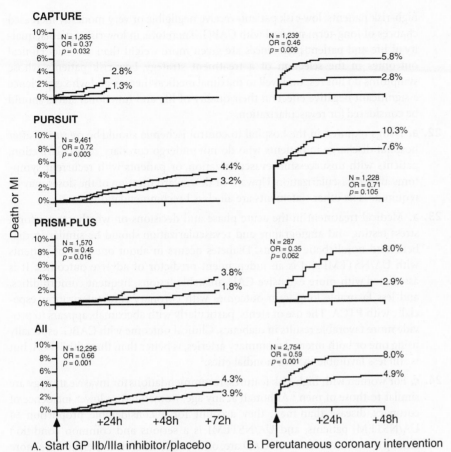

**FIGURE 4–15** Kaplan-Meier curves showing cumulative incidence of death or MI in patients randomly assigned to platelet GP IIb/IIIa receptor antagonist *(bold line)* or placebo. Data are derived from the CAPTURE, PURSUIT, and PRISM-PLUS trials. **(Left)** Events during the initial period of medical treatment until the moment of PCI or CABG. In the CAPTURE trial, abciximab was administered for 18 to 24 hours before the PCI was performed in almost all patients as per study design; abciximab was discontinued 1 hour after the intervention. In PURSUIT, a PCI was performed in 11.2% of patients during a period of medical therapy with eptifibatide that lasted 72 hours and for 24 hours after the intervention. In PRISM-PLUS, an intervention was performed in 30.2% of patients after a 48-hour period of medical therapy with tirofiban, and the drug infusion was maintained for 12 to 24 hours after an intervention. **(Right)** Events occurring at the time of PCI and the next 48 hours, with the event rates reset to 0% before the intervention. CK or CK-MB elevations exceeding two times the upper limit of normal were considered as infarction during medical management and exceeding three times the upper limit of normal for PCI-related events. OR, odds ratio. (Adapted from Boersma E, Akkerhuis KM, Theroux P, et al. Platelet glycoprotein IIb/IIIa receptor inhibition in non–ST-elevation acute coronary syndromes: early benefit during medical treatment only, with additional protection during percutaneous coronary intervention. *Circulation.* 1999;100:2045–2048, with permission.)

anticoagulant and oral antiplatelet therapy may be reasonable for high-risk UA/NSTEMI patients (class IIb recommendation). There is no evidence to support routine use of GP IIb/IIIa in all patients with UA/NSTEMI.

21. **b.** PCI or CABG for patients with one- or two-vessel CAD without significant proximal left anterior descending CAD is indicated in patients with a large area of viable myocardium and high-risk criteria on noninvasive testing.[2] In general, the indications for PCI and CABG in UA/NSTEMI are similar to those in stable angina. High-risk patients with LV systolic dysfunction, two-vessel disease with severe proximal LAD involvement, severe three-vessel disease, or left main disease should be considered for CABG. Many other patients will have less severe CAD that does not put them at high risk for cardiac death. However, even less severe disease can have a substantial negative effect on the quality of life. Compared with

high-risk patients, low-risk patients receive negligible or very modestly increased chances of long-term survival with CABG. Therefore, in low-risk patients, quality of life and patient preferences are given more weight than are strict clinical outcomes in the selection of a treatment strategy. Low-risk patients whose symptoms do not respond well to maximal medical therapy and who experience a significant negative effect on their quality of life and functional status should be considered for revascularization.

22. **a.** Drugs required in the hospital to control ischemia should be *continued* after hospital discharge in patients who do not undergo coronary revascularization, patients with unsuccessful revascularization, or patients with recurrent symptoms after revascularization. Upward or downward titration of the doses may be required.[2] The other statements are all class I recommendations.

23. **a.** Medical treatment in the acute phase and decisions on whether to perform stress testing and angiography and revascularization should be similar in diabetic and nondiabetic patients. Diabetes occurs in about one fifth of patients with UA/NSTEMI and is an independent predictor of adverse outcomes. It is associated with more extensive CAD, unstable lesions, frequent comorbidities, and less favorable long-term outcomes with coronary revascularization, especially with PTCA. The use of stents, particularly with abciximab, appears to provide more favorable results in diabetics. Clinical outcome with CABG, especially using one or both internal mammary arteries, is better than that with PTCA, but is still less favorable than in nondiabetics.[2]

24. **c.** For women with high-risk features, recommendations for invasive strategy are similar to those of men.[2] Although at any age, women have a lower incidence of coronary disease than men, they account for a considerable proportion of UA/NSTEMI patients, and UA/NSTEMI is a serious and common condition among women. Women with CAD are, on average, older than men and are more likely to have comorbidities such as hypertension, diabetes mellitus, and heart failure with preserved systolic function; to manifest angina rather than MI; and, among angina and MI patients, to have atypical symptoms. The BARI trial of 1,829 patients compared PTCA and CABG, primarily in patients with UA, and showed that the results of revascularization were, if anything, better in women than men when corrected for other factors.[22]

25. **a.** A class I indication for coronary angiography in these patients is disabling (Canadian Cardiovascular Society [CCS] classes III and IV) chronic stable angina *despite* medical therapy. Patients identified as having increased risk on the basis of an assessment of clinical data and noninvasive testing are generally referred for coronary arteriography even if their symptoms are not severe. Noninvasive testing that is used appropriately is less costly than coronary angiography and has an acceptable predictive value for adverse events. This is most true when the pretest probability of severe CAD is low. When the pretest probability of severe CAD is high, direct referral for coronary angiography without noninvasive testing is probably most cost-effective because the total number of tests is reduced. Coronary angiography, the traditional "gold standard" for clinical assessment of coronary atherosclerosis, has limitations. It is not a reliable indicator of the functional significance of a coronary stenosis and is insensitive in detection of a thrombus (an indicator of disease activity). More importantly, coronary angiography is ineffective in determining which plaques have characteristics likely to lead to acute coronary events, that is, the vulnerable plaque with large lipid core, thin fibrous cap, and increased inflammatory content. Serial angiographic studies performed before and after acute events and early after MI suggest that plaques resulting in unstable angina and MI commonly produced <50% stenosis before the acute event and were therefore angiographically "silent." Despite these limitations of coronary angiography, the extent and severity of coronary disease and LV dysfunction identified on angiography are the

most powerful predictors of long-term patient outcome. Several prognostic indexes have been used to relate disease severity to the risk of subsequent cardiac events; the simplest and most widely used is the classification of disease into one-, two-, or three-vessel or left main coronary artery disease. In the Coronary Artery Surgery Study (CASS) registry of medically treated patients, the 12-year survival rate of patients with normal coronary arteries was 91% compared with 74% for those with one-vessel disease, 59% for those with two-vessel disease, and 40% for those with three-vessel disease. It has been known for many years that patients with significant stenosis of the left main coronary artery have a poor prognosis when treated medically. The impact of LV dysfunction on survival was quite dramatic. In the CASS registry, the 12-year survival rate was 73% for patients with an ejection fraction between 50% and 100%, 54% for those with an ejection fraction between 35% and 49%, and only 21% for those with an ejection fraction <35%.[23]

26. **b.** Proximal LAD stenosis with one-vessel disease is a class IIa indication.[23] Proximal LAD stenosis with two-vessel disease becomes class I if ischemia is documented by noninvasive study and/or an LVEF <0.50.

27. **d.** Exercise ECG without imaging is a reasonable option stress test in a patient with a normal rest ECG who is not taking digoxin and is a class IIa indication. The rest are all class I recommendations.[23]

28. **d.** An analysis of 2,974 consecutive patients to evaluate the correlates and long-term outcomes of all patients who presented with angiographically proven stent thrombosis (ST) after drug-eluting stent (DES) implantation demonstrated that ST occurred in more complex subsets of patients and lesions and was associated with significantly higher mortality rates at 1 and 6 months compared with those without ST. Treatment of bifurcation lesions, in-stent restenosis lesions, renal failure, and lack of clopidogrel therapy were detected as independent predictors of ST.[24] Most ST was seen in the first 30 days after DES implantation. The incidence of ST was similar for sirolimus-eluting and paclitaxel-eluting stents. Several studies have suggested diabetes as a predictor for stent thrombosis.[25–27] Reference diameter or vessel size has not been an independent predictor of ST.

29. **b.** Stroke is a leading cause of death and disability. Although clinical trials of the early lipid-lowering therapies did not demonstrate a reduction in the rates of stroke, data from recently completed statin trials strongly suggest benefit. The effect of pravastatin 40 mg/day on stroke events was investigated in a prospectively defined pooled analysis of three large, placebo-controlled, randomized trials that included 19,768 patients with 102,559 person-years of follow-up. In all, 598 participants had a stroke during approximately 5 years of follow-up. The two secondary prevention trials (CARE [Cholesterol and Recurrent Events] and LIPID [Long-term Intervention with Pravastatin in Ischemic Disease]) individually demonstrated reductions in nonfatal and total stroke rates. When the 13,173 patients from CARE and LIPID were combined, there was a 22% reduction in total strokes (95% CI, 7% to 35%, $p = 0.01$) and a 25% reduction in nonfatal stroke (95% CI, 10% to 38%). The beneficial effect of pravastatin on total stroke was observed across a wide range of patient characteristics. WOSCOPS (West of Scotland Coronary Prevention Study, a primary prevention trial in hypercholesterolemic men) exhibited a similar, although smaller, trend for a reduction in total stroke. Among the CARE/LIPID participants, pravastatin was associated with a 23% reduction in nonhemorrhagic strokes (95% CI, 6% to 37%), but there was no statistical treatment group difference in hemorrhagic or unknown type.[28]

30. **c.** The Post-CABG trial was done to assess patients after CABG and determine prognostic factors for atherosclerosis progression. Saphenous vein grafts (SVGs) are effective in relieving angina and, in certain patient subsets, in prolonging life. However, the progression of atherosclerosis in many of these grafts limits their

usefulness. The Post-CABG trial studied moderate versus aggressive lipid-lowering and low-dose warfarin versus placebo in patients with a history of coronary artery bypass surgery and found that more aggressive lipid lowering was effective in preventing progression of atherosclerosis in SVGs, but warfarin had no effect. Using variables measured at baseline, we sought the independent prognostic factors for atherosclerosis progression in SVGs, employing the statistical method of generalized estimating equations with a logit-link function. Twelve independent prognostic factors for atherosclerosis progression were found. In the order of their importance they were: maximum stenosis of the graft at baseline angiography, years post-SVG placement; the moderate low-density lipoprotein-cholesterol (LDL-C) lowering strategy; prior myocardial infarction; high triglyceride level; small minimum graft diameter; low high-density lipoprotein-cholesterol (HDL-C); high LDL-C; high mean arterial pressure; low ejection fraction; male gender; and current smoking.[29]

31. **c.** Percutaneous coronary revascularization is widely used in improving symptoms and exercise performance in patients with ischemic heart disease and stable angina pectoris. In the AVERT study, the investigators compared percutaneous coronary revascularization with lipid-lowering treatment for reducing the incidence of ischemic events. They studied 341 patients with stable coronary artery disease, relatively normal left ventricular function, asymptomatic or mild to moderate angina, and a serum level of low-density lipoprotein (LDL) cholesterol of at least 115 mg/dL (3.0 mmol/L) who were referred for percutaneous revascularization. The patients were randomly assigned either to receive medical treatment with atorvastatin, at 80 mg/day (164 patients), or to undergo the recommended percutaneous revascularization procedure (angioplasty) followed by usual care, which could include lipid-lowering treatment (177 patients). The follow-up period was 18 months. Twenty-two (13%) of the patients who received aggressive lipid-lowering treatment with atorvastatin (resulting in a 46% reduction in the mean serum LDL cholesterol level, to 77 mg/dL [2.0 mmol/L]) had ischemic events, as compared with 37 (21%) of the patients who underwent angioplasty (who had an 18% reduction in the mean serum LDL cholesterol level, to 119 mg/dL [3.0 mmol/L]). The incidence of ischemic events was thus 36% lower in the atorvastatin group over an 18-month period ($p = 0.048$, which was not statistically significant after adjustment for interim analyses). This reduction in events was a result of a smaller number of angioplasty procedures, coronary-artery bypass operations, and hospitalizations for worsening angina. As compared with the patients who were treated with angioplasty and usual care, the patients who received atorvastatin had a significantly longer time to the first ischemic event ($p = 0.03$). In low-risk patients with stable coronary artery disease, aggressive lipid-lowering therapy is at least as effective as angioplasty and usual care in reducing the incidence of ischemic events.[30]

32. **c.** The 4S trial was designed to evaluate the effect of lowering cholesterol with simvastatin on mortality and morbidity in patients with coronary heart disease (CHD). Four thousand four hundred and forty-four patients with angina pectoris or previous myocardial infarction and serum cholesterol 5.5 to 8.0 mmol/L on a lipid-lowering diet were randomized to double-blind treatment with simvastatin or placebo. Over the 5.4-year median follow-up period, simvastatin produced mean changes in total cholesterol, low-density-lipoprotein cholesterol, and high-density-lipoprotein cholesterol of −25%, −35%, and +8%, respectively, with few adverse effects. Two hundred and fifty-six patients (12%) in the placebo group died, compared with 182 (8%) in the simvastatin group. The relative risk of death in the simvastatin group was 0.70 (95% CI, 0.58 to 0.85, $p = 0.0003$). The 6-year probabilities of survival in the placebo and simvastatin groups were 87.6% and 91.3%, respectively. There were 189 coronary deaths in the placebo group and 111 in the simvastatin group (relative risk 0.58, 95% CI,

0.46 to 0.73), while noncardiovascular causes accounted for 49 and 46 deaths, respectively. Six hundred and twenty-two patients (28%) in the placebo group and 431 (19%) in the simvastatin group had one or more major coronary events. The relative risk was 0.66 (95% CI, 0.59 to 0.75, $p$ <0.00001), and the respective probabilities of escaping such events were 70.5% and 79.6%. This risk was also significantly reduced in subgroups consisting of women and patients of both sexes aged 60 or more. Other benefits of treatment included a 37% reduction ($p$ <0.00001) in the risk of undergoing myocardial revascularisation procedures. This study showed that long-term treatment with simvastatin is safe and improves survival in CHD patients.[31]

**33. b.** The objective of this trial was to compare lovastatin with placebo for prevention of the first acute major coronary event in men and women without clinically evident atherosclerotic cardiovascular disease with average total cholesterol (TC) and LDL-C levels and below-average high-density lipoprotein cholesterol (HDL-C) levels. A randomized, double-blind, placebo-controlled trial was the design of this trial in the setting of outpatient clinics in Texas. A total of 5,608 men and 997 women with average TC and LDL-C and below-average HDL-C (as characterized by lipid percentiles for an age- and sex-matched cohort without cardiovascular disease from the National Health and Nutrition Examination Survey [NHANES] III) were studied. Mean (SD) TC level was 5.71 (0.54) mmol/L (221 [21] mg/dL) (51st percentile), mean (SD) LDL-C level was 3.89 (0.43) mmol/L (150 [17] mg/dL) (60th percentile), mean (SD) HDL-C level was 0.94 (0.14) mmol/L (36 [5] mg/dL) for men and 1.03 (0.14) mmol/L (40 [5] mg/dL) for women (25th and 16th percentiles, respectively), and median (SD) triglyceride levels were 1.78 (0.86) mmol/L (158 [76] mg/dL) (63rd percentile). Lovastatin (20 to 40 mg daily) or placebo in addition to a low-saturated-fat, low-cholesterol diet was studied. The main outcome measure was first acute major coronary event defined as fatal or nonfatal myocardial infarction, unstable angina, or sudden cardiac death. After an average follow-up of 5.2 years, lovastatin reduced the incidence of first acute major coronary events (83 vs. 116 first events; RR, 0.63; 95% CI, 0.50 to 0.79; $p$ <0.001), myocardial infarction (95 vs. 57 myocardial infarctions; RR, 0.60; 95% CI, 0.43 to 0.83; $p$ = 0.002), unstable angina (87 vs. 60 first unstable angina events; RR, 0.68; 95% CI, 0.49 to 0.95; $p$ = 0.02), coronary revascularization procedures (157 vs. 106 procedures; RR, 0.67; 95% CI, 0.52 to 0.85; $p$ = 0.001), coronary events (215 vs. 163 coronary events; RR, 0.75; 95% CI, 0.61 to 0.92; $p$ = 0.006), and cardiovascular events (255 vs. 194 cardiovascular events; RR, 0.75; 95% CI, 0.62 to 0.91; $p$ = 0.003). Lovastatin (20 to 40 mg daily) reduced LDL-C by 25% to 2.96 mmol/L (115 mg/dL) and increased HDL-C by 6% to 1.02 mmol/L (39 mg/dL). There were no clinically relevant differences in safety parameters between treatment groups. Lovastatin reduced the risk for the first acute major coronary event in men and women with average TC and LDL-C levels and below-average HDL-C levels.[32]

**34. b.** The WOSCOPS was a primary prevention trial that demonstrated the effectiveness of pravastatin (40 mg/day) in reducing morbidity and mortality from coronary heart disease (CHD) in moderately hypercholesterolemic men. The authors examined the extent to which differences in LDL and other plasma lipids both at baseline and on treatment influenced CHD risk reduction. Relationships between baseline lipid concentrations and incidence of all cardiovascular events and between on-treatment lipid concentrations and risk reduction in patients taking pravastatin were examined by use of Cox regression models and by division of the cohort into quintiles. Variation in plasma lipids at baseline did not influence the relative risk reduction generated by pravastatin therapy. Fall in LDL level in the pravastatin-treated group did not correlate with CHD risk reduction in multivariate regression. Furthermore, maximum benefit of an approximately 45% risk reduction was observed in the middle quintile of

LDL reduction (mean 24% fall); further mean decrements in LDL (up to 39%) were not associated with a greater decrease in CHD risk. Comparison of event rates between placebo- and pravastatin-treated subjects with the same LDL cholesterol level provided evidence for an apparent treatment effect that was independent of LDL. The investigators concluded that the treatment effect of 40 mg/day of pravastatin is proportionally the same regardless of baseline lipid phenotype. There is no CHD risk reduction unless LDL levels are reduced, but a fall in the range of 24% is sufficient to produce the full benefit in patients taking this dose of pravastatin. LDL reduction alone did not appear to account entirely for the benefits of pravastatin therapy.[33]

**35. b.** Patients with treated diabetes in the randomized-trial segment of the BARI study who were randomized to initial revascularization with PTCA had significantly worse 5-year survival than patients assigned to CABG. This treatment difference was not seen among diabetic patients eligible for BARI who opted to select their mode of revascularization. Among diabetics taking insulin or oral hypoglycemic drugs at entry, angiographic and clinical presentations were comparable between randomized and registry patients. The 5-year all-cause mortality rate was 34.5% in randomized diabetic patients assigned to PTCA versus 19.4% in CABG patients ($p = 0.0024$; RR = 1.87); corresponding cardiac mortality rates were 23.4% and 8.2%, respectively ($p = 0.0002$; RR = 3.10). The CABG benefit was more apparent among patients requiring insulin. In the registry, all-cause mortality was 14.4% for PTCA versus 14.9% for CABG ($p = 0.86$, RR = 1.10), with corresponding cardiac mortality rates of 7.5% and 6.0%, respectively ($p = 0.73$; RR = 1.07). These RRs in the registry increased to 1.29 and 1.41, respectively, after adjustment for all known differences between treatment groups. BARI registry results were consistent with the finding in the randomized trial that initial CABG is associated with better long-term survival than PTCA in treated diabetic patients with multivessel coronary disease suitable for either surgical or catheter-based revascularization.[34]

**36. b.** Cigarette smoking has been causally linked to coronary heart disease. To investigate the effect of smoking on the activity of ischemic heart disease, 65 patients with chronic stable manifestations of coronary disease and a positive exercise tolerance test underwent continuous ambulatory monitoring to quantify the amount of ischemic ST-segment depression during daily life. Twenty-four smokers were compared with 41 nonsmokers for frequency and duration of electrocardiographic signs of ischemia during 24 hours. A total of 4,968 hours of ambulatory monitoring were analyzed. The frequency of episodes was three times as often (median) and the duration of ischemia was 12 times longer (median duration, 24 minutes vs. 2 minutes per 24 hours) in smokers than nonsmokers. This finding remained statistically significant when a number of potentially confounding factors were controlled by means of logistic regression. This study showed that patients with coronary artery disease who smoke have significantly and substantially more active myocardial ischemia during daily life than patients who do not.[35]

**37. b.** The leading cause of death in patients hospitalized for acute myocardial infarction is cardiogenic shock. The SHOCK investigators conducted a randomized trial to evaluate early revascularization in patients with cardiogenic shock. Patients with shock caused by left ventricular failure complicating myocardial infarction were randomly assigned to emergency revascularization (152 patients) or initial medical stabilization (150 patients). Revascularization was accomplished by either coronary-artery bypass grafting or angioplasty. Intra-aortic balloon counterpulsation was performed in 86% of the patients in both groups. The primary end point was mortality from all causes at 30 days. Six-month survival was a secondary end point. The mean age of the patients was 66 +/− 10 years; 32% were women and 55% were transferred from other hospitals.

The median time to the onset of shock was 5.6 hours after infarction, and most infarcts were anterior in location. Ninety-seven percent of the patients assigned to revascularization underwent early coronary angiography, and 87% underwent revascularization; only 2.7% of the patients assigned to medical therapy crossed over to early revascularization without clinical indication. Overall mortality at 30 days (primary end point) did not differ significantly between the revascularization and medical-therapy groups (46.7% and 56.0%, respectively; difference, $-9.3$%; 95% CI for the difference, $-20.5$% to 1.9%; $p = 0.11$). However, at 6 months mortality was lower in the revascularization group than in the medical-therapy group (50.3% vs. 63.1%, $p = 0.027$).[36]

**38. a.** Califf et al. analyzed the clinical outcomes in 688 patients with isolated stenosis of one major coronary artery. The survival rate among patients with disease of the right coronary artery (RCA) was higher than that among patients with left anterior descending (LAD) or left circumflex coronary artery (LCA) disease. The survival rate among patients in all three anatomic subgroups exceeded 90% at 5 years. The presence of a lesion proximal to the first septal perforator of the LAD was associated with decreased survival compared with the presence of a more distal lesion. For the entire group of one-vessel-disease patients, total ischemic events (death and nonfatal infarction) occurred at similar rates regardless of the anatomic location of the lesion. Left ventricular ejection fraction was the baseline descriptor most strongly associated with survival, and the characteristics of the angina had the strongest relationship with nonfatal myocardial infarction. No differences in survival or total cardiac event rates were found with surgical or nonsurgical therapy. The relief of angina was superior with surgical therapy, although the majority of nonsurgically treated patients had significant relief of angina. The survival rate of patients with one-vessel coronary disease is excellent, and the risk of nonfatal infarction is low.[37]

**39. c.** Iskandrian et al. examined the ability of SPECT imaging with thallium-201 during adenosine-induced coronary hyperemia to detect high-risk patients with left main or three-vessel CAD. There were 339 patients: 102 with either left main or three-vessel CAD (group 1) and 237 with no CAD, one-, or two-vessel disease (group 2). By means of univariate analysis, several variables were found to differ between groups 1 and 2: Q wave myocardial infarction (35% vs. 25%, $p < 0.05$), ST-segment depression on resting ECG (35% vs. 19%, $p < 0.001$), age (67 $+/-$ 9 vs. 62 $+/-$ 10 years, $p < 0.001$), resting systolic blood pressure (142 $+/-$ 22 vs. 135 $+/-$ 20 mm Hg, $p < 0.01$), abnormal thallium images (95% vs. 74%, $p < 0.0001$), multivessel thallium abnormality (76% vs. 39%, $p < 0.0001$), extent of thallium abnormality (24 $+/-$ 11% vs. 19 $+/-$ 13%, $p < 0.0001$), and increased lung thallium uptake (39% vs. 15%, $p < 0.01$). According to step-wise discriminate analysis, only three variables were predictors of high risk: multivessel thallium abnormality (chi 2 = 27), increased lung thallium uptake (chi 2 = 10), and ST depression (chi 2 = 5). On the basis of these variables, patients were divided into three groups with different prevalence rates for left main and three-vessel CAD: 63% in 68 patients, 30% in 137 patients, and 13% in 137 patients.[38]

**40. a.** Abciximab, a potent inhibitor of the platelet glycoprotein IIb/IIIa receptor, reduces thrombotic complications in patients undergoing percutaneous coronary intervention (PCI). Because of its potent inhibition of platelet aggregation, the effect of abciximab on risk of stroke, and particularly of hemorrhagic stroke, is a concern. To determine whether abciximab use among patients undergoing PCI is associated with an increased risk of stroke, Akkerhuis et al. combined analysis of data from four double-blind, placebo-controlled, randomized trials (EPIC, CAPTURE, EPILOG, and EPISTENT) conducted between November 1991 and October 1997 at a total of 257 academic and community hospitals in the United States and Europe. A total of 8,555 patients undergoing PCI with or without stent deployment for a variety of indications were randomly assigned to receive a bolus and infusion of abciximab (n = 5,476) or matching placebo (n = 3,079). Risk of hemorrhagic and nonhemorrhagic stroke within 30 days of treatment among abciximab and placebo groups was analyzed. No significant difference in stroke rate was observed between patients assigned abciximab (n = 22 [0.40%]) and those assigned placebo (n = 9 [0.29%]; *p* = 0.46). Excluding the EPIC abciximab bolus-only group, there were nine strokes (0.30%) among 3,023 patients who received placebo and 15 (0.32%) in 4,680 patients treated with abciximab bolus plus infusion, a difference of 0.02% (95% CI, −0.23% to 0.28%). The rate of nonhemorrhagic stroke was 0.17% in patients treated with abciximab and 0.20% in patients treated with placebo (difference, −0.03%; 95% CI, −0.23% to 0.17%), and the rates of hemorrhagic stroke were 0.15% and 0.10%, respectively (difference, 0.05%; 95% CI, −0.11% to 0.21%). Among patients treated with abciximab, the rate of hemorrhagic stroke in patients receiving standard-dose heparin in EPIC, CAPTURE, and EPILOG was higher than in those receiving low-dose heparin in the EPILOG and EPISTENT trials (0.27% vs. 0.04%; *p* = 0.057). Abciximab in addition to aspirin and heparin does not increase the risk of stroke in patients undergoing PCI.[39]

41. **c.** Despite the significant survival benefit associated with successful reperfusion therapy for acute myocardial infarction, global indices of outcome left ventricular function, such as ejection fraction, have often demonstrated little or no improvement. Although these measurements are confounded by numerous clinical, physiologic, and angiographic variables, no comprehensive analysis of this issue in a large series of patients is available. Lundergan et al. used the Global Utilization of Streptokinase and Tissue Plasminogen Activator for Occluded Coronary Arteries (GUSTO-I) database to better understand this phenomenon by determining independent predictors of left ventricular function and their interplay with regard to outcome ventricular function and improvement in function during the initial postinfarction week. Ninety-minute and 5- to 7-day post-treatment global and regional indices derived from left ventriculograms were analyzed from a population of 676 patients. These observations were combined with clinical data to describe independent determinants of ventricular function outcome. Clinical factors predictive of global and regional ventricular function as well as improvement in function between 90 minutes and 5 to 7 days included time to treatment, early infarct-related artery flow grade, and body mass index. Conversely, age was not found to be predictive. These same factors contribute significantly to compensatory hyperkinesis of the noninfarct zone, which is critical to maintenance of global ventricular function during this time period. The ventricular function benefits of early complete reperfusion after myocardial infarction are readily demonstrable after adjustment for multiple covariables and include (a) maintenance of global ventricular function and (b) prevention or delay in ventricular dilatation.[40]

42. **e.** Stone et al. analyzed the Thrombolysis in Myocardial Ischemia (TIMI) IIIB database to determine if certain baseline characteristics are predictive of patients who fail medical therapy, since such patients could then be expeditiously directed to a more invasive strategy in a cost-effective manner. The study cohort consisted of the 733 patients who were randomized to conservative strategy within the trial. Patients were to be treated with bedrest, anti-ischemic medications, aspirin, and heparin, and were to undergo risk-stratifying tests, consisting of an exercise test with ECG and thallium scintigraphy, scheduled to be performed within 3 days prior to, or 5 days after, hospital discharge and 24-hour Holter monitoring scheduled to begin 2 to 5 days after randomization. Baseline clinical and ECG characteristics were compared between patients who "failed" medical therapy and those who did not "fail." Failure was defined using clinical end points (death, myocardial infarction, or spontaneous ischemia by 6 weeks after randomization) or a strongly positive risk-stratifying test. For each test an

ordered failure profile of results was calculated and consisted of death, myocardial infarction, or rest ischemia occurring prior to performance of the test, a markedly abnormal test result, and no abnormality. Clinical end points occurred in 241 (33%) patients and were more likely to occur in patients who at presentation were older, had ST-segment depression on the qualifying ECG, or were being treated with heparin or aspirin. Characteristics independently predictive of developing a clinical event or an abnormal exercise treadmill test included ST-segment depression on the qualifying ECG, history of prior angina, family history of premature coronary disease (i.e., onset <55 years of age), prior use of heparin or aspirin, and increasing age. By combining these baseline risk characteristics for each outcome, the incidence of developing a clinical event ranged from 8% if none was present to 63% if all six were present, and of developing a markedly abnormal risk stratifying test from 8% to 21% if none were present to approximately 90% if all six were present. Patients with these characteristics are appropriate candidates for expeditious cardiac catheterization and consideration for revascularization, while patients without them may be suitable for medical management alone.[41]

**43. d.** For persons with coronary heart disease (CHD) and CHD risk equivalents, LDL-lowering therapy greatly reduces risk for major coronary events and stroke and yields highly favorable cost-effectiveness ratios. The cut points for initiating lifestyle and drug therapies are shown in Table 4–2.[42] *If baseline LDL cholesterol is 130 mg/dL*, intensive lifestyle therapy and maximal control of other risk factors should be started. Moreover, for most patients, an LDL-lowering drug will be required to achieve an LDL cholesterol level of <100 mg/dL; thus an LDL-cholesterol lowering drug can be started simultaneously with lifestyle changes (TLC) to attain the goal of therapy.

*In high-risk persons, the recommended LDL-C goal is <100 mg/dL.*

An LDL-C goal of <70 mg/dL is a therapeutic option on the basis of available clinical trial evidence, especially for patients at very high risk.

If LDL-C is ≥100 mg/dL, an LDL-lowering drug is indicated simultaneously with lifestyle changes.

If baseline LDL-C is <100 mg/dL, institution of an LDL-lowering drug to achieve an LDL-C level <70 mg/dL is a therapeutic option on the basis of available clinical trial evidence.[42]

**44. c.** Two phase III trials of enoxaparin (LMWH) for unstable angina/non-Q-wave myocardial infarction have shown it to be superior to unfractionated heparin for preventing a composite of death and cardiac ischemic events. A prospectively planned meta-analysis was performed to provide a more precise estimate of the effects of enoxaparin on multiple end points. Event rates for death, the composite end points of death/nonfatal myocardial infarction and death/nonfatal myocardial infarction/urgent revascularization, and major hemorrhage were extracted from the TIMI 11B and ESSENCE databases. Treatment effects at days 2, 8, 14, and 43 were expressed as the OR (and 95% CI) for enoxaparin versus unfractionated heparin. All heterogeneity tests for efficacy end points were negative, which suggests comparability of the findings in TIMI 11B and ESSENCE. Enoxaparin was associated with a 20% reduction in death and serious cardiac ischemic events that appeared within the first few days of treatment, and this benefit was sustained through 43 days. Enoxaparin's treatment benefit was not associated with an increase in major hemorrhage during the acute phase of therapy, but there was an increase in the rate of minor hemorrhage. The accumulated evidence, coupled with the simplicity of subcutaneous administration and elimination of the need for anticoagulation monitoring, indicates that enoxaparin should be considered as a replacement for unfractionated heparin as the

**TABLE 4–2   ATP III LDL-C Goals and Cut Points for TLC and Drug Therapy in Different Risk Categories and Proposed Modifications Based on Recent Clinical Trial Evidence**

| Risk Category | LDL-C Goal | Initiate TLC | Consider Drug Therapy[a] |
|---|---|---|---|
| *High risk:* CHD[b] or CHD risk equivalents[c] (10-year risk >20%) | <100 mg/dL (optional goal: <70 mg/dL)[d] | ≥100 mg/dL[e] | ≥100 mg/dL[f] (<100mg/dL: consider drug options)[a] |
| *Moderately high risk:* 2+ risk factors[g] (10-year risk 10% to 20%)[h] | <130 mg/dL[i] | ≥130 mg/dL[e] | ≥130 mg/dL (100–129 mg/dL; consider drug options)[j] |
| *Moderate risk:* 2+ risk factors[g] (10-year risk <10%)[h] | <130 mg/dL | ≥130 mg/dL | ≥160 mg/dL |
| *Lower risk:* 0–1 risk factor[k] | <160 mg/dL | ≥160 mg/dL | ≥190 mg/dL (160–189 mg/dL: LDL-lowering drug optional) |

[a]When LDL-lowering drug therapy is employed, it is advised that intensity of therapy be sufficient to achieve at least a 30% to 40% reduction in LDL-C levels.

[b]CHD includes history of myocardial infarction, unstable angina, stable angina, coronary artery procedures (angioplasty or bypass surgery), or evidence of clinically significant myocardial ischemia.

[c]CHD risk equivalents include clinical manifestations of noncoronary forms of atherosclerotic disease (peripheral arterial disease, abdominal aortic aneurysm, and carotid artery disease [transient ischemic attacks or stroke of carotid origin or >50% obstruction of a carotid artery]), diabetes, and 2+ risk factors with 10-year risk for hard CHD >20%.

[d]Very high risk favors the optional LDL-C goal of <70 mg/dL, and in patients with high triglycerides, non-HDL-C <100 mg/dL.

[e]Any person at high risk or moderately high risk who has lifestyle-related risk factors (e.g., obesity, physical inactivity, elevated triglyceride, low HDL-C, or metabolic syndrome) is a candidate for therapeutic lifestyle changes to modify these risk factors regardless of LDL-C level.

[f]If baseline LDL-C is <100 mg/dL, institution of an LDL-lowering drug is a therapeutic option on the basis of available clinical trial results. If a high-risk person has high triglycerides or low HDL-C, combining a fibrate or nicotinic acid with an LDL-lowering drug can be considered.

[g]Risk factors include cigarette smoking, hypertension (BP ≥140/90 mm Hg or on antihypertensive medication), low HDL cholesterol (<40 mg/dL), family history of premature CHD (CHD in male first-degree relative <55 years of age; CHD in female first-degree relative <65 years of age), and age (men ≥45 years; women ≥55 years).

[h]Electronic 10-year risk calculators are available at www.nhlbi.nih.gov/guidelines/cholesterol.

[i]Optional LDL-C goal <100 mg/dL.

[j]For moderately high-risk persons, when LDL-C level is 100 to 129 mg/dL, at baseline or on lifestyle therapy, initiation of an LDL-lowering drug to achieve an LDL-C level <100 mg/dL is a therapeutic option on the basis of available clinical trial results.

[k]Almost all people with zero or one risk factor have a 10-year risk <10%, and 10-year risk assessment in people with zero or one risk factor is thus not necessary.

From Grundy SM, Cleeman JI, Merz CN, et al. Implications of recent clinical trials for the National Cholesterol Education Program Adult Treatment Panel III guidelines. *Circulation.* 2004;110: 227–239, with permission.

antithrombin for the acute phase of management of patients with high-risk unstable angina/non-Q-wave myocardial infarction.[43]

**45. c.** A proportion of patients who present with suspected acute coronary syndrome (ACS) are found to have insignificant coronary artery disease (CAD) during coronary angiography. Of the 5,767 patients with non–ST-segment elevation ACS who were enrolled in the Platelet Glycoprotein IIb/IIIa in Unstable Angina: Receptor Suppression Using Integrilin (Eptifibatide) Therapy (PURSUIT) trial and who underwent in-hospital angiography, 88% had significant CAD (any stenosis >50%), 6% had mild CAD (any stenosis >0% to ≤50%), and 6% had no CAD (no stenosis identified). Overall, 12% of the patients had nonsignificant coronary artery disease.[44]

**46. b.** Hirudin is a naturally occurring anticoagulant secreted by the salivary glands of the leech *Hirudo medicinalis*. It is a potent and specific anticoagulant and exerts its action by binding directly to the active catalytic site of thrombin. Unlike heparin, it does not require a cofactor (antithrombin) and does not appear to cause immune-mediated thrombocytopenia. It is also a more potent inhibitor of platelet function than heparin, probably because of a direct inhibitory effect on thrombin. Recently, recombinant hirudin has been used as an adjunct to thrombolytic agents and as an anticoagulant during percutaneous transluminal coronary angioplasty. Unlike heparin, which is readily neutralized by protamine or platelet factor 4, a specific agent useful in reversing the effects of hirudin is unavailable. Irani et al. demonstrated the first clinical experience suggesting benefit from prothrombin complex concentrate in neutralizing the effect of r-hirudin. Although the specific mechanism of action remains unclear, the generation of additional thrombin probably plays a role. Also, epinephrine-induced platelet aggregation in hirudinized platelet-rich plasma is restored by addition of prothrombin complex concentrate, most probably by additional thrombin generation. Adverse effects of prothrombin complex concentrate include intravascular thrombosis, particularly in patients with liver disease and possible viral hepatitis. The concentrate is made from human plasma and is heated to 80°C for 24 hours to inactivate viruses, particularly hepatitis C virus. However, because the product contains some activated clotting factors (II, VII, IX, and X) and has thrombogenic potential, it should be used as a last resort, especially in patients with liver disease. Clinical experience suggests that prothrombin complex concentrate in a dose of 25 to 30 U/kg can be considered for patients with life-threatening hemorrhage caused by hirudin.[45]

**47. c.** Patients with prior coronary bypass surgery with acute ST-segment elevation myocardial infarction (MI) pose an increasingly common clinical problem. Labinaz et al. assessed the characteristics and outcomes of such patients undergoing thrombolysis for acute MI. They compared the characteristics and outcomes of patients in the Global Utilization of Streptokinase and Tissue Plasminogen Activator for Occluded Coronary Arteries trial (GUSTO-I) who had had prior bypass (n = 1,784, 4% of the population) with those without prior coronary artery bypass grafting (CABG), all of whom were randomized to receive one of four thrombolytic strategies. Patients with prior bypass were older with significantly more prior MI and angina. Overall, 30-day mortality was significantly higher in patients with prior bypass (10.7% vs. 6.7% for no prior bypass, $p < 0.001$); these patients also had significantly more pulmonary edema, sustained hypotension, or cardiogenic shock. Patients with prior bypass showed a 12.5% relative reduction (95% CI, 0% to 41.9%) in 30-day mortality with accelerated alteplase over the streptokinase monotherapies. In the 62% of patients with prior CABG who underwent coronary angiography, the infarct-related vessel was a native coronary artery in 61.9% and a bypass graft in 38.1% of cases. The Thrombolysis in Myocardial Infarction (TIMI)-3 flow rate was 30.5% for culprit native coronary arteries and 31.7% for culprit bypass grafts. Patients with prior bypass had more severe infarct-vessel stenoses (99% [90%, 100%] vs. 90% [80%, 99%], $p < 0.001$). Mortality in patients with prior CABG remained high (16.7%) at 1 year. These results are at least partially explained by the higher baseline risk of these patients and by the lower rate of patency of the infarct-related artery.[46]

**48. b.** Stone et al. sought to characterize the presenting characteristics of patients with previous coronary artery bypass graft surgery (CABG) and acute myocardial infarction (AMI) and to determine the angiographic success rate and clinical outcomes of a primary percutaneous transluminal coronary angioplasty

(PTCA) strategy. Patients who have had previous CABG and AMI comprise a high-risk group with decreased reperfusion success and increased mortality after thrombolytic therapy. Little is known about the efficacy of primary PTCA in AMI. Early cardiac catheterization was performed in 1,100 patients within 12 hours of onset of AMI at 34 centers in the prospective, controlled Second Primary Angioplasty in Myocardial Infarction (PAMI-2) trial, followed by primary PTCA when appropriate. Data were collected by independent study monitors, end points were adjudicated, and films were read at an independent core laboratory. Of 1,100 patients with AMI, 58 (5.3%) had undergone previous CABG. The infarct-related vessel in these patients was a bypass graft in 32 patients (55%) and a native coronary artery in 26 patients. Compared with patients without previous CABG, patients with previous CABG were older and more frequently had a previous myocardial infarction and triple-vessel disease. Coronary angioplasty was less likely to be performed when the infarct-related vessel was a bypass graft rather than a native coronary artery (71.9% vs. 89.8%, $p = 0.001$); Thrombolysis in Myocardial Infarction trial (TIMI) flow grade 3 was less frequently achieved (70.2% vs. 94.3%, $p < 0.0001$); and in-hospital mortality was increased (9.4% vs. 2.6%, $p = 0.02$). Mortality at six months was significantly higher in patients with (14.3%) versus without previous CABG (4.1%) ($p < 0.001$). By multivariate analysis, independent determinants of late mortality in the entire study group were advanced age, triple-vessel disease, Killip class, and post-PTCA TIMI flow grade <3. Reperfusion success of a primary PTCA strategy in patients with previous CABG, although favorable with respect to historic control studies, is reduced as compared with that in patients without previous CABG.[47]

**49. d.** The clinical triad of hypotension, clear lung fields, and elevated jugular venous pressure, occurring in <10% of patients presenting with acute inferior myocardial infarction, is characteristic of right ventricular infarction.

**50. d.** To determine whether primary angioplasty improves right ventricular function and the clinical outcome in patients with right ventricular infarction, Bowers et al. performed echocardiographic studies before and after angioplasty in 53 patients with acute right ventricular infarction. Complete reperfusion, defined as normal flow in the right main coronary artery and its major right ventricular branches, was achieved in 41 patients (77%), leading to prompt and striking recovery of right ventricular function (mean [+/( SE] score for free-wall motion, 3.0 +/− 0.1 at baseline, and 1.4 +/− 0.1 at 3 days; $p < 0.001$). Twelve patients (23%) had unsuccessful reperfusion, defined as the failure to restore right ventricular branch flow, with or without patency of the right main coronary artery. Unsuccessful reperfusion was associated with lack of recovery of right ventricular function (score for free-wall motion, 3.2 +/− 0.2 at baseline and 3.0 +/− 0.9 at 3 days; $p = 0.55$), as well as persistent hypotension and low cardiac output (in 83% of the patients vs. 12% of those with successful reperfusion; $p = 0.002$) and a high mortality rate (58% vs. 2% for those with successful reperfusion; $p = 0.001$). In patients with right ventricular infarction, complete reperfusion of the right coronary artery by angioplasty resulted in the dramatic recovery of right ventricular performance and an excellent clinical outcome.[48] Another recent cohort analysis demonstrated that intensive medical therapy that includes restoring blood flow into the right coronary artery, including the major RV branch, may improve clinical outcomes in right ventricular infarction.[49]

**51. c.** Papillary muscle rupture leading to acute mitral regurgitation and ventricular septal rupture are well-recognized complications of acute myocardial infarction. A systolic murmur is usually audible in both these cases. Dynamic left ventricular outflow tract (LVOT) obstruction has traditionally been associated with hypertrophic obstructive cardiomyopathy. Recently, acute dynamic LVOT obstruction has been described as a complication of myocardial infarction (MI). Haley et al. described cases of three patients, all of whom presented with a systolic murmur and electrocardiographic evidence of MI. All three patients developed cardiogenic shock and were subsequently found by echocardiography to manifest an acute dynamic LVOT obstruction. Cardiogenic shock persisted until therapy was directed toward decreasing the degree of the dynamic LVOT obstruction. The treatment of acute coronary syndromes in the presence of a dynamic LVOT obstruction differs from the traditional treatment of acute coronary syndromes and includes the use of beta-blockers and alpha-1 agonists, as well as the avoidance of therapies that aggravate the magnitude of the LVOT obstructive gradient, including nitrates, inotropic agents, and agents reducing the afterload. The development of a systolic murmur in the setting of acute MI complicated by cardiogenic shock with only a small elevation in creatine kinase suggests the presence of a dynamic LVOT obstruction, as well as the classical mechanical complications of MI, namely, ventricular septal rupture and papillary muscle rupture. The presence of a dynamic LVOT obstruction is reliably detected by transthoracic echocardiography or by transesophageal echocardiography if transthoracic image quality is suboptimal.[50]

**52. c.** Numerous clinical trials have established the benefits of intravenous glycoprotein IIb/IIIa inhibition in the management of coronary artery disease. In contrast, the recent large-scale, placebo-controlled, randomized trials of the oral glycoprotein IIb/IIIa antagonists have failed to provide commensurate reductions in late composite ischemic end points despite potent inhibition of platelet aggregation. The odds ratios (ORs) for death, myocardial infarction, urgent revascularization, and major bleeding from the four large-scale, placebo-controlled, randomized trials with oral glycoprotein IIb/IIIa inhibitors were recently calculated and combined. Stratification by low-dose or high-dose therapy and the use of concurrent aspirin was also undertaken. In 33,326 patients followed for >30 days, a consistent and statistically significant increase in mortality was observed with oral glycoprotein IIb/IIIa therapy (OR, 1.37; 95% CI, 1.13 to 1.66; $p = 0.001$). This effect was evident regardless of aspirin coadministration and treatment with either low-dose or high-dose therapy. Although a reduction in urgent revascularization was observed with oral glycoprotein IIb/IIIa inhibition, pooled analysis favored an increase in myocardial infarction that did not demonstrate statistical significance. Chew et al. found a highly significant excess in mortality consistent across four trials with three different oral glycoprotein IIb/IIIa inhibitor agents, and this was associated with a reduction in the need for urgent revascularization and no increase in myocardial infarction. These findings suggest the potential for a direct toxic effect with these agents and argue against a prothrombotic mechanism.[51]

**53. b.** Many clinical trials have evaluated the benefit of long-term use of antiplatelet drugs in reducing the risk of clinical thrombotic events. Aspirin and ticlopidine have been shown to be effective, but both have potentially serious adverse effects. Clopidogrel, a new thienopyridine derivative similar to ticlopidine, is an inhibitor of platelet aggregation induced by adenosine diphosphate. CAPRIE was a randomized, blinded, international trial designed to assess the relative efficacy of clopidogrel (75 mg once daily) and aspirin (325 mg once daily) in reducing the risk of a composite outcome cluster of ischemic stroke, myocardial infarction, or vascular death; their relative safety was also assessed. The population studied comprised subgroups of patients with atherosclerotic vascular disease manifested as recent ischemic stroke, recent myocardial infarction, or symptomatic peripheral arterial disease. Patients were followed for 1 to 3 years. Nineteen thousand one hundred and eighty-five patients, with more than 6,300 in each of the clinical subgroups, were recruited over 3 years, with a mean follow-up of 1.91 years. There were 1,960 first events included in the outcome cluster on which an intention-to-treat analysis showed that patients treated with clopidogrel had an annual 5.32% risk of ischemic stroke, myocardial infarction, or vascular death compared with 5.83% with aspirin. These rates reflect a statistically significant ($p = 0.043$) relative-risk reduction of 8.7% in favor of clopidogrel (95% CI, 0.3 to 16.5). Corresponding on-treatment analysis yielded a relative-risk reduction of 9.4%. There were no major differences in terms of safety. Reported adverse experiences in the clopidogrel and aspirin groups judged to be severe included rash (0.26% vs. 0.10%), diarrhea (0.23% vs. 0.11%), upper gastrointestinal discomfort (0.97% vs. 1.22%), intracranial hemorrhage (0.33% vs. 0.47%), and gastrointestinal hemorrhage (0.52% vs. 0.72%), respectively. There were ten (0.10%) patients in the clopidogrel group with significant reductions in neutrophils ($<1.2 \times 10[9]/L$) and 16 (0.17%) in the aspirin group. Long-term administration of clopidogrel to patients with atherosclerotic vascular disease is more effective than aspirin in reducing the combined risk of ischemic stroke, myocardial infarction, or vascular death. The overall safety profile of clopidogrel is at least as good as that of medium-dose aspirin.[52]

**54. a.** Antiplatelet therapy with aspirin and systematic anticoagulation with warfarin reduce cardiovascular morbidity and mortality after myocardial infarction when given alone. In the Coumadin Aspirin Reinfarction Study (CARS), the investigators aimed to find out whether a combination of low-dose warfarin and low-dose aspirin would give superior results to standard aspirin monotherapy without excessive bleeding risk. Using a randomized double-blind study design, they randomly assigned 8,803 patients, who had had myocardial infarction, treatment with 160 mg aspirin, treatment with 3 mg warfarin with 80 mg aspirin, or treatment with 1 mg warfarin with 80 mg aspirin. Patients took a single tablet daily, and attended for prothrombin time (PT) measurements at weeks 1, 2, 3, 4, 6, and 12, and then every 3 months. Patients were followed up for a maximum of 33 months (median 14 months). The primary event was first occurrence of reinfarction, nonfatal ischemic stroke, or cardiovascular death. One-year life-table estimates for the primary event were 8.6% (95% CI, 7.6 to 9.6) for 160 mg aspirin, 8.4% (7.4 to 9.4) for 3 mg warfarin with 80 mg aspirin, and 8.8% (7.6 to 10) for 1 mg warfarin with 80 mg aspirin. Primary comparisons were done with all follow-up data. The relative risk of the primary event for the 160 mg aspirin group compared with the 3 mg warfarin with 80 mg aspirin group was 0.95 (0.81 to 1.12, $p = 0.57$). For spontaneous major hemorrhage (not procedure related), 1-year life-table estimates were 0.74% (0.43 to 1.1) in the 160 mg aspirin group and 1.4% (0.94 to 1.8) in the 3 mg warfarin with 80 mg aspirin group ($p = 0.014$ log rank on follow-up). For the 3,382 patients assigned 3 mg warfarin with 80 mg aspirin, the international normalized ratio (INR) results were: at week 1 (n = 2,985) median 1.51 (interquartile range [IQR] 1.23 to 2.13); at week 4 (n = 2,701) 1.27 (1.13- to 1.64); at month 6 (n = 2,145) 1.19 (1.08 to 1.44). Low, fixed-dose warfarin (1 mg or 3 mg) combined with low-dose aspirin (80 mg) in patients who have had myocardial infarction does not provide clinical benefit beyond that achievable with 160 mg aspirin monotherapy.[53]

**55. a.** The Brockenbrough response includes an increase in left ventricular systolic pressure; a decrease in aortic systolic pressure, an increase in left ventricular to aortic gradient, and diminished aortic pulse pressure.

**56. c.** The angiogram clearly shows severe ostial and moderate distal left main trunk stenosis.

**57. a.** The recent recognition that coronary-artery stenting has improved the short- and long-term outcomes of patients treated with angioplasty made it necessary to re-evaluate the relative benefits of bypass surgery and percutaneous interventions in patients with multivessel disease. Serruys et al. studied a total of 1,205 patients who were randomly assigned to undergo stent implantation or bypass surgery when a cardiac surgeon and an interventional cardiologist agreed that the same extent of revascularization could be achieved by either technique. The primary clinical end point was freedom from major adverse cardiac and cerebrovascular events at 1 year. The costs of hospital resources used were also determined. At 1 year, there was no significant difference between the two groups in terms of the rates of death, stroke, or myocardial infarction. Among patients who survived without a stroke or a myocardial infarction, 16.8% of those in the stenting group underwent a second revascularization, as compared with 3.5% of those in the surgery group. The rate of event-free survival at 1 year was 73.8% among the patients who received stents and 87.8% among those who underwent bypass surgery ($p <0.001$ by the log-rank test). The costs for the initial procedure were $4,212 less for patients assigned to stenting than for those assigned to bypass surgery, but this difference was reduced during follow-up because of the increased need for repeated revascularization; after 1 year, the net difference in favor of stenting was estimated to be $2,973 per patient. The authors concluded, as measured 1 year after the procedure, that coronary stenting for multivessel disease is less expensive than bypass surgery and offers the same degree of protection against death, stroke, and myocardial infarction. However, stenting is associated with a greater need for repeated revascularization.[54]

58. **c.** Kawasaki disease is a leading cause of acquired heart disease in children in the United States. An acute vasculitis of unknown etiology, it occurs predominantly in infancy and early childhood, and more rarely in teenagers. Coronary artery aneurysms or ectasia develop in approximately 15% to 25% of children with the disease. Treatment with intravenous gamma globulin, 2 g/kg, in the acute phase reduces this risk threefold to fivefold. Angiographic resolution occurs in approximately one half of aneurysmal arterial segments, but these show persistent histologic and functional abnormalities. The remainder continues to be aneurysmal, often with development of progressive stenosis or occlusion. The worst prognosis occurs in children with so-called "giant aneurysms," i.e., those with a maximum diameter >8 mm, because thrombosis is promoted both by sluggish blood flow within the massively dilated vascular space and by the frequent development of stenotic lesions. Serial stress tests with myocardial imaging are mandatory in the management of patients with Kawasaki disease and significant coronary artery disease to determine the need for coronary angiography and transcatheter interventions or coronary bypass surgery. Continued long-term surveillance in patients with and without detected coronary abnormalities is necessary to determine the natural history of Kawasaki disease.[55]

59. **b.** The coronary angiogram reveals large coronary A-V fistula involving the right coronary artery. Patient underwent surgical ligation of the fistula with resolution of her symptoms.

60. **c.** The angiogram reveals severe ostial and proximal left circumflex artery stenosis.

61. **c.** The coronary angiogram reveals anomalous origin of the left circumflex coronary artery from the right sinus. A multipurpose catheter is the catheter of choice to cannulate a left circumflex artery arising from this site.

62. **a.** Angiogram reveals large angiographically visible thrombus in the mid portion of the right coronary artery distal to a severe stenosis.

63. **a.** The angiogram reveals anomalous origin of the left main trunk from the right coronary sinus with a course anterior to the pulmonary artery.

64. **d.** The angiogram reveals anomalous common origin of the left anterior descending artery and the right coronary artery.

65. **c.** The angiogram demonstrates extravasation of contrast caused by perforation of the right coronary artery.

66. **b.** The maximum coronary vasodilator capacity after intravenous dipyridamole (0.14 mg/kg/min $\times$ 4 minutes) was studied in seven patients with primary scleroderma myocardial disease and compared to that of seven control subjects by Nitenberg et al. Hemodynamic data and left ventricular angiographic data were

not different in the two groups. The coronary flow reserve was evaluated by the dipyridamole/basal coronary sinus blood flow ratio (D/B CSBF) and the coronary resistance reserve by the dipyridamole/basal coronary resistance ratio (D/B CR). Coronary reserve was greatly impaired in the group with primary scleroderma myocardial disease: D/B CSBF was lower than in the control group (2.54 +/− 1.37 vs. 4.01 +/− 0.56, respectively; $p$ <0.05) and D/B CR was higher than in the control group (0.47 +/− 0.25 vs. 0.23 +/− 0.04, respectively; $p$ <0.05). Such a decreased coronary flow and resistance reserve in patients with primary scleroderma myocardial disease was not explained by an alteration of left ventricular function. The authors concluded that this may be an important contributing factor in the pathogenesis of primary scleroderma myocardial disease.[56]

**67. b.** An excessive rate of cardiac death is a well-known feature of renal failure. Coronary heart disease is frequent and the possibility has been raised that the natural history of the coronary plaque is different in uremic patients. Schwarz et al. assessed the morphology of coronary arteries in patients with end-stage renal failure and compared them with coronary arteries of matched nonuremic control patients. Fifty-four cases were identified at autopsy who met the inclusion criteria: cases, end-stage renal disease (n = 27); controls, nonrenal patients with coronary artery disease (n = 27). At autopsy all three coronary arteries were prepared at corresponding sites for investigations: (i) qualitative analysis (after Stary), (ii) quantitative measurements of intima and media thickness (by planimetry), (iii) immunohistochemical analysis of the coronary plaques, and (iv) x-ray diffraction of selected calcified plaques. Qualitative analysis of the coronary arteries showed significantly more calcified plaques of coronary arteries in patients with end-stage renal failure. Plaques of nonuremic patients were mostly fibroatheromatous. Media thickness of coronary arteries was significantly higher in uremic patients and intima thickness tended to be higher, but this difference was not statistically significant. Plaque area was comparable in both groups. Lumen area, however, was significantly lower in end-stage renal patients. Immunohistochemical analysis of the cellular infiltrate in coronary arteries showed no major differences in these advanced plaques of uremic and nonuremic subjects. Coronary plaques in patients with end-stage renal failure were characterized by increased media thickness and marked calcification. In contrast to the previous opinion, the authors demonstrated that the most marked difference compared to nonuremic controls does not concern the size, but the composition of the plaque.[57] Deposition of calcium within the plaques may contribute to the high complication rate in uremic patients.

**68. b.** Plasma homocysteine (tHCY) has been associated with coronary artery disease (CAD). Anderson et al. tested whether tHCY also increases secondary risk, after initial CAD diagnosis, and whether it is independent of traditional risk factors, C-reactive protein (CRP), and methylenetetrahydrofolate reductase (MTHFR) genotype. Blood samples were collected from 1,412 patients with severe angiographically defined CAD (stenosis ≥70%). Plasma tHCY was measured by fluorescence polarization immunoassay. The study cohort was evaluated for survival after a mean of 3.0 +/− 1.0 years of follow-up (minimum 1.5 years, maximum 5.0 years). The average age of the patients was 65 +/− 11 years, 77% were males, and 166 died during follow-up. Mortality was greater in patients with tHCY in tertile 3 than in tertiles 1 and 2 (mortality 15.7% versus 9.6%, $p$ = 0.001 [log-rank test], hazard ratio [HR] 1.63). The relative hazard increased 16% for each 5-$\mu$mol/L increase in tHCY ($p$ <0.001). In multivariate Cox regression analysis, controlling for univariate clinical and laboratory predictors, elevated tHCY remained predictive of mortality (HR 1.64, $p$ = 0.009), together with age (HR 1.72 per 10-year increment, $p$ <0.0001), ejection fraction (HR 0.84 per 10% increment, $p$ = 0.0001), diabetes (HR 1.98, $p$ = 0.001), CRP (HR 1.42 per tertile, $p = 0.004$), and hyperlipidemia. Homozygosity for the MTHFR variant was weakly predictive of tHCY levels but not mortality. The authors concluded that in patients with angiographically defined CAD, tHCY is a significant predictor of mortality, independent of traditional risk factors, CRP, and MTHFR genotype.[58]

**69. c.** The coronary angiogram of the left circulation in the postero-anterior (PA) cranial view shows severe left anterior descending artery stenosis after the takeoff of the first septal artery.

**70. b.** The OAT study showed high rates of procedural success with PCI and sustained patency but no clinical benefit during an average 3-year follow-up with respect to death, reinfarction, or heart failure.[59] There was, in fact, a trend toward excess nonfatal reinfarction when routine PCI was performed in stable patients who were found to have occlusion of the infarct-related artery 3 to 28 days after myocardial infarction. A strategy of CABG was not tested in the OAT trial.

**71. a.** In this large trial of 15,603 patients with established atherothrombotic disease or at high risk for such disease, there was no significant benefit associated with clopidogrel plus aspirin as compared with placebo plus aspirin in reducing the incidence of the primary end point of myocardial infarction, stroke, or death from cardiovascular causes, and clopidogrel was associated with a significant increase in the rate of moderate bleeding.[60]

**72. a.** The coronary angiogram of the left circulation in the right anterior oblique (RAO) caudal view shows severe proximal left circumflex artery stenosis explaining the lateral ischemia.

**73. b.** A cohort study of ~1,400 patients demonstrated that the use of combination evidence-based medical therapies was independently and strongly associated with lower 6-month mortality in patients with acute coronary syndromes.[61] Furthermore, there was a gradient of benefit across the different TIMI risk groups with higher risk patients obtaining higher absolute benefit.[62]

**74. b.** The COURAGE trial compared optimal medical therapy alone or in combination with PCI as an initial management strategy in patients with stable coronary artery disease. Although the addition of PCI to optimal medical therapy reduced the prevalence of angina, it did not reduce long-term rates of death, nonfatal myocardial infarction, and hospitalization for acute coronary syndromes.[63]

**75. d.** The coronary angiogram in the RAO view shows severe mid right coronary artery stenosis explaining the inferior ischemia.

**76. c.** Although in the initial randomized clinical trials dual antiplatelet therapy followed by aspirin only was recommended for 2 to 3 months for sirolimus-eluting (Cypher) and 6 months paclitaxel-eluting (TAXUS) stents, it has been common practice in many centers to administer dual antiplatelet therapy for a longer period of time. The FDA recommendation is consistent with the ACC/AHA/SCAI PCI Practice Guidelines, which recommend that patients receive aspirin indefinitely plus a minimum of 3 months (for Cypher patients) or 6 months (for TAXUS patients) of clopidogrel, with therapy extended to 12 months in patients at a low risk of bleeding.[64] A science advisory from the American Heart Association, American College of Cardiology, Society for Cardiovascular Angiography and Interventions, American College of Surgeons, and American Dental Association, with representation from the American College of Physicians, recommended 12 months of dual antiplatelet therapy after placement of a drug-eluting stent and educating the patient and health care providers about hazards of premature discontinuation.[65]

**77. c.** The implantation of DES may be avoided in patients with an absolute indication for oral anticoagulation as triple therapy may significantly increase bleeding.[66] In this patient, dual antiplatelet therapy in association with oral anticoagulation should be administered for at least 6 months and preferably 12 months. Dual antiplatelet therapy is mandatory to protect for DES thrombosis. From the early bare-metal stent (BMS) trials it is known that the association of aspirin and oral anticoagulation is not protective against stent thrombosis. The regimen of clopidogrel and oral anticoagulation has never been tested with respect to stent thrombosis, either with DES or with BMS.

**78. a.** The coronary angiogram of the left circulation in the RAO caudal view shows severe mid left circumflex coronary artery stenosis.

**79. e.** In patients scheduled for noncardiac surgery in the year following percutaneous coronary intervention (PCI), the implantation of DESs should be avoided. Accordingly, one of the most frequent predisposing conditions to DES thrombosis is the (partial or total) discontinuation of dual antiplatelet therapy because of urgent or elective noncardiac surgery.[67] Although preliminary data suggest that continuation of dual antiplatelet therapy during surgery may be protective of DES thrombosis, no recommendation can be made at this time. Conceptually, the potential for stent thrombosis remains because of the intrinsic prothrombotic state related to surgery. Thrombosis of a BMS implanted shortly prior to noncardiac surgery has been described and associated with prohibitive morbidity and mortality. Therefore, whenever possible, noncardiac surgery should be postponed for at least 6 weeks following implantation of a BMS.

**80. d.** Currently there are no data to support an extension of dual antiplatelet therapy beyond 12 months. Nevertheless, it remains the decision of the treating physicians to administer aspirin and clopidogrel for a longer period of time in individual high-risk cases, such as the one described. The CHARISMA study did show a benefit of prolonged aspirin and clopidogrel therapy over aspirin only in the secondary prevention setting, but did not specifically address the PCI population.

# References

1. Cannon CP, Weintraub WS, Demopoulos LA, et al. Comparison of early invasive and conservative strategies in patients with unstable coronary syndromes treated with the glycoprotein IIb/IIIa inhibitor tirofiban. *N Engl J Med.* 2001;344:1879–1887.

2. Anderson JL, Adams CD, Antman EM, et al. ACC/AHA 2007 guidelines for the management of patients with unstable angina/non-ST-Elevation myocardial infarction: a report of the American College of Cardiology/American Heart Association Task Force on Practice Guidelines (Writing Committee to Revise the 2002 Guidelines for the Management of Patients with Unstable Angina/Non-ST-Elevation Myocardial Infarction) developed in collaboration with the American College of Emergency Physicians, the Society for Cardiovascular Angiography and Interventions, and the Society of Thoracic Surgeons endorsed by the American Association of Cardiovascular and Pulmonary Rehabilitation and the Society for Academic Emergency Medicine. *J Am Coll Cardiol.* 2007;50:e1–e157.

3. Belardinelli R, Paolini I, Cianci G, et al. Exercise training intervention after coronary angioplasty: the ETICA trial. *J Am Coll Cardiol.* 2001;37:1891–1900.

4. Koenig W, Sund M, Frohlich M, et al. C-Reactive protein, a sensitive marker of inflammation, predicts future risk of coronary heart disease in initially healthy middle-aged men: results from the MONICA (Monitoring Trends and Determinants in Cardiovascular Disease) Augsburg Cohort Study, 1984 to 1992. *Circulation.* 1999;99:237–242.

5. Ridker PM, Glynn RJ, Hennekens CH. C-reactive protein adds to the predictive value of total and HDL cholesterol in determining risk of first myocardial infarction. *Circulation.* 1998;97:2007–2011.

6. Stone GW, Ellis SG, O'Shaughnessy CD, et al. Paclitaxel-eluting stents vs vascular brachytherapy for in-stent restenosis within bare-metal stents: the TAXUS V ISR randomized trial. *JAMA.* 2006;295:1253–1263.

7. Holmes DR, Jr., Teirstein P, Satler L, et al. Sirolimus-eluting stents vs vascular brachytherapy for in-stent restenosis within bare-metal stents: the SISR randomized trial. *JAMA.* 2006;295:1264–1273.

8. Mukherjee D, Moliterno DJ. Brachytherapy for in-stent restenosis: a distant second choice to drug-eluting stent placement. *JAMA.* 2006;295:1307–1309.

9. Yusuf S, Sleight P, Pogue J, et al. Effects of an angiotensin-converting-enzyme inhibitor, ramipril, on cardiovascular events in high-risk patients. The Heart Outcomes Prevention Evaluation Study Investigators. *N Engl J Med.* 2000;342:145–153.

10. Fuster V, Lewis A. Conner Memorial Lecture. Mechanisms leading to myocardial infarction: insights from studies of vascular biology. *Circulation.* 1994;90:2126–2146.

11. Hoffman JI. Transmural myocardial perfusion. *Prog Cardiovasc Dis.* 1987;29:429–464.

12. Adams JE, 3rd, Abendschein DR, Jaffe AS. Biochemical markers of myocardial injury. Is MB creatine kinase the choice for the 1990s? *Circulation.* 1993;88:750–763.

13. The GUSTO Angiographic Investigators. The effects of tissue plasminogen activator, streptokinase, or both on coronary-artery patency, ventricular function, and survival after acute myocardial infarction. *N Engl J Med.* 1993;329:1615–1622.

14. The GUSTO investigators. An international randomized trial comparing four thrombolytic strategies for acute myocardial infarction. *N Engl J Med.* 1993;329:673–682.

15. Lee KL, Woodlief LH, Topol EJ, et al. Predictors of 30-day mortality in the era of reperfusion for acute myocardial infarction. Results from an international trial of 41,021 patients. GUSTO-I Investigators. *Circulation.* 1995;91:1659–1668.

16. Beller GA. Current status of nuclear cardiology techniques. *Curr Probl Cardiol.* 1991;16:451–535.

17. Rogers WJ, Bourassa MG, Andrews TC, et al. Asymptomatic Cardiac Ischemia Pilot (ACIP) study: outcome at 1 year for patients with asymptomatic cardiac ischemia randomized to medical therapy or revascularization. The ACIP Investigators. *J Am Coll Cardiol.* 1995;26:594–605.

18. Davies RF, Goldberg AD, Forman S, et al. Asymptomatic Cardiac Ischemia Pilot (ACIP) study two-year follow-up: outcomes of patients randomized to initial strategies of medical therapy versus revascularization. *Circulation.* 1997;95:2037–2043.

19. Mukherjee D, Nissen SE, Topol EJ. Risk of cardiovascular events associated with selective COX-2 inhibitors. *JAMA.* 2001;286:954–959.

20. Boersma E, Akkerhuis KM, Theroux P, et al. Platelet glycoprotein IIb/IIIa receptor inhibition in non-ST-elevation acute coronary syndromes: early benefit during medical treatment only, with additional protection during percutaneous coronary intervention. *Circulation.* 1999;100:2045–2048.

21. Boersma E, Harrington RA, Moliterno DJ, et al. Platelet glycoprotein IIb/IIIa inhibitors in acute coronary syndromes: a meta-analysis of all major randomized clinical trials. *Lancet.* 2002;359:189–198.

22. Jacobs AK, Kelsey SF, Yeh W, et al. Documentation of decline in morbidity in women undergoing coronary angioplasty (a report from the 1993-94 NHLBI Percutaneous Transluminal Coronary Angioplasty Registry). National Heart, Lung, and Blood Institute. *Am J Cardiol.* 1997;80:979–984.

23. Gibbons RJ, Abrams J, Chatterjee K, et al. ACC/AHA 2002 guideline update for the management of patients with chronic stable angina—summary article: a report of the American College of Cardiology/American Heart Association Task Force on practice guidelines (Committee on the Management of Patients With Chronic Stable Angina). *J Am Coll Cardiol.* 2003;41:159–168.

24. Kuchulakanti PK, Chu WW, Torguson R, et al. Correlates and long-term outcomes of angiographically proven stent thrombosis with sirolimus- and paclitaxel-eluting stents. *Circulation.* 2006;113:1108–1113.

25. Daemen J, Wenaweser P, Tsuchida K, et al. Early and late coronary stent thrombosis of sirolimus-eluting and paclitaxel-eluting stents in routine clinical practice: data from a large two-institutional cohort study. *Lancet.* 2007;369:667–678.

26. Iakovou I, Schmidt T, Bonizzoni E, et al. Incidence, predictors, and outcome of thrombosis after successful implantation of drug-eluting stents. *JAMA.* 2005;293:2126–2130.

27. Urban P, Gershlick AH, Guagliumi G, et al. Safety of coronary sirolimus-eluting stents in daily clinical practice: one-year follow-up of the e-Cypher registry. *Circulation.* 2006;113:1434–1441.

28. Byington RP, Davis BR, Plehn JF, et al. Reduction of stroke events with pravastatin: the Prospective Pravastatin Pooling (PPP) Project. *Circulation.* 2001;103:387–392.

29. Domanski MJ, Borkowf CB, Campeau L, et al. Prognostic factors for atherosclerosis progression in saphenous vein grafts: the postcoronary artery bypass graft (Post-CABG) trial. Post-CABG Trial Investigators. *J Am Coll Cardiol.* 2000;36:1877–1883.

**NOTES**

**NOTES**

30. Pitt B, Waters D, Brown WV, et al. Aggressive lipid-lowering therapy compared with angioplasty in stable coronary artery disease. Atorvastatin versus Revascularization Treatment Investigators. *N Engl J Med.* 1999;341:70–76.

31. Randomised trial of cholesterol lowering in 4444 patients with coronary heart disease: the Scandinavian Simvastatin Survival Study (4S). *Lancet.* 1994;344:1383–1389.

32. Downs JR, Clearfield M, Weis S, et al. Primary prevention of acute coronary events with lovastatin in men and women with average cholesterol levels: results of AFCAPS/TexCAPS. Air Force/Texas Coronary Atherosclerosis Prevention Study. *JAMA.* 1998;279:1615–1622.

33. Influence of pravastatin and plasma lipids on clinical events in the West of Scotland Coronary Prevention Study (WOSCOPS). *Circulation.* 1998;97:1440–1445.

34. Detre KM, Guo P, Holubkov R, et al. Coronary revascularization in diabetic patients: a comparison of the randomized and observational components of the Bypass Angioplasty Revascularization Investigation (BARI). *Circulation.* 1999;99:633–640.

35. Barry J, Mead K, Nabel EG, et al. Effect of smoking on the activity of ischemic heart disease. *JAMA.* 1989;261:398–402.

36. Hochman JS, Sleeper LA, Webb JG, et al. Early revascularization in acute myocardial infarction complicated by cardiogenic shock. SHOCK Investigators. Should We Emergently Revascularize Occluded Coronaries for Cardiogenic Shock. *N Engl J Med.* 1999;341:625–634.

37. Califf RM, Tomabechi Y, Lee KL, et al. Outcome in one-vessel coronary artery disease. *Circulation.* 1983;67:283–290.

38. Iskandrian AS, Heo J, Lemlek J, et al. Identification of high-risk patients with left main and three-vessel coronary artery disease by adenosine-single photon emission computed tomographic thallium imaging. *Am Heart J.* 1993;125:1130–1135.

39. Akkerhuis KM, Deckers JW, Lincoff AM, et al. Risk of stroke associated with abciximab among patients undergoing percutaneous coronary intervention. *JAMA.* 2001;286:78–82.

40. Lundergan CF, Ross AM, McCarthy WF, et al. Predictors of left ventricular function after acute myocardial infarction: effects of time to treatment, patency, and body mass index: the GUSTO-I angiographic experience. *Am Heart J.* 2001;142:43–50.

41. Stone PH, Thompson B, Zaret BL, et al. Factors associated with failure of medical therapy in patients with unstable angina and non-Q wave myocardial infarction. A TIMI-IIIB database study. *Eur Heart J.* 1999;20:1084–1093.

42. Grundy SM, Cleeman JI, Merz CN, et al. Implications of recent clinical trials for the National Cholesterol Education Program Adult Treatment Panel III guidelines. *Circulation.* 2004;110:227–239.

43. Antman EM, Cohen M, Radley D, et al. Assessment of the treatment effect of enoxaparin for unstable angina/non-Q-wave myocardial infarction. TIMI 11B-ESSENCE meta-analysis. *Circulation.* 1999;100:1602–1608.

44. Roe MT, Harrington RA, Prosper DM, et al. Clinical and therapeutic profile of patients presenting with acute coronary syndromes who do not have significant coronary artery disease. The Platelet Glycoprotein IIb/IIIa in Unstable Angina: Receptor Suppression Using Integrilin Therapy (PURSUIT) Trial Investigators. *Circulation.* 2000;102:1101–1106.

45. Irani MS, White HJ, Jr., Sexon RG. Reversal of hirudin-induced bleeding diathesis by prothrombin complex concentrate. *Am J Cardiol.* 1995;75:422–423.

46. Labinaz M, Sketch MH, Jr., Ellis SG, et al. Outcome of acute ST-segment elevation myocardial infarction in patients with prior coronary artery bypass surgery receiving thrombolytic therapy. *Am Heart J.* 2001;141:469–477.

47. Stone GW, Brodie BR, Griffin JJ, et al. Clinical and angiographic outcomes in patients with previous coronary artery bypass graft surgery treated with primary balloon angioplasty for acute myocardial infarction. Second Primary Angioplasty in Myocardial Infarction Trial (PAMI-2) Investigators. *J Am Coll Cardiol.* 2000;35:605–611.

48. Bowers TR, O'Neill WW, Grines C, et al. Effect of reperfusion on biventricular function and survival after right ventricular infarction. *N Engl J Med.* 1998;338:933–940.

49. Assali AR, Teplitsky I, Ben-Dor I, et al. Prognostic importance of right ventricular infarction in an acute myocardial infarction cohort referred for contemporary percutaneous reperfusion therapy. *Am Heart J.* 2007;153:231–237.

50. Haley JH, Sinak LJ, Tajik AJ, et al. Dynamic left ventricular outflow tract obstruction in acute coronary syndromes: an important cause of new systolic murmur and cardiogenic shock. *Mayo Clin Proc.* 1999;74:901–906.

51. Chew DP, Bhatt DL, Sapp S, et al. Increased mortality with oral platelet glycoprotein IIb/IIIa antagonists: a meta-analysis of phase III multicenter randomized trials. *Circulation.* 2001;103:201–206.

52. CAPRIE Steering Committee. A randomized, blinded, trial of clopidogrel versus aspirin in patients at risk of ischemic events (CAPRIE). *Lancet.* 1996;348:1329–1339.

53. Coumadin Aspirin Reinfarction Study (CARS) Investigators. Randomised double-blind trial of fixed low-dose warfarin with aspirin after myocardial infarction. *Lancet.* 1997;350:389–396.

54. Serruys PW, Unger F, Sousa JE, et al. Comparison of coronary-artery bypass surgery and stenting for the treatment of multivessel disease. *N Engl J Med.* 2001;344:1117–1124.

55. Newburger JW, Burns JC. Kawasaki disease. *Vasc Med.* 1999;4:187–202.

56. Nitenberg A, Foult JM, Kahan A, et al. Reduced coronary flow and resistance reserve in primary scleroderma myocardial disease. *Am Heart J.* 1986;112:309–315.

57. Schwarz U, Buzello M, Ritz E, et al. Morphology of coronary atherosclerotic lesions in patients with end-stage renal failure. *Nephrol Dial Transplant.* 2000;15:218–223.

58. Anderson JL, Muhlestein JB, Horne BD, et al. Plasma homocysteine predicts mortality independently of traditional risk factors and C-reactive protein in patients with angiographically defined coronary artery disease. *Circulation.* 2000;102:1227–1232.

59. Hochman JS, Lamas GA, Buller CE, et al. Coronary intervention for persistent occlusion after myocardial infarction. *N Engl J Med.* 2006;355:2395–2407.

60. Bhatt DL, Fox KA, Hacke W, et al. Clopidogrel and aspirin versus aspirin alone for the prevention of atherothrombotic events. *N Engl J Med.* 2006;354:1706–1717.

61. Mukherjee D, Fang J, Chetcuti S, et al. Impact of combination evidence-based medical therapy on mortality in patients with acute coronary syndromes. *Circulation.* 2004;109:745–749.

62. Mukherjee D, Fang J, Kline-Rogers E, et al. Impact of combination evidence based medical treatment in patients with acute coronary syndromes in various TIMI risk groups. *Heart.* 2005;91:381–382.

63. Boden WE, O'Rourke RA, Teo KK, et al. Optimal medical therapy with or without PCI for stable coronary disease. *N Engl J Med.* 2007;356:1503–1516.

64. Smith SC, Jr., Feldman TE, Hirshfeld JW, et al. ACC/AHA/SCAI 2005 guideline update for percutaneous coronary intervention: a report of the American College of Cardiology/American Heart Association Task Force on Practice Guidelines (ACC/AHA/SCAI Writing Committee to Update 2001 Guidelines for Percutaneous Coronary Intervention). *Circulation.* 2006;113:e166–e286.

65. Grines CL, Bonow RO, Casey DE, Jr., et al. Prevention of premature discontinuation of dual antiplatelet therapy in patients with coronary artery stents: a science advisory from the American Heart Association, American College of Cardiology, Society for Cardiovascular Angiography and Interventions, American College of Surgeons, and American Dental Association, with representation from the American College of Physicians. *J Am Coll Cardiol.* 2007;49:734–739.

66. Orford JL, Fasseas P, Melby S, et al. Safety and efficacy of aspirin, clopidogrel, and warfarin after coronary stent placement in patients with an indication for anticoagulation. *Am Heart J.* 2004;147:463–467.

67. Schouten O, van Domburg RT, Bax JJ, et al. Noncardiac surgery after coronary stenting: early surgery and interruption of antiplatelet therapy are associated with an increase in major adverse cardiac events. *J Am Coll Cardiol.* 2007;49:122–124.

**NOTES**

# chapter 5

# Pharmacology

MICHAEL A. MILITELLO · JODIE M. FINK

## QUESTIONS

### Pharmacokinetics and Pharmacodynamics

1. P. M. is admitted to the coronary intensive care unit (ICU) with atrial fibrillation (AFib) and rapid ventricular rate. After controlling the ventricular rate with metoprolol, it is decided to initiate procainamide by intravenous (IV) infusion. P. M. weighs 80 kg. How much of a loading dose would be required to target a level of 8 µg/L? The average steady-state volume of distribution (Vd) for procainamide is 2 L/kg. The bioavailability of the IV formulation is 100%, whereas the oral (PO) form is only 83%.

   a. 1,000 mg
   b. 1,300 mg
   c. 1,500 mg
   d. 1,700 mg

2. L. M. has been receiving digoxin 0.25 mg PO tablets daily. Her serum drug level is 1.8 ng/mL. She is no longer able to take PO medications and needs to receive digoxin IV. By what percentage do you need to decrease the dose to maintain the current digoxin level?

   a. 10%
   b. 25%
   c. 40%
   d. 50%

3. What two pharmacokinetic parameters alter the half-life of medications?

   a. loading dose and clearance
   b. absorption and clearance
   c. Vd and clearance
   d. absorption and Vd

4. What is the relationship between drug concentration and pharmacologic effect known as?

   a. pharmacokinetics
   b. pharmacogenetics
   c. pharmacology
   d. pharmacodynamics

5. Each line in Figure 5–1 represents a beta-blocker in development. Which beta-blocker is the most potent?

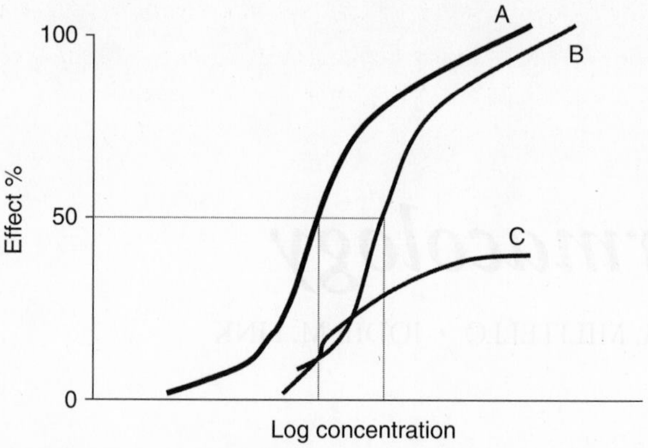

**FIGURE 5–1** Relationship between drug concentration and effect.

 a. A
 b. B
 c. C
 d. Potency cannot be determined from the above graph.

6. F. R. is a 56-year-old (y/o) man with a history of AFib treated with amiodarone 200 mg PO daily. He is also on warfarin, and you would like to start a statin to lower his LDL cholesterol. Which of the following statins is least likely to interact with amiodarone?

 a. simvastatin
 b. lovastatin
 c. atorvastatin
 d. pravastatin

7. Ethanol alters the metabolism of warfarin. Two types of ethanol abuse are chronic ethanol abuse and binge ethanol drinking. How do these types of ethanol use alter warfarin metabolism? Chronic ethanol use _____ and binge ethanol drinking _____.

 a. decreases warfarin metabolism, increases warfarin metabolism
 b. decreases warfarin metabolism, decreases warfarin metabolism
 c. increases warfarin metabolism, decreases warfarin metabolism
 d. increases warfarin metabolism, increases warfarin metabolism

8. Which of the following drugs can significantly increase digoxin concentrations?

 a. amiodarone
 b. metoprolol
 c. simvastatin
 d. fenofibrate

9. Which of the following drugs is the *least* likely to enhance the effects of warfarin?

 a. amiodarone
 b. cholestyramine
 c. metronidazole
 d. erythromycin

## Angiotensin-Converting Enzyme (ACE) Inhibitors

10. Which of the following ACE inhibitors are *not* prodrugs?

 a. captopril, lisinopril, ramipril
 b. lisinopril, enalapril, benazepril
 c. captopril, lisinopril, enalaprilat
 d. moexipril, captopril, lisinopril

11. Which of the following statements is *true* with regard to ACE inhibitors?

    a. Mortality benefit in heart failure (HF) patients is a class effect with ACE inhibitors, and all are FDA approved for this indication.
    b. ACE inhibitor dose is negligible in HF with regard to mortality benefit.
    c. Sodium depletion is an important factor in the development of renal insufficiency associated with ACE inhibitors.
    d. ACE inhibitor–associated potassium retention is related to the increase in feedback that leads to aldosterone release.

12. All of the following are contraindications to the use of ACE inhibitors *except*

    a. bilateral renal artery stenosis
    b. pregnancy
    c. angioedema
    d. cough

## Angiotensin II-Receptor Blockers (ARBs)

13. Which of the following statements is false regarding ARBs?

    a. Valsartan, candesartan, and losartan are the only ARBs indicated for HF.
    b. ARBs may be considered as an alternative for patients who developed angioedema while on an ACE inhibitor.
    c. Renal dysfunction, hyperkalemia, and hypotension are side effects shared by ACE inhibitors and ARBs.
    d. None of the above.

14. Which of the following statements is true?

    a. Angiotensin II serum concentrations may remain elevated despite ACE inhibitor therapy at target doses.
    b. It is reasonable to add beta-blocker therapy before target doses of ARBs are achieved in stable patients.
    c. It is reasonable to consider the addition of an ARB to conventional treatment in persistently symptomatic HF patients.
    d. All of the above.

## Beta-blockers

15. Match the properties with the associated beta-blocking agents.

    1. pindolol           i. alpha-blockade
    2. propranolol      ii. intrinsic sympathomimetic activity (ISA)
    3. labetalol         iii. membrane-stabilizing activity
    4. bisoprolol        iv. $\beta_1$-selectivity

    a. (1) iv; (2) ii; (3) iii; (4) i
    b. (1) iii; (2) i; (3) ii; (4) iv
    c. (1) ii; (2) iii; (3) i; (4) iv
    d. (1) ii; (2) iv; (3) iii; (4) i

## Calcium Channel Blockers (CCBs)

16. By which of the following mechanisms do diltiazem and verapamil slow ventricular rate in patients with AFib?

    a. They decrease the conduction velocity within the AV node.
    b. They decrease the refractory period of nodal tissue.
    c. They stimulate vagal tone.
    d. They prolong the refractory period of atrial tissue.

**17.** Short-acting dihydropyridine CCBs possess all of the following properties *except*

  **a.** They cause peripheral edema.
  **b.** They cause reflex tachycardia.
  **c.** They cause flushing.
  **d.** They slow ventricular response in patients with AFib.

**18.** Which of the following CCBs is indicated in patients presenting with a subarachnoid hemorrhage?

  **a.** verapamil
  **b.** diltiazem
  **c.** isradipine
  **d.** nimodipine

## Nitroglycerin

**19.** All of the following are suggested mechanisms of nitrate tolerance *except*

  **a.** sulfhydryl-group depletion
  **b.** plasma volume expansion
  **c.** free radical depletion
  **d.** neurohormonal stimulation

## Diuretics

**20.** T. P. is a 45 y/o female with dilated cardiomyopathy and is admitted with shortness of breath caused by fluid overload. Her home HF regimen consists of furosemide 80 mg PO twice daily, lisinopril 20 mg PO daily, carvedilol 12.5 mg PO twice daily. On admission, her serum creatinine is 2.0 mg/dL, and despite changing furosemide to 80 mg IV twice daily, she has not achieved adequate diuresis. All of the following regimens would be appropriate to address diuretic resistance, *except*

  **a.** initiate continuous infusion furosemide 20 mg/hr
  **b.** add metolazone 5 mg PO daily
  **c.** add chlorothiazide 500 mg IV daily
  **d.** change furosemide dose to 40 mg IV four times daily

**21.** Which of the following loop diuretics is a *not* a sulfonamide and can, therefore, be given to a patient with a sulfonamide allergy?

  **a.** ethacrynic acid
  **b.** bumetanide
  **c.** torsemide
  **d.** furosemide

**22.** All of the following metabolic or electrolyte abnormalities occur with thiazide diuretics *except*

  **a.** hypokalemia
  **b.** hypocalcemia
  **c.** hyperuricemia
  **d.** hypomagnesemia

**23.** True or False: Conivaptan is indicated for the treatment of hyponatremia for patients with underlying HF.

  **a.** true
  **b.** false

## Inotropic Agents

**24.** How does digoxin improve myocardial contractility?

  **a.** inhibition of the $Na^+/K^+$–adenosine triphosphatase
  **b.** inhibition of the breakdown of cyclic adenosine monophosphate (cAMP)

c. increases intracellular $K^+$, leading to the opening of calcium channels

d. directly stimulates calcium release from the sarcoplasmic reticulum

25. F. F. is a 75 y/o man with a history of HF and AFib and was initiated on amiodarone and warfarin. He has been treated for many years with captopril, furosemide, potassium, amlodipine, and digoxin. After 3 days in the hospital, the patient was sent home. One week after discharge, he developed nausea, vomiting, confusion, and symptomatic VT. His serum digoxin concentration was 3.9 ng/mL, and his serum potassium level was 5.8 mmol/L. The rhythm was treated with lidocaine, and the patient is now having episodes of nonsustained VT with a BP of 80/40 mm Hg during each episode. What should be your next course of action?

    a. discontinue the amiodarone and digoxin and observe

    b. discontinue the digoxin and administer digoxin-specific antibodies

    c. decrease the dose of digoxin

    d. discontinue digoxin and observe

26. N. M. is a 75-year-old woman with a long-standing history of HF secondary to viral cardiomyopathy. She presents to the outpatient clinic for routine follow-up. On examination, she was short of breath and reported increasing orthopnea. She was admitted to the ICU for right-heart catheterization. Initial readings show a cardiac index of 1.8 L/minute/$m^2$, elevated pulmonary capillary wedge pressure (25 mm Hg), and high pulmonary pressures (72/45 mm Hg). Her initial BP was 105/55 mm Hg, and she had a heart rate of 105 beats per minute (bpm). Home medications include captopril, spironolactone, metoprolol XL, and furosemide. Which of the following inotropic agents would be most appropriate?

    a. dopamine

    b. dobutamine

    c. milrinone

    d. isoproterenol

## Anticoagulation

27. Which of the following agents bind only to factor Xa?

    a. enoxaparin

    b. fondaparinux

    c. bivalirudin

    d. unfractionated heparin

28. A. F. is a 52 y/o man with a history of AFib, transient ischemic attacks (TIAs), hypertension (HTN), and rheumatic heart disease. The recommendations from the Sixth American College of Chest Physicians (ACCP) Consensus Conference on Antithrombotic Therapy suggest that this patient be initiated on _____ for antithrombotic therapy because of AFib.

    a. aspirin, 81 mg daily

    b. aspirin, 325 mg daily

    c. warfarin, with a target-goal INR of 2.5

    d. warfarin, with a target-goal INR of 3.5

29. The patient above is going to be electively cardioverted. What is the timing of PO anticoagulant therapy?

    a. warfarin with a target INR of 3.5 for 4 weeks before cardioversion and continued for 6 weeks after cardioversion

    b. warfarin with a target INR of 3.5 for 3 weeks before cardioversion and continued for 6 weeks after cardioversion

    c. warfarin with a target INR of 2.5 for 3 weeks before cardioversion and continued for 4 weeks after cardioversion

    d. warfarin with a target INR of 2.5 for 6 weeks before cardioversion and continued for 6 weeks after cardioversion

30. Heparin must first bind to _____ to exert its anticoagulant activity.
    a. antithrombin
    b. thrombin
    c. factor X
    d. protein C

31. J. M. was initiated on heparin and was given a 5,000-unit bolus. Five minutes after the loading dose of heparin, she began to have bloody emesis, and her systolic pressure dropped to 80 mm Hg. How much protamine will she require?
    a. 25 mg
    b. 50 mg
    c. 75 mg
    d. 100 mg

32. All of the following factors increase the risk of severe allergic reactions to protamine *except*
    a. allergy to fish
    b. use of neutral protamine Hagedorn (NPH) insulin
    c. use of regular insulin
    d. vasectomized males

33. Patients who develop heparin-induced thrombocytopenia have an in vitro cross-reactivity with LMWH by what percent?
    a. 90% to 100%
    b. 60% to 70%
    c. 25% to 45%
    d. 5% to 10%

34. A patient with a recent history of heparin-associated antibodies presents with new-onset symptomatic AFib and requires anticoagulation. Other significant past medical history includes severe renal failure secondary to long-standing HTN. The patient's baseline serum creatinine is 4 mg/dL, with an estimated creatinine clearance of 10 mL/minute. Which of the following choices is the best initial therapy?
    a. lepirudin, 0.4 mg/kg bolus, then 0.15 mg/kg/hour
    b. lepirudin, 0.2 mg/kg bolus, then 0.15 mg/kg/hour
    c. argatroban, 2 mcg/kg/minute
    d. enoxaparin, 1 mg/kg SC daily

35. Which of the following direct thrombin inhibitors is *not* a reversible inhibitor of thrombin?
    a. bivalirudin
    b. lepirudin
    c. argatroban
    d. melagatran

36. Of the following clinical conditions, all require long-term systemic anticoagulation *except*
    a. mitral valve regurgitation with a history of systemic embolism
    b. mitral valve prolapse with documented unexplained TIAs
    c. infective endocarditis with a mechanical prosthetic valve
    d. mitral annular calcification and systemic embolism not documented to be a calcific embolism

## Antiplatelet Agents

37. Which of the following side effects differentiate ticlopidine from clopidogrel?
    a. diarrhea
    b. rash

**c.** neutropenia

**d.** thrombotic thrombocytopenic purpura

**38.** By which of the following mechanisms do clopidogrel and ticlopidine exert their antiplatelet effects?

    **a.** cyclo-oxygenase inhibitor

    **b.** glycoprotein IIb/IIIa inhibitor

    **c.** adenosine diphosphate (ADP) inhibitor

    **d.** direct thrombin inhibitor

**39.** All of the following are considered contraindications to abciximab administration *except*

    **a.** readministration of abciximab

    **b.** thrombocytopenia with a platelet count of less than 100,000 cells/μL

    **c.** active internal bleeding

    **d.** intracranial tumor, arteriovenous malformation, or aneurysm

**40.** Which of the following glycoprotein IIb/IIIa inhibitors has the highest incidence of severe thrombocytopenia?

    **a.** tirofiban

    **b.** abciximab

    **c.** eptifibatide

    **d.** The incidence is not different between the different agents.

**41.** Which of the following glycoprotein IIb/IIIa inhibitors has the shortest half-life but the longest duration of therapy?

    **a.** tirofiban

    **b.** eptifibatide

    **c.** abciximab

    **d.** lamifiban

## Antiarrhythmic Agents

**42.** Which of the following agents is effective for converting AFib to sinus rhythm and for maintaining sinus rhythm after it is restored?

    **a.** digoxin

    **b.** amiodarone

    **c.** diltiazem

    **d.** propranolol

**43.** A. R. is a 65 y/o man with a history of AFib, MI, status post coronary artery bypass graft (CABG) 5 years ago, HTN, deep venous thrombosis (DVT), and hypercholesterolemia, who presented to the emergency department with AFib and a rapid ventricular rate. After initiation of beta-blockers, his rate was well controlled (heart rate, 80 bpm). A. R. has been on warfarin for a DVT that developed after a fall. He has not been on antiarrhythmic therapy. All of the following are appropriate choices *except*

    **a.** amiodarone

    **b.** sotalol

    **c.** procainamide

    **d.** flecainide

**44.** M. G., a 50 y/o man, collapsed at home after shoveling his sidewalk. His son initiated cardiopulmonary resuscitation immediately, and an emergency medical service was called. When the squad arrived, it was determined that M. G. was in ventricular fibrillation (VF), and he was cardioverted with 200 J, 300 J, and 360 J. Epinephrine was given, and M. G. was shocked again. M. G. was still in VF. It was decided to initiate antiarrhythmic therapy. Choose the most appropriate agent from the list below.

    **a.** lidocaine
    **b.** amiodarone
    **c.** procainamide
    **d.** bretylium

**45.** All of the following drugs are contraindicated when coadministered with dofetilide *except*

    **a.** diltiazem
    **b.** verapamil
    **c.** trimethoprim
    **d.** ketoconazole

**46.** All of the following side effects may occur during amiodarone therapy *except*

    **a.** pulmonary toxicity
    **b.** hyperthyroidism
    **c.** peripheral neuropathy
    **d.** diarrhea

## Acute Coronary Syndromes

**47.** G. M. is a 45 y/o man presenting with a non–ST-segment-elevation myocardial infarction (MI). His creatinine clearance is estimated to be 30 mL/minute. You would like to initiate eptifibatide. Which of the following doses would be the best choice?

    **a.** loading dose of 180 μg/kg and a maintenance of 2 μg/kg/minute
    **b.** loading dose of 90 μg/kg/minute and a maintenance dose of 2 μg/kg/minute
    **c.** loading dose of 180 μg/kg and a maintenance dose of 1 μg/kg/minute
    **d.** loading dose of 90 μg/kg/minute and a maintenance dose of 1 μg/kg/minute

**48.** M. M. is a 39 y/o male with an inferior wall non–ST-segment-elevation MI. He has a history of poorly controlled HTN and diabetes mellitus (DM). You initiate aspirin, clopidogrel, and atorvastatin. His baseline serum creatinine is 3.4 mg/dL and you estimate his creatinine clearance to be 25 mL/minute. What dose of enoxaparin would you choose?

    **a.** 1 mg/kg every 12 hours
    **b.** 1 mg/kg daily
    **c.** enoxaparin is not indicated at this time
    **d.** fondaparinux is safer to use in M. M.

**49.** B. B. is a 77 y/o male who presents with typical chest pain and pressure. He has ST elevations in lead $V_{2-4}$. He is 80 kg with a serum creatinine of 0.7 mg/dL with an estimate creatinine clearance of 75 mL/minute. You initiate aspirin, clopidogrel, metoprolol, and atorvastatin. You want to initiate enoxaparin and reteplase. What is the enoxaparin dose for this patient?

    **a.** loading dose of 30 mg IV once followed immediately by 1 mg/kg every 12 hours
    **b.** loading dose of 30 mg IV once followed by 0.75 mg/kg every 12 hours
    **c.** 1 mg/kg daily
    **d.** 0.75 mg/kg every 12 hours

**50.** Which of the following is *not* a contraindication to thrombolytic therapy?

    **a.** acute pericarditis
    **b.** aortic dissection
    **c.** intracranial neoplasm
    **d.** diabetic retinopathy

**51.** Which of the following is *not* a risk factor for intracranial hemorrhage in patients receiving fibrinolytic therapy in the treatment of ST-segment-elevation MI?

  **a.** HTN
  **b.** body weight
  **c.** age
  **d.** time to presentation

**52.** R. M. is a 65 y/o man presenting to the emergency department with an ST-segment-elevation MI. It is decided to initiate thrombolytic therapy to induce reperfusion. The patient weighs 72 kg. What is the most effective dose of alteplase for this patient?

  **a.** 0.9 mg/kg, with a maximum of 90 mg
  **b.** 15 mg bolus; then 54 mg over 30 minutes; then 36 mg over 60 minutes
  **c.** 15 mg bolus; then 50 mg over 30 minutes; then 35 mg over 60 minutes
  **d.** 60 mg over 1 hour; then 20 mg per hour for 2 hours

## Hyperlipidemia

**53.** M. R. is a 74 y/o male with a history of hypercholesterolemia treated with simvastatin. Two months ago he had a permanent pacemaker placed for sick sinus syndrome. He now presents with a 1-month history of fever, chills, and unexplained weight loss. On physical exam he has a new tricuspid regurgitation murmur. A transesophageal echocardiogram confirms your suspicion of endocarditis. Which of the following antibiotics increases the risk of rhabdomyolysis when given with simvastatin?

  **a.** ceftriaxone
  **b.** vancomycin
  **c.** daptomycin
  **d.** linezolid

**54.** Put the following regimens in order according to their LDL-lowering ability.

  atorvastatin, 10 mg daily (A)
  cholestyramine, 8 g daily (C)
  pravastatin, 20 mg daily (P)
  gemfibrozil, 600 mg twice daily (G)

  **a.** A > P > C > G
  **b.** P > A > G > C
  **c.** A > P > G > C
  **d.** A > C > P > G

**55.** D. L. is a 76 y/o white man with a past medical history significant for DM type 2 and HTN. Chronic AFib was recently diagnosed with coronary artery disease (CAD) and hypercholesterolemia and he was initiated on gemfibrozil 600 mg two times daily and atorvastatin 40 mg daily. His other medications include glyburide, metoprolol, furosemide, levothyroxine, insulin, and aspirin. Two weeks later, he began to experience pain in his right calf, with pain and stiffness throughout his back, buttocks, and thigh. After another week, he was admitted to the hospital with similar heightened symptoms. On admission, his BUN was elevated, and the urinalysis showed orange, cloudy urine; protein, greater than 300; glucose, greater than 1,000; ketones, 2+; hemoglobin, 3+; red blood cell count, 6 to 10; and myoglobin, 1,367. Which of the following statements is *true*?

  **a.** The patient is experiencing rhabdomyolysis secondary to the drug interaction of atorvastatin and glyburide.
  **b.** Forced diuresis with urine alkalinization and discontinuation of gemfibrozil and atorvastatin are indicated for this patient.
  **c.** Atorvastatin is contraindicated in a patient with diabetes mellitus type 2 and HTN.
  **d.** If nicotinic acid, rather than gemfibrozil, had been used for hypercholesterolemia, this reaction would have been prevented.

**56.** All of the following drugs adversely affect the lipid profiles *except*

a. thiazide diuretics
b. beta-blockers
c. protease inhibitors
d. ACE inhibitors

## Hypertension

**57.** N. H. is a 57 y/o man status post MI with a BP of 150/88 mm Hg and a heart rate of 87 bpm. He is currently on aspirin, clopidogrel, atorvastatin, and lisinopril. Which agent would be the most appropriate addition for treatment of his HTN?

a. hydrochlorothiazide
b. metoprolol
c. clonidine
d. losartan

**58.** B. T. is a 56 y/o woman with long-standing HTN that is difficult to control. She is currently being treated with amlodipine 10 mg daily, lisinopril 40 mg daily, hydrochlorothiazide 25 mg daily, and clonidine 0.4 mg three times daily. She presented to the emergency room, and her initial BP was 200/110 mm Hg. She states she had run out of one of her medications. Which one of her medications would most likely be implicated in causing hypertensive urgency?

a. amlodipine
b. lisinopril
c. hydrochlorothiazide
d. clonidine

**59.** C. P. is a 46 y/o white man admitted with worsening headache, and nausea and vomiting over 48 hours. The patient is status post single-lung transplant secondary to alpha$_1$-antitrypsin deficiency. His immunosuppression regimen includes cyclosporine, prednisone, and azathioprine. As a result of the cyclosporine, he has HTN and renal dysfunction (baseline serum creatinine, 1.9 mg/dL). His BP is controlled with clonidine 0.2 mg twice daily, and metoprolol tartrate 25 mg twice daily. Two months ago, he was changed to metoprolol from amlodipine because of peripheral edema. The patient was in his usual state of health until approximately 1 week ago, when he experienced diarrhea, which has since resolved. On admission, his BP was 208/110 mm Hg, and his serum creatinine was 3.8 mg/dL. What is the most appropriate regimen to control this patient's BP?

a. change back to amlodipine 10 mg daily
b. initiate nitroprusside drip and give IV fluids
c. add captopril to the regimen and titrate to effect
d. give sublingual nifedipine

## Heart Failure

**60.** ACE inhibitors have benefits on systolic dysfunction that include all of the following *except*

a. they decrease ventricular dilation and cardiac remodeling
b. they prevent the growth effects of angiotensin II on myocytes
c. they increase preload and decrease afterload
d. they attenuate aldosterone-induced cardiac fibrosis

**61.** R. W. is a 60 y/o female with HF (left ventricular ejection fraction <30%) who has hypertension with a blood pressure of 152/90 mm Hg. Her potassium is 4.0 mg/dL and serum creatinine is stable at 1.5 mg/dL. She is currently on digoxin and furosemide. Which regimen is most appropriate to initiate in this patient?

a. hydralazine 25 mg four times daily
b. metoprolol tartrate 12.5 mg twice daily
c. valsartan 20 mg twice daily
d. lisinopril 5 mg daily

62. A. V. is a 49 y/o female with a history of HF presenting to the emergency department (ED) for the second time in a month with acutely decompensated HF. She has dyspnea at rest and 3+ edema in her lower extremities. Her serum creatinine is 1.8 mg/dL and blood pressure is 90/60 mm Hg. Her home regimen includes enalapril 20 mg twice daily, carvedilol 3.125 mg twice daily, and furosemide 40 mg PO daily. Which of the following is most appropriate for this patient?

a. admit her to the hospital for IV furosemide therapy and hemodynamic monitoring
b. admit her to the hospital for diuresis with nesiritide
c. initiate an infusion of nesiritide in the ED and reassess in 4 hours
d. schedule intermittent outpatient infusions of nesiritide

63. The mechanisms of benefit for HF of beta-blockers include all of the following *except*

a. increased ventricular pressure
b. blockade of sympathetic stimulation of cell growth
c. antiarrhythmic activity
d. decreased programmed cell death

64. A patient with New York Heart Association class III HF was hospitalized 2 months ago for an exacerbation of his HF. The patient was discharged on lisinopril, furosemide, and digoxin. His lungs are clear, and his vitals are as follows: BP, 105/56 mm Hg; heart rate, 84 bpm; and respiration rate, 18. Which regimen is most appropriate to initiate in this patient?

a. atenolol 50 mg daily
b. carvedilol 3.125 mg twice daily
c. carvedilol 25 mg twice daily
d. metoprolol tartrate 50 mg twice daily

65. Which beta-blockers are recommended for use for patients with HF?

a. metoprolol tartrate, pindolol, propranolol
b. carvedilol, metoprolol succinate, bisoprolol
c. metoprolol succinate, metoprolol tartrate, carvedilol
d. metoprolol tartrate, carvedilol, bisoprolol

66. All of the following medications used to treat HF have been shown to improve survival *except*

a. captopril
b. prazosin
c. hydralazine and isosorbide dinitrate (ISDN)
d. metoprolol

67. Y. J. is a 67 y/o African American male with HF who has been treated with lisinopril 20 mg daily, metoprolol succinate 25 mg daily, furosemide 40 mg twice daily, and spironolactone 12.5 mg daily. Despite his current therapy, he still complains of shortness of breath while conducting usual daily activities. What is the most appropriate change that should be made to his regimen?

a. increase spironolactone
b. start hydralazine
c. initiate isosorbide dinitrate and hydralazine
d. increase lisinopril

NOTES

68. Which of the following statements is *true*?
    a. Serum levels are used to guide the selection of the dose of digoxin.
    b. Because spironolactone was found to have mortality benefit in the Randomized Aldactone Evaluation Study (RALES), the addition of spironolactone should be considered for all HF patients.
    c. The benefit of long-term IV inotropic therapy may outweigh the increased mortality risk in refractory patients unable to be weaned from IV inotropic support.
    d. Digoxin exhibits both symptomatic and mortality benefit in patients with HF.

## Endocarditis

69. One month ago, a 37 y/o female with sinus infection responded well to a 14-day course of amoxicillin/clavulanate 875/125 mg twice daily. She is scheduled for a root canal in 1 week. In the past, her dentist had prescribed one dose of clindamycin 600 mg, 1 hour prior to any dental work, for endocarditis prophylaxis because of her history of mitral valve prolapse. Realizing she has not received her prescription, the patient calls the dentist's office for an antibiotic. What prophylaxis is indicated for this patient?
    a. amoxicillin 2 g PO 1 hour before the procedure
    b. clindamycin 600 mg PO 1 hour before the procedure
    c. azithromycin 500 mg PO 1 hour before the procedure
    d. no prophylaxis recommended in this patient

70. S. C. is a 59 y/o woman diagnosed with enterococcal endocarditis. She has no known drug allergies. Which of the following would exhibit standard therapy?
    a. penicillin G, 5 million units IV every 4 hours for 4 to 6 weeks, plus gentamicin, 2.5 mg/kg IV every 8 hours for 4 to 6 weeks
    b. ampicillin, 2 g IV every 4 hours for 4 to 6 weeks, plus gentamicin, 1 mg/kg IV every 8 hours for 4 to 6 weeks
    c. ampicillin, 2 g IV every 4 hours for 4 to 6 weeks, plus gentamicin, 1 mg/kg IV every 8 hours for 3 to 5 days
    d. vancomycin, 30 mg/kg per 24 hours in two equally divided doses for 4 to 6 weeks

# Answers

1. **b.** 1,300 mg. To determine the loading dose of a one-compartment drug, three items are needed: (a) the drug's Vd (L/kg), (b) the desired steady-state concentration (Cpss [mg/L]), and (c) the patient's weight. Loading dose = Vd × Cpss. Kilograms and liters cancel, and you are left with the loading dose in milligrams.

2. **b.** 25%. The bioavailability of digoxin tablets is 75%. Therefore, when converting from PO to IV administration (bioavailability of 100%), there is a 25% increase in bioavailability. Without altering the dose of digoxin, this patient would most likely have an increase in digoxin level to approximately 2.4 ng/mL. This could lead to potential digoxin toxicity.

3. **c.** Half-life is a function of both clearance (Cl) and Vd. The elimination-rate constant ($k_{el}$) is determined by two independent factors: Cl and Vd. $k_{el} = $ Cl/Vd. Half-life is determined by the equation $0.693/k_{el}$. Therefore, as the apparent Vd and Cl change, the half-life of a drug may change.

4. **d.** Pharmacodynamics. Pharmacodynamics has been defined as the study of the biologic effects resulting from the interaction between drugs and biologic systems. Pharmacokinetic principles consider drug distribution, metabolism, clearance, and bioavailability, whereas pharmacodynamic principles take this one step further and relate these factors to pharmacologic response. Pharmacogenetics is the study of heredity on variations in drug response among individuals and populations. Pharmacogenetic studies have established that genetics play an important role in the dose-concentration-response relationships of medications, whereas pharmacology is simply the study of drugs.

5. **a.** Drug A is the most potent agent. This is based on the fact that at any given concentration of this agent, the effect is greater than that of the other drugs at similar concentrations. Drug B has the same maximal effect; however, it occurs at a higher concentration. Drug C is similar to drug B; however, it is less efficacious, because its maximal effect occurs at a concentration that is 50% lower than that of drug B.

6. **d.** Pravastatin, unlike simvastatin, lovastatin, and atorvastatin, is not metabolized to a large extent by the cytochrome P450 enzyme system. Amiodarone is an inhibitor of this enzyme system and can increase the levels of simvastatin, lovastatin, and atorvastatin. However, amiodarone does not increase the levels of pravastatin.

7. **c.** Increases warfarin metabolism, decreases warfarin metabolism. Chronic ethanol consumption can lead to increased hepatic metabolism of many medications that are cleared through the liver. Increased hepatic metabolism is related to enhanced enzyme function. Therefore, chronic ethanol users typically need higher-than-usual doses of warfarin to achieve therapeutic INRs. Acute ingestion of large amounts of ethanol at a time may inhibit warfarin metabolism. This may lead to elevated INRs and increase the risk of hemorrhagic complications. Moderate ingestion of ethanol does not seem to affect the metabolism of warfarin.

8. **a.** Amiodarone significantly increases the levels of digoxin. Amiodarone decreases the clearance of digoxin and inhibits p-glycoprotein. Amiodarone can increase digoxin levels by 50% to 70%. This interaction can occur in the first days of therapy and a 50% dosage reduction is required immediately. Metoprolol does not increase the levels of digoxin; however, it can have synergistic effects on lowering heart rate and should be monitored closely. Simvastatin and fenofibrate do not alter the levels of digoxin.

9. **b.** Cholestyramine is least likely to enhance the effects of warfarin. Amiodarone, metronidazole, and erythromycin all enhance warfarin's effects by decreasing the

clearance of warfarin. Amiodarone may also alter protein binding of warfarin. Cholestyramine decreases the absorption and prevents the enterohepatic recycling of warfarin, thus decreasing the effectiveness of warfarin. It is recommended that the dose of warfarin be separated from the cholestyramine dose by at least 2 hours before or 2 hours after warfarin. In addition, more frequent monitoring should be done when initiating, discontinuing, or changing the dose of cholestyramine.

10. **c.** All ACE inhibitors, except for captopril, lisinopril, and enalaprilat, are prodrugs that require hepatic activation for pharmacologic activity.

11. **c.** Sodium depletion is an important factor in the development of renal insufficiency associated with ACE inhibitors. Patients with hyponatremia, dehydration, and severe HF are most dependent on the maintenance of renal perfusion by angiotensin II–mediated vasoconstriction of the efferent arteriole. Prevention of hyponatremia by decreasing diuretics can reduce such risk. Numerous studies, including the Studies of Left Ventricular Dysfunction (SOLVD) treatment trial, Veterans' Administration Heart Failure Trial (V-HeFT) II, and Cooperative North Scandinavian Enalapril Survival Study (CONSENSUS), have shown ACE inhibitors to reduce mortality in patients with ischemic and nonischemic cardiomyopathy and mild to moderate HF. ACE inhibitors are considered to be associated with a class benefit; however, not all ACE inhibitors carry the FDA indication for HF. The ACE inhibitors that are approved for the treatment of HF include captopril, enalapril, lisinopril, quinapril, fosinopril, and ramipril. In 1998, the Assessment of Treatment with Lisinopril and Survival (ATLAS) trial showed that high doses of lisinopril were superior to low doses in decreasing risk of death or hospitalization. Therefore, an effort to use target doses used in clinical trials is important (e.g., captopril 50 mg three times daily, enalapril 10 mg twice daily, lisinopril 20 mg daily). Potassium retention of ACE inhibitors is caused by a reduction in the feedback of angiotensin II to stimulate aldosterone release. Caution is necessary when initiating a potassium supplement in a patient on ACE-inhibitor therapy.

12. **d.** Cough is a common side effect of ACE inhibitors. It is not a contraindication to initiate patients on ACE inhibitors if they have pre-existing cough. ACE inhibitor–associated cough is difficult at times to differentiate from cough associated with HF. Also, cough is not life threatening and is considered an annoyance. In many patients, the cough is such a nuisance that cessation of therapy will be required. Patients with bilateral renal artery stenosis are at high risk of developing acute renal failure with the use of ACE inhibitors. ACE inhibitors preferentially dilate the efferent arteriole in the nephron, and in the presence of decreased afferent arterial pressures lead to a decrease in glomerular filtration. This can lead to acute renal failure and is typically reversible if the ACE inhibitor is discontinued early. In the second and third trimesters of pregnancy, ACE inhibitors can lead to oligohydramnios, fetal calvarial hypoplasia, fetal pulmonary hypoplasia, fetal growth retardation, and fetal death. Therefore, these agents should be used with extreme caution in women of childbearing potential. Finally, angioedema is a rare but potentially fatal adverse event that can occur with ACE inhibitors. Angioedema typically occurs within the first few doses; however, it may develop after years of therapy. ACE inhibitors are considered contraindicated in patients with a prior history of angioedema.

13. **a.** Valsartan and candesartan are the only ARBs approved for the treatment of HF. The results of Val-HEFT and CHARM trials led to the recommendation for use of ARBs in patients with HF symptoms and reduced LVEF who are intolerant to ACE inhibitors, including those with angioedema. The incidence of ARB-induced angioedema is reduced compared to ACE inhibitors; however, caution is necessary because of the seriousness of this adverse effect.

**14. d.** All of the statements are true. The rationale for combination ACE inhibitor and ARB therapy is to further reduce the effects of the renin-angiotensin-aldosterone system since serum concentrations of angiotensin II may remain elevated while on ACE inhibitor therapy. In symptomatic patients with reduced LVEF, ARBs may be added to conventional therapy. However, because of insufficient data and risk of hyperkalemia, the addition of an ARB in patients already on ACE inhibitor and an aldosterone antagonist is not recommended. As for the addition of a beta-blocker to therapy, the American College of Cardiology and American Heart Association (ACC/AHA) Guideline for the Diagnosis and Management of Chronic Heart Failure recommend that the addition of beta-blockers may be added before target doses of ACE inhibitors or ARBs are achieved.

**15. c.** (1) ii; (2) iii; (3) i; (4) iv. Agents exhibiting alpha-blockade include labetalol and carvedilol. Agents with ISA are pindolol, penbutolol, carteolol, and acebutolol. Agents with membrane-stabilizing activity are propranolol, labetalol, and acebutolol. Beta$_1$-selective agents include bisoprolol, betaxolol, atenolol, acebutolol, and metoprolol.

**16. a.** Diltiazem and verapamil decrease conduction velocity within the AV node and increase refractory period of nodal tissue. This then causes slowing of ventricular rate.

**17. d.** Dihydropyridines are more selective for vascular smooth-muscle calcium channels than for myocardial calcium channels. Dihydropyridine CCBs do not slow AV-nodal conduction. Unlike verapamil and diltiazem, dihydropyridine CCBs cause a reflex tachycardia and do not increase AV-nodal refractory period. Pedal edema is one of the most common side effects of dihydropyridine-type CCBs and is associated with short half-life, short-acting agents. Because of their ability to produce such profound vasodilation, these agents can produce flushing as well.

**18. d.** Nimodipine. Nimodipine is the only agent indicated for patients with subarachnoid hemorrhage. Nimodipine decreases the influx of extracellular calcium, thus preventing vasospasm.

**19. c.** Free radical depletion is not a suggested mechanism. Long-term administration of nitroglycerin without a nitrate-free interval may lead to nitrate tolerance. Although the exact mechanism of this effect is not fully understood, there are a number of hypotheses, including volume expansion, sulfhydryl-group depletion, reflex vasoconstriction, and free-radical production. The mechanism for volume depletion causing tolerance is unknown. Additionally, there is a lack of evidence suggesting that the depletion of sulfhydryl groups, which are necessary for intracellular biotransformation of nitrates to nitric oxide, is responsible for tolerance. A neurohormonal hypothesis associates the administration of nitrates with a reflexive release of vasoconstrictor hormones that decrease the vasodilating effects of nitrates; however, this has not been consistently observed. Finally, free-radical production, specifically superoxide anion, leads to nitrate tolerance in animal trials and has been reversed with the administration of antioxidants.

**20. d.** Increasing the frequency of the same diuretic dose is not a successful method to overcome diuretic resistance. Limiting sodium intake, management of underlying disease, discontinuing interacting medications, switching to a more potent agent (e.g., loops over thiazides), and improving bioavailability (e.g., IV administration) are all ways to improve diuresis. Additionally, higher doses to achieve diuretic thresholds and combination regimens with agents acting at different segments of the nephron (e.g., loop + thiazide) are effective strategies to overcome resistance. Finally, continuous infusions of loop diuretics expose the kidney to constant drug concentrations, thereby preventing sodium reabsorption that can occur between intermittent doses.

21. **a.** Ethacrynic acid is the only loop diuretic that is not a sulfonamide. It is used only in patients allergic to other either loop or thiazide diuretics. Disadvantages of ethacrynic acid include GI intolerance and a narrower dose-response curve.

22. **b.** Hypocalcemia. Thiazide diuretics retain calcium by increasing reabsorption in the proximal tubule. Therefore, these agents need to be avoided in patients with hypercalcemia, in contrast to loop diuretics, which are used to treat hypercalcemia. Like loop diuretics, thiazide diuretics cause hypokalemia, hyperuricemia, and hypomagnesemia. Hyperuricemia is not typically problematic; however, it can produce gout attacks.

23. **b.** False. Conivaptan is a dual vasopressin antagonist indicated for the treatment of euvolemic and hypervolemic hyponatremia. Its predominant pharmacodynamic effect is through the V2 antagonism of vasopressin in the renal collecting ducts that results in excretion of free water. Because of the limited number of HF patients with hypervolemic hyponatremia treated with conivaptan, safety in HF patients has not been established; therefore, its use in HF patients may be considered only when the clinical benefit outweighs the risk of adverse effects.

24. **a.** Inhibition of the $Na^+/K^+$–adenosine triphosphatase. Digoxin inhibits the $Na^+/K^+$–adenosine triphosphatase pump on the myocardial cell surface. This inhibits the ability of the cell to exchange potassium for sodium and thus leads to an increase in intracellular sodium. This increase in intracellular sodium leads to exchange of sodium for calcium, increasing intracellular calcium concentrations. Increased intracellular calcium enhances contraction coupling.

25. **b.** Discontinue the digoxin and administer digoxin-specific antibodies. Digoxin-immune Fab is indicated for patients with life-threatening ventricular arrhythmias relating to digoxin toxicity. It is also indicated in patients with progressive bradyarrhythmias, such as severe sinus bradycardia or second- or third-degree heart block not responsive to atropine. It should not be used for milder forms of digoxin toxicity. Also, in the setting of hyperkalemia and digitalis intoxication, digoxin-immune Fab fragment is indicated. Digoxin-immune Fab fragment is ovine derived; there is a potential for hypersensitivity reactions, and there are no data available in regard to readministration.

26. **c.** Milrinone. Milrinone is a phosphodiesterase inhibitor classified as inodilator. Thus, milrinone produces positive inotropic effects and vasodilation. Milrinone inhibits the phosphodiesterase III enzyme, leading to an increase in intracellular cAMP, thus causing increased intracellular levels of calcium. In addition, milrinone will decrease pulmonary pressures and LV end-diastolic pressures more predictably than the other agents listed. These combined effects lead to minimal increases in myocardial $O_2$ consumption. Also, milrinone may be useful in this patient secondary to chronic metoprolol therapy.

27. **b.** Fondaparinux, a pentasaccharide, selectively inhibits activated Xa through its binding to antithrombin. Enoxaparin and unfractionated heparin (UFH) bind to both thrombin (IIa) and activated Xa, whereas bivalirudin binds directly to thrombin. UFH binds to thrombin and activated Factor Xa in a 1:1 ratio, whereas low-molecular-weight heparins vary in their binding ratios.

28. **c.** Warfarin, with a target goal INR of 2.5. This patient is at high risk for a thromboembolic event. Recommendations for antithrombotic therapy include risk stratification. Risks are stratified into high, moderate, and low. High-risk patients include patients with prior stroke or TIA or systemic embolus, history of HTN, poor LV systolic function, age older than 75 years, rheumatic mitral valve disease, and a prosthetic heart valve. Moderate risk factors include age between 65 and 75 years, diabetes mellitus, and CAD with preserved LV systolic function. Low-risk patients are those younger than 65 years old with no clinical or TTE evidence of cardiovascular disease.

29. **c.** Warfarin with a target INR of 2.5 for 3 weeks before cardioversion and continued for 4 weeks after cardioversion. Recommendations from the Sixth ACCP Consensus Conference on Antithrombotic Therapy state that patients undergoing elective cardioversion for AFib should be initiated on oral anticoagulant therapy for 3 weeks before and at least 4 weeks after elective DC cardioversion. The grade of evidence is 1C+. Also, an alternative approach would be to initiate anticoagulation, have the patients undergo a TEE, and have the cardioversion performed if no thrombi are seen. Warfarin should be continued for at least 4 weeks, as long as the patient maintains NSR. This is a grade 1C recommendation.

30. **a.** Antithrombin. Heparin must first bind to antithrombin to exert is anticoagulant effect. This complex accelerates antithrombin effect. Heparin potentiates antithrombin's effect by binding to a glucosamine unit within a pentasaccharide sequence.

31. **b.** 50 mg. Every 1 mg of protamine will antagonize approximately 100 units of heparin. Because this patient just received the bolus, she would require 50 mg of protamine. If she had received the dose 30 to 60 minutes ago, then a dose of 0.50 to 0.75 mg of protamine per 100 units of heparin would be required. If she had been on a continuous infusion of heparin, then the dosing would be dependent on the time and dose of the last bolus of heparin and the rate of infusion. In this scenario, most patients require approximately 25 to 50 mg of protamine.

32. **c.** Use of regular insulin. Severe hypersensitivity reactions can occur with the administration of protamine. Patients at risk include those with fish allergies, those who use NPH insulin, those who have had prior protamine exposure (other than NPH insulin), and vasectomized men. Protamine is derived from fish. Originally, it was discovered in salmon testes. The commercially available product is still made from fish. Fifty percent of diabetic patients using NPH insulin may develop antibodies to protamine and are at risk of developing hypersensitivity reactions to protamine. Vasectomized males develop protamine antibodies approximately one third of the time and are also at risk for developing a hypersensitivity reaction after the administration of protamine. Regular insulin does not contain protamine and, therefore, diabetic patients receiving only regular insulin are not at risk.

33. **a.** 90% to 100%. There have been several reports of patients who have heparin-induced thrombocytopenia being treated with LMWH. However, the cross-reactivity in vitro approaches 100%. The use of LMWH should be considered a contraindication unless there is a documented negative test for antibodies against LMWH.

34. **c.** Argatroban, 2 mcg/kg/minute. Argatroban is hepatically cleared and, therefore, does not require dosing adjustment for patients with renal dysfunction and may be a safer alternative for anticoagulation. Lepirudin is reasonable as well; however, patients with significant renal dysfunction require appropriate dosing adjustments. Continuous infusion should not be used in patients with a creatinine clearance less than 15 mL/minute because of accumulation of drug. LMWHs have a high likelihood for in vitro and in vivo cross-reactivity of 80% to 100%, and there is a potential for an increase in thrombotic complications.

35. **b.** Lepirudin is not a reversible inhibitor of thrombin. Hirudin and recombinant derivatives bind to both the catalytic site and substrate-recognition site of thrombin irreversibly. Bivalirudin, a synthetic hirudin derivative, contains two covalently linked groups that bind to the catalytic site and the substrate site of thrombin. This bivalent binding is both reversible and transient. Argatroban and melagatran bind only to the catalytic site of thrombin. They bind by competitive inhibition and are reversible.

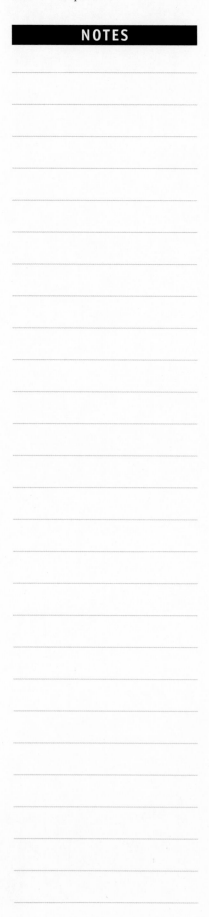

**36. b.** Mitral valve prolapse with documented unexplained TIAs does not require long-term systemic anticoagulation. The recommendations from the Sixth Consensus Conference on Antithrombotic Therapy from the ACCP state that patients with mitral valve prolapse and unexplained TIAs need long-term aspirin therapy, 50 to 162 mg daily. This is a grade 1A recommendation.

**37. c.** Neutropenia. Ticlopidine causes neutropenia in 2.4% of patients who are initiated on therapy. Nearly 1% of patients develop severe neutropenia. Therefore, a complete blood count is required every 2 weeks during initiation of therapy for the first 3 months of therapy. Both agents can cause diarrhea and rash. Structurally, these two drugs are so similar that allergic cross-reactivity is expected. Thrombotic thrombocytopenic purpura has been reported with both agents. There have been >100 cases of thrombotic thrombocytopenic purpura reported with the use of ticlopidine and clopidogrel.

**38. c.** ADP inhibitor. ADP is released from red blood cells, activated platelets, and damaged endothelial cells, leading to platelet adhesion and aggregation. However, the precise mechanism of their action has not been completely identified. ADP blockade decreases the expression of the glycoprotein IIb/IIIa receptor. Platelet inhibition occurs at maximal effect within 3 to 5 days and produces approximately 40% to 50% platelet inhibition. The onset and degree of platelet inhibition can be expedited with use of loading doses (300 to 600 mg).

**39. a.** Readministration of abciximab is not a contraindication. Concerns regarding the readministration of abciximab relate to the development of antibodies to abciximab. This may lead to increases in hypersensitivity reactions, decrease or loss of effectiveness, and the development of thrombocytopenia. Recently, published data from the ReoPro readministration registry show that the risk of thrombocytopenia is similar to that for abciximab-naïve patients. However, there was an increase in the number of patients who developed severe thrombocytopenia and also in cases of delayed-onset thrombocytopenia. There were no cases of hypersensitivity, and clinical outcomes were also unchanged.

**40. b.** Abciximab. All glycoprotein IIb/IIIa inhibitors may cause thrombocytopenia. However, abciximab has the highest rate of all, based on the clinical trials.

**41. c.** Abciximab. Abciximab has a serum half-life of 10 to 30 minutes; however, because of its high binding affinity to the glycoprotein IIb/IIIa receptor, it maintains its activity for many hours after discontinuation of therapy, and abciximab can be detected in the serum for longer than 2 weeks. The short-acting inhibitors have half-lives of approximately 2 hours, depending on renal function; however, because of their competitive inhibiting nature, once the infusion is discontinued, their effects wane relatively quickly.

**42. b.** Amiodarone. Although amiodarone does not carry an FDA indication for the treatment of AFib, it can convert to and maintain normal sinus rhythm. The other agents listed are only used for rate control when used for AFib.

**43. d.** Flecainide is not an appropriate choice. In general, antiarrhythmic agents are proarrhythmic and possess myocardial-depressant effects. Flecainide, encainide, and moricizine were evaluated in the Cardiac Arrhythmia Suppression Trial I or II. These agents were evaluated in patients with multiple PVCs after MI. By suppressing ventricular ectopy, it was felt that there would be a decrease in mortality. However, there was an increase in mortality in all groups despite suppression of initial arrhythmia. At this time, class IC antiarrhythmics are indicated for life-threatening sustained VT and paroxysmal SVT, including Wolff-Parkinson-White syndrome and AFib or flutter in patients without structural heart disease.

**44. b.** Amiodarone. The most recent advanced cardiac life support guidelines recommend that amiodarone be the first-line agent in patients with pulseless VT/VF. This recommendation is based on the Amiodarone for Resuscitation After Out-of-Hospital Cardiac Arrest due to Ventricular Fibrillation (ARREST) trial, which showed that amiodarone increased the likelihood of admission to the hospital after an out-of-hospital arrest. This is further supported by the recently presented Amiodarone versus Lidocaine in Pre-Hospital Refractory Ventricular Fibrillation Evaluation (ALIVE) trial. Lidocaine is now considered Class Indeterminate based on the lack of controlled trials supporting its use in pulseless VT/VF. Procainamide administration is prolonged and not suitable for rapid administration. Bretylium is no longer available secondary to lack of raw materials.

45. **a.** Diltiazem is not contraindicated when coadministered with dofetilide. There are seven medications that are contraindicated to give with dofetilide; these include verapamil, trimethoprim, ketoconazole, itraconazole, cimetidine, hydrochorothiazine, and prochlorperazine. In general, medications that inhibit the cation transport system within the kidneys interfere with elimination of dofetilide. Dofetilide is primarily eliminated by the kidneys, and only 20% of elimination occurs via hepatic metabolism through the CYP3A4 enzyme system. Therefore, coadministration of contraindicated medications increases the risk of developing drug-induced arrhythmias, specifically torsades de pointes.

46. **d.** Diarrhea is not a side effect. Pulmonary toxicity in the form of pulmonary fibrosis and hypersensitivity pneumonitis occurs in approximately 3% to 17% of patients on amiodarone therapy. Pulmonary toxicity occurs primarily with doses greater than 400 mg daily and after several months to years. Pulmonary toxicity is very difficult to diagnose, because symptoms and signs are similar to HF and pneumonia. Patient self-reporting is the most effective way to identify pulmonary toxicity early. Thyroid dysfunction occurs in approximately 10% of patients on amiodarone. Patients can present with either hyperthyroidism or hypothyroidism and should be evaluated at baseline and every 6 months thereafter. Neuropathy and other neurologic side effects can occur in up to 20% of patients on chronic amiodarone therapy. Most frequently, amiodarone causes constipation in long-term administration.

47. **c.** Loading dose of 180 mcg/kg and a maintenance dose of 1 mcg/kg/minute. Based on product information, eptifibatide loading dose should not be changed and the maintenance infusion should be initiated at 1 mcg/kg/minute. Eptifibatide is contraindicated in patients on dialysis and there is limited experience using this agent in this patient population. Tirofiban is not contraindicated in patients on dialysis; however, there is limited data to support its use in dialysis patients.

48. **b.** Enoxaparin 1 mg/kg daily. Enoxaparin is approved for both ST-segment-elevation and non–STsegment-elevation MI. In patients with a creatinine clearance greater than 30 mL/minute then the standard dose of 1 mg/kg every 12 hours is appropriate. However, when the creatinine clearance is less than 30 mL/minute then the dose should be reduced to 1 mg/kg once daily. Fondaparinux is contraindicated in patients with a creatinine clearance less then 30 mL/minute.

49. **d.** 0.75 mg/kg every 12 hours. Enoxaparin recently was approved for the treatment of ST-segment-elevation MI with fibrinolysis based on the ExTRACT-TIMI 25 trial. In the older patients, lower enoxaparin doses were used to minimize bleeding. There was a lower risk of the primary end point in those that received enoxaprin versus those receiving unfractionated heparin. There was no difference in intracranial hemorrhage; however, there was a significantly higher rate of major bleeding with enoxaparin (2.1% vs. 1.4%).

50. **d.** Diabetic retinopathy is not a contraindication to thrombolytic therapy. A review of large clinical trials did not show an increase in the rates of intraocular hemorrhage in patients with diabetic proliferative retinopathy. Other absolute contraindications include previous hemorrhagic stroke, other strokes or cerebrovascular events within 1 year, and active bleeding.

**51. d.** Time to presentation is not a risk factor for intracranial hemorrhage in patients receiving thrombolytic therapy. In clinical trials, the risks for intracranial hemorrhage included age older than 65 years, low body weight (less than 70 kg), HTN on hospital admission, and the use of alteplase. Also, the levels of concomitant anticoagulation can also increase the risk of intracranial hemorrhage.

**52. c.** 15 mg bolus; then 50 mg over 30 minutes; then 35 mg over 60 minutes. Based on the first GUSTO trial, the most effective dosing for acute ST-segment-elevation MI is front-loaded tPA. The maximum dose should be 100 mg and, therefore, answer B may increase the risk of major bleeding, specifically intracranial hemorrhage. Answer D is standard dosing of recombinant tissue-type plasminogen activator and was found inferior to front loading. Finally, answer A is the recommended dosing for acute ischemic stroke.

**53. c.** Daptomycin may cause elevations in creatine phosphokinase (CPK) levels. The product literature for daptomycin recommends temporary discontinuation of medications that can raise CPK levels when a patient is receiving this antibiotic. Even though this adverse reaction is rare, CPK levels should be monitored weekly in patients receiving daptomycin alone and more frequently if statin therapy is continued.

**54. a.** A > P > C > G. HMG-CoA reductase inhibitors decrease LDL by 18% to 55%. Atorvastatin is the most potent agent statin of the group. Bile-acid sequestrants decreased LDL by 15% to 30%. Fibrates decrease LDL by 5% to 20%.

**55. b.** Forced diuresis with urine alkalinization and discontinuation of gemfibrozil and atorvastatin are indicated for this patient. Rhabdomyolysis secondary to the interaction of atorvastatin and gemfibrozil is responsible for this clinical picture. Rhabdomyolysis is defined as the disintegration of muscle, associated with the excretion of myoglobin in the urine. Clinical signs and symptoms include myalgias, elevated creatine kinase, elevated urine and serum myoglobin, and dark urine. Complications of rhabdomyolysis are numerous and may include renal failure, disseminated intravascular coagulation, metabolic acidosis, and cardiomyopathy. HMG-CoA reductase inhibitors (statins) can be considered direct myotoxins and may induce rhabdomyolysis when used alone. However, the risk of toxicity increases when statins are used in combination with fibric acid derivatives (gemfibrozil or fenofibrate), nicotinic acid, cyclosporine, itraconazole, or erythromycin, to name a few. Treatment of the underlying cause, in this case discontinuation of the offending agents, is necessary. In addition, renal failure caused by products of tissue degradation must be combated with urinary alkalinization and maintenance of a high urine volume.

**56. d.** ACE inhibitors have no effect on the lipid profile. Beta-blockers and thiazide diuretics typically have the most effect on raising TG levels. Beta-blockers may decrease HDL levels, whereas thiazide diuretics may increase LDL and total cholesterol. Protease inhibitors have the most effect on TGs and total cholesterol and cause adipose tissue redistribution.

**57. b.** Metoprolol. The ACC and AHA recommend the use of beta-blockers in patients after surviving an MI to decrease mortality, sudden death, and reinfarction. Therefore, if this patient is not already on a beta-blocker, one would be indicated, not only for his HTN but also for secondary prevention.

**58. d.** Clonidine. Abrupt withdrawal of an alpha-2 agonist is the most likely cause of severe rebound HTN. Typically, this is seen within 24 to 48 hours of discontinuation of clonidine and typically occurs in patients taking large doses for longer than 3 months. The best treatment for this is to restart clonidine. Beta-blockers could make the situation worse by causing unopposed alpha-1 stimulation.

**59. b.** Initiate nitroprusside drip and give IV fluids. Hypertensive emergencies are defined by the presence of end-organ damage in the face of high BP. This patient was dehydrated from the diarrhea and had uncontrolled BP because of the medication change that occurred. Use of nitroprusside would be most appropriate in this patient because of the emergent situation of the renal insufficiency and possible cerebrovascular involvement exhibited by the headache. Typically, parenteral antihypertensive agents are initiated for hypertensive emergencies. In addition, it is necessary to correct the underlying cause of the hypertensive episode, if it can be identified; therefore, rehydration in this patient is prudent. Nitroprusside is the drug of choice because it has a quick onset of action yet is easily titratable. Sublingual nifedipine is no longer advocated because of the precipitous drop in BP and the subsequent adverse effects.

60. **c.** Because angiotensin II can alter cardiac structure by hemodynamically and nonhemodynamically mediated mechanisms, ACE inhibitors are beneficial in HF A hemodynamic benefit, however, is reduction in both preload and afterload.

61. **d.** Lisinopril 5 mg daily. Because the patient is not already receiving ACE-inhibitor therapy, an ACE inhibitor is indicated in patients with HF and a reduced EF (less than 35% to 45%) to decrease morbidity and mortality, as shown in the SOLVD, V-HeFT, and CONSENSUS trials. The patient has no contraindications to such therapy. If the patient's renal function were changing, thereby making an ACE inhibitor inappropriate, then hydralazine plus a nitrate would be indicated, because V-HeFT I showed mortality benefit compared to placebo and an alpha-blocker. An ARB, like valsartan, would be indicated if the patient were intolerant to ACE inhibitors in the past. Both ACE inhibitors and ARB should be initiated at low doses, and titrated (as tolerated) to doses proven in clinical trials to reduce cardiovascular events.

62. **a.** Nesiritide is contraindicated for use in patients with systolic blood pressure <90 mm Hg. However, based on meta-analyses that raised questions of increased renal dysfunction and mortality associated with nesiritide, the FDA convened a panel to assess available data and provide recommendations regarding appropriate use of nesiritide. These recommendations state that nesiritide should be limited to hospitalized patients with decompensated HF with dyspnea at rest and it should not be used to replace diuretics. Furthermore, because of insufficient evidence, nesiritide should not be used for intermittent outpatient infusions, for scheduled repetitive use, to improve renal function, or to enhance diuresis. A large-scale clinical trial to assess outcomes and further assess the risks of nesiritide versus standard therapy is currently being conducted.

63. **a.** Increased ventricular pressure is not a mechanism of benefit. Beta-blockers interfere with neurohormonal actions of the sympathetic nervous system. Sympathetic activity causes an increase in ventricular volume, thereby increasing ventricular pressure as a result of peripheral vasoconstriction. Norepinephrine and sympathetic activity can lead to arrhythmias, cardiac hypertrophy, and apoptosis (programmed cell death). By administering beta-blockers, these activities are inhibited, thereby causing positive effects in patients with HF, as exhibited in several clinical trials, including Cardiac Insufficiency Bisoprolol Study (CIBIS) I, CIBIS II, Metoprolol CR/XL Controlled Release Randomized Intervention Trial in Heart Failure (MERIT-HF), and others.

64. **b.** Carvedilol 3.125 mg twice daily. All patients with stable, class II or III HF should be initiated on a beta-blocker, unless a contraindication (bronchospastic disease, symptomatic bradycardia, or advanced heart block) or intolerance is exhibited. Initiation of beta-blocker therapy is recommended in stable patients with mild to moderate HF and a low EF (less than 35% to 40%). The mortality benefit of beta-blocker use was seen when added to a pre-existing regimen of an ACE inhibitor and diuretic, with or without digoxin. It should be noted that beta-blockers must be initiated at very low doses and only gradually increased if low doses have been well tolerated.

**65. b.** Overwhelming mortality benefit in patients with chronic HF has been proven in clinical trials for carvedilol, metoprolol succinate, and bisoprolol when added to standard HF therapy. These agents are specifically recommended in the ACC/AHA Guidelines for the Management of Chronic Heart Failure. Despite survival benefit with each of these beta-blockers, a class-effect with all beta-blockers should not be assumed as demonstrated by the Carvedilol or Metoprolol European Trail (COMET). The COMET trial compared carvedilol to metoprolol tartrate in HF patients, and concluded that carvedilol exhibited superior mortality benefit. Beta-blockers with ISA should not be used on patients with HF. Pindolol and others with ISA (such as penbutolol, carteolol, and acebutolol) are partial beta agonists and can maintain normal sympathetic tone. This activity prevents the benefits seen with the reduced heart rate, cardiac output, and peripheral blood flow caused by other beta-blockers.

**66. b.** Prazosin has not been shown to improve survival. Multiple trials have shown that ACE inhibitors, beta-blockers, and the combination of hydralazine and ISDN improve survival in patients who have HF. In the V-HeFT-I trial, prazosin was compared to placebo and the combination of hydralazine and ISDN; in those patients who received prazosin, there was no significant difference in mortality when compared with placebo.

**67. c.** The ACC/AHA guidelines recommend the initiation of isosorbide dinitrate and hydralazine as a reasonable addition to standard therapy in blacks with NYHA class III/IV HF. The A-HeFT trial evaluated a proprietary drug combination (hydralazine 37.5 mg and isosorbide dinitrate 20 mg per tablet) in African Americans with HF along with standard treatment; because of significant mortality benefit, the study was prematurely discontinued.

**68. c.** The benefit of long-term IV inotropic therapy may outweigh the increased mortality risk in refractory patients unable to be weaned from IV inotropic support. Because long-term IV positive inotropic therapy may cause an increased risk of death, such therapy is not regularly recommended. This risk, however, may be outweighed in patients who cannot be weaned from continuous support. Such patients with refractory HF may experience an improved quality of life because of the relative clinical stability afforded by the inotrope; therefore, IV positive inotropic therapy may be considered as a palliative measure in end-stage HF. The DIG (Digitalis Investigation Group) trial showed that digoxin's benefit in HF was the alleviation of symptoms and improvement in clinical status. These findings were associated with a decreased morbidity (fewer hospitalizations) but not mortality. Because digoxin has negligible effect on survival, it is recommended that digoxin be used in conjunction with diuretics, ACE inhibitors, and beta-blockers to decrease the clinical symptoms of HF. Furthermore, little evidence supports the practice of dosing digoxin according to serum levels. This is because of the lack of data exhibiting a relationship between digoxin serum concentrations and therapeutic effect. In the RALES trial, spironolactone was shown to be associated with reduced mortality and morbidity. However, the patients who were included in this trial were patients with class IV HF. Therefore, it would only be prudent to consider spironolactone in patients with recent or current severe HF symptoms. Efficacy and safety of spironolactone's use in patients with mild to moderate HF is yet to be determined.

**69. d.** No prophylaxis is recommended in this patient. The recommendations according to the 2007 Guidelines for Prevention of Infective Endocarditis no longer recommend prophylactic antibiotics prior to dental procedures for people with mitral valve prolapse, rheumatic heart disease, bicuspid valve disease, calcified aortic stenosis, or congenital heart conditions such as ventricular septal defect, atrial septal defect, and hypertrophic cardiomyopathy.

**70. b.** Ampicillin, 2 g IV every 4 hours for 4 to 6 weeks, plus gentamicin, 1 mg/kg IV every 8 hours for 4 to 6 weeks. Treatment of enterococcal endocarditis is complicated because of the high levels of resistance to penicillin, extended-spectrum penicillins, and vancomycin. However, penicillin, ampicillin, or vancomycin in combination with an aminoglycoside causes synergistic bactericidal effect on these organisms. Treatment with an aminoglycoside for the full 4 to 6 weeks at a synergistic dose (1 mg/kg IV every 8 hours) in addition to the penicillin agent or vancomycin is required.

## Suggested Reading

Anderson JL, Adams CD, Antman EM, et al. ACC/AHA 2007 guidelines for the management of patients with unstable angina/non–ST-elevation myocardial infarction: a report of the American College of Cardiology/American Heart Association Task Force on Practice Guidelines (Writing Committee to Revise the 2002 Guidelines for the Management of Patients with Unstable Angina/Non–ST-Elevation Myocardial Infarction): developed in collaboration with the American College of Emergency Physicians, American College of Physicians, Society for Academic Emergency Medicine, Society for Cardiovascular Angiography and Interventions, and Society of Thoracic Surgeons. *J Am Coll Cardiol.* 2007;50:e1–157.

Antman EM, Hand M, Armstrong PW, et al. 2007 focused update of the ACC/AHA 2004 Guidelines for the Management of Patients with ST-Elevation Myocardial Infarction: a report of the American College of Cardiology/American Heart Association Task Force on Practice Guidelines (Writing Group to Review New Evidence and Update the ACC/AHA 2004 Guidelines for the Management of Patients with ST-Elevation Myocardial Infarction). *Circulation.* 2008;117:296–329.

Expert Panel of Detection, Evaluation, and Treatment of High Blood Cholesterol in Adults. Executive summary of the third report of the National Cholesterol Education Program (NCEP) Expert Panel on Detection, Evaluation, and Treatment of High Blood Cholesterol in Adults (Adult Treatment Panel III). *JAMA.* 2001;285:2486–2497.

Hunt SA, Abraham WT, Chin MH, et al. ACC/AHA 2005 guideline update for the diagnosis and management of chronic heart failure in the adult: a report of the American College of Cardiology/American Heart Association Task Force on Practice Guidelines (Writing Committee to Update the 2001 Guidelines for the Evaluation and Management of Heart Failure). American College of Cardiology Web Site. Available at: http://www.acc.org/clinical/guidelines/failure//index.pdf.

The Sixth Report of the National Committee on Detection, Evaluation, and Treatment of High Blood Pressure (JNC-VI). *Arch Intern Med.* 1997;157:2413–2446.

Wilson W, Taubert KA, Gewitz M, et al. Prevention of infective endocarditis: guidelines from the American Heart Association: a guideline from the American Heart Association Rheumatic Fever, Endocarditis, and Kawasaki Disease Committee, Council on Cardiovascular Disease in the Young, and the Council on Clinical Cardiology, Council on Cardiovascular Surgery and Anesthesia, and the Quality of Care and Outcomes Research Interdisciplinary Working Group, published online on April 19, 2007 (DOI: 10.1161/CIRCULATIONAHA.106.183095). Circulation 2007;116:1736—54. Available at http://circ.ahajournals.org/cgi/content/full/116/15/1736

# chapter 6

# Aorta

CRAIG R. ASHER • GIAN M. NOVARO

## QUESTIONS

### Case 1 (Questions 1–3)

A 72-year-old woman is referred to the cardiology clinic for further evaluation and management of aortic regurgitation. A review of systems is notable only for recent onset of headaches and myalgia. The patient has no cardiac risk factors, except mild hypertension (HTN), and has not previously undergone any cardiac testing.

#### Physical Examination

BP is 138/78 mm Hg in both arms.

Pulse is 62 bpm and regular.

The funduscopic examination reveals no changes consistent with hypertensive retinopathy. The heart examination is notable for a normal $S_1$ and increased intensity $S_2$ $(A_2)$. There was an $S_4$ gallop; a II/IV diastolic decrescendo murmur, heard best at the right sternal border; and a II/IV early-peaking systolic ejection murmur, heard at the left sternal border. There was no systolic ejection click. The pulses were strong and equal in both the upper and lower extremities.

An ECG reveals sinus rhythm with nonspecific ST changes.

1. What is the most likely cause of the patient's heart murmur?

   a. a bicuspid aortic valve with aortic regurgitation
   b. degenerative severe aortic valve stenosis and regurgitation
   c. aortic dilation caused by HTN
   d. aortic dilation caused by an aortic aneurysm

2. Subsequently, a TTE is performed. It shows normal LV and RV size and function. The aortic valve anatomy could not be clearly determined. The aorta was dilated at the aortic sinuses to 4.0 cm, the sinotubular junction to 4.4 cm, and the ascending aorta to 4.5 cm. There was moderate effacement of the sinotubular junction. The peak and mean aortic gradients were 22/13 mm Hg, and there was grade 2+ aortic regurgitation. A small circumferential pericardial effusion was also detected. Laboratory tests revealed an erythrocyte sedimentation rate of 74. What additional test would be most helpful in determining the etiology of the patient's aortic regurgitation?

   a. cardiac catheterization
   b. MRI of the aorta and magnetic resonance angiography (MRA) of the great vessels
   c. CT scan of the aorta
   d. CXR

3. MRI and MRA were performed. They showed enlargement of the aorta, as noted on the TTE, with uniform thickening of the aortic walls. There was sparing of the upper extremity branch vessels. What is the most likely diagnosis for the patient's aortic regurgitation and aortic enlargement?

   **a.** Takayasu's arteritis
   **b.** annuloaortic ectasia
   **c.** hypertensive heart disease
   **d.** giant cell arteritis

## Case 2 (Questions 4 and 5)

An 18-year-old woman presents for her annual physical examination. She had a brother with Marfan syndrome who was 24 years old when he died suddenly. She also has a history of steroid-dependent asthma.

### Physical Examination

The patient is 5 ft 7 in tall and 150 lb.
Her arm-span—to—height ratio is greater than 1.05.
The head and neck examination is notable for a high-arched palate, and a slit-lamp examination shows ectopia lentis. The musculoskeletal examination is notable for a pectus carinatum and a positive wrist and thumb sign. The cardiac examination is notable for a mitral valve click and a soft murmur of mitral regurgitation.

4. What additional testing is needed to determine whether this woman has Marfan syndrome?

   **a.** a TTE
   **b.** an ECG
   **c.** a chest CT of the aorta
   **d.** no additional testing

5. A TTE is performed that shows mitral valve prolapse with grade 1+ mitral regurgitation. The aortic sinuses are dilated at 5.5 cm, with moderate effacement of the sinotubular junction. The ascending aorta is measured at 3.6 cm. There is no aortic regurgitation. See Figure 6–1 for the TEE from a patient with a similar finding. What is the most appropriate recommendation to be made to this patient after the TTE?

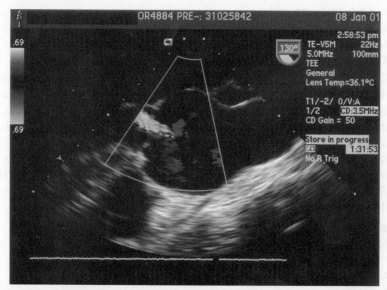

**FIGURE 6–1**    TEE. Long-axis view in a patient with Marfan syndrome, showing dilation of the aortic sinuses, effacement of the sinotubular junction, and normal ascending aortic dimension. Mild aortic regurgitation is also seen because of annular dilation.

a. repeat the TTE in 6 months
b. initiate a beta-blocker
c. no treatment; avoid strenuous exertion or contact sports
d. elective aortic replacement surgery

## Case 3 (Questions 6–8)

A 67-year-old man with long-standing HTN presents to the emergency room (ER) with sudden-onset chest pain, described as ripping in quality, which has subsided since its onset. He underwent a cardiac catheterization 1 year previously because of an abnormal treadmill ECG that showed only a 50% lesion in the mid–left anterior descending coronary artery. His medications include aspirin, gemfibrozil, and nifedipine. Other medical problems include $O_2$-dependent chronic obstructive pulmonary disease.

### Physical Examination

He appears diaphoretic. BP is 106/54 mm Hg in the right arm and 72/35 mm Hg in the left arm. The jugular venous pressure is elevated. The heart sounds are muffled, and there is no audible systolic or diastolic murmur. The pulses are absent in the left arm.

The ECG on presentation shows ST elevation in the inferior leads and very low voltage. The CXR shows cardiomegaly, with a globular-shaped heart and interstitial edema.

6. What is the first medication that should be given to this patient?

   a. thrombolytic therapy
   b. sodium nitroprusside
   c. IV ganglionic blocking agent
   d. none of the above

7. Which of the following is the first diagnostic test that should be performed?

   a. cardiac enzymes
   b. MRI of the aorta
   c. CT of the chest
   d. TTE or TEE
   e. cardiac catheterization

8. A TTE was performed, confirming a pericardial effusion and signs of cardiac tamponade. What interventions should be performed next for the management of this patient?

   a. cardiac catheterization
   b. emergent aortic surgery
   c. Swan-Ganz catheterization
   d. pericardiocentesis

9. A 36-year-old man with a known bicuspid aortic valve develops sudden onset of headache, mental status changes, and unequal pupils. He is rushed to an ER, and a CT scan is done that shows an intracerebral bleed. Except for a known history of HTN, he has no known medical problems and no history of drug abuse. A visit to his physician's office 1 week before this event revealed a BP of 120/75 mm Hg on metoprolol and ramipril and a negative review of systems. What is the most likely reason for the patient's intracerebral bleed?

   a. hypertensive crisis
   b. aortic dissection
   c. cerebral aneurysm rupture
   d. mycotic aneurysm associated with endocarditis

## Case 4 (Questions 10 and 11)

A 74-year-old man presents to the ER with lower back pain ongoing for 3 hours. The pain is described as sharp, occurring at rest. He has no associated symptoms of shortness of breath, chest pain, or presyncope. His past medical history is notable for a coronary artery bypass graft (CABG) 5 years ago, HTN, and continued tobacco use. At the time of his CABG, he was noted to have a 4.5-cm ascending aortic aneurysm. His medications include aspirin, an ACE inhibitor, and a beta-blocker.

### Physical Examination

BP is 180/110 mm Hg.

Pulse rate is 90 bpm.

The lung and cardiac examinations are unremarkable, and no cardiac murmur is heard. The abdomen is mildly tender. No bruit is audible. The pulses are equal but diminished in the lower extremities.

The ECG shows sinus rhythm with nonspecific ST changes and an old inferior MI. A panel of laboratory tests, including liver function tests, amylase, and lipase, is normal.

10. What is the most appropriate diagnostic procedure to perform next?

    a. TTE
    b. TEE
    c. CT of the chest and abdomen
    d. aortography

11. The patient has presented to a community hospital that has access to a cardiac catheterization laboratory but not immediate access to a CT scan or TEE. Therefore, a cardiac catheterization and aortography are performed. The catheterization shows patent grafts and adequate filling of the distal native coronaries. Aortography demonstrates an ascending aortic aneurysm of 4.8 cm and a descending aortic aneurysm of 5.3 cm but no evidence of dissection. The patient continues to have ongoing pain despite high doses of beta-blockers and sodium nitroprusside as well as opioid analgesics. What is most appropriate next decision for management?

    a. discharge, with no further interventions or testing required
    b. CT of the abdomen in the morning
    c. intensifying the medical regimen of beta-blockers and afterload reduction
    d. transfer the patient to a nearby facility for CT of the aorta, including the chest and abdomen

12. A 62-year-old man presents for a routine annual examination. He has a history of HTN that is managed with nifedipine. He is active and has no symptoms. BP is 162/88 mm Hg in both arms. Pulse rate is 70 bpm. The heart and lung examination is unremarkable. His abdominal examination reveals a pulsatile mass. An ECG shows sinus rhythm and a complete RBBB. An abdominal ultrasound finds an infrarenal abdominal aortic aneurysm of 3.9 cm. What is the most appropriate management step?

    a. initiate a beta-blocker and repeat ultrasound in 6 months
    b. refer for abdominal aortic aneurysm surgery
    c. refer for aortic stenting
    d. repeat ultrasound in 2 years

## Case 5 (Questions 13–15)

A 76-year-old man presents to the ER with severe sharp chest pain that began 2 hours previously. He has a history of HTN; had CABG 2 years ago, after an MI; and continues to smoke. The CABG was performed off-pump because of severe atheroma of the ascending aorta seen by intraoperative TEE. The patient's pain has not subsided with the initiation of IV heparin, nitroglycerin, and beta-blockers. The pain is different in character from the pain before his MI.

### Physical Examination

BP is 160/94 mm Hg.
Pulse is 76 bpm.
The lung and heart sounds are normal. The pulses are diminished in the lower extremities.
The ECG shows a chronic left anterior hemiblock and RBBB. The initial set of cardiac enzymes is negative.

**13.** What diagnostic test is *least* appropriate to perform next?

  **a.** cardiac catheterization
  **b.** aortogram
  **c.** TEE
  **d.** MRI

**14.** Despite the severe atheroma in the aorta, the physician taking care of the patient is not convinced that he does not have an acute coronary syndrome and so performs a cardiac catheterization. It shows that the grafts are patent, and there is no culprit lesion of the native vessels. He then decides to perform aortography, and a focal outpouching is seen in the aortic wall in the proximal ascending aorta at the site of a large atheroma (Fig. 6–2). Contrast dye collects slowly in this region. The patient's chest pain is intensifying. What is the most appropriate management step to take next?

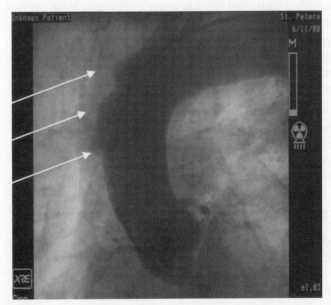

**FIGURE 6–2**  (Image compliments of Dr. Wael Jaber, Cleveland Clinic Foundation.)

  **a.** medical management with beta-blockers and afterload reduction only
  **b.** medical management and transfer to the operating room immediately; do intraoperative TEE
  **c.** medical management and obtain an MR or CT in the morning
  **d.** medical management and obtain a TEE in the morning

**15.** What is the most likely diagnosis?

    **a.** aortic dissection

    **b.** aortic aneurysm

    **c.** intramural hematoma

    **d.** penetrating aortic ulcer

## Case 6 (Questions 16–18)

A 60-year-old European woman presents to her physician with new-onset claudication in her left leg, dizziness, headache, and a cold right hand. She has no chest pain or shortness of breath. There is no significant past medical history. She does not smoke and has no cardiac risk factors.

### Physical Examination

BP is 170/82 mm Hg in the left arm and 140/68 mm Hg in the right arm.
Lung sounds are clear. The cardiac examination is notable for a normal $S_1$ and $S_2$ and II/IV diastolic decrescendo murmur at the left sternal border. The right brachial pulse is diminished. A bruit is heard over the left carotid artery and right subclavian artery. The lower extremity pulses are diminished.

**16.** What is the best test for diagnosing the patient's condition?

    **a.** TEE

    **b.** carotid duplex ultrasound

    **c.** MRI of the head and carotid vessels

    **d.** angiography

**17.** Angiography is performed and shows a long segment of narrowing involving the right subclavian and left common carotid artery. There is also a segment of distal descending aortic and left iliac artery obstruction. What medical therapy is *least* appropriate?

    **a.** warfarin

    **b.** methotrexate or cyclophosphamide

    **c.** corticosteroids

    **d.** antihypertensive agents

**18.** What is the most likely diagnosis?

    **a.** Behçet's disease

    **b.** relapsing polychondritis

    **c.** giant cell arteritis

    **d.** Takayasu's arteritis

## Case 7 (Questions 19 and 20)

A 78-year-old man is seen by his primary care physician for a routine physical examination. He has a history of HTN and underwent CABG 7 years before. His cholesterol levels remain >200, despite lipid-lowering agents. His medications include aspirin, gemfibrozil, atenolol, captopril, and hydralazine.

### Physical Examination

BP is 188/94 mm Hg in the left arm.
The clinician performs a maneuver whereby the cuff is inflated to obliterate the brachial and radial pulse and palpates a rigid, noncompressible radial artery on the same side.

**19.** What is the most likely explanation for this finding?

    **a.** peripheral embolism

    **b.** noncompliant peripheral vessels

c. brachial artery dissection with collateral circulation
d. brachial artery occlusion with collateral circulation

**20.** What is the significance of this finding?

a. overestimation of the intra-arterial BP
b. underestimation of the intra-arterial BP
c. no difference between the cuff and intra-arterial BP

## Case 8 (Questions 21 and 22)

A 45-year-old man is referred to a tertiary facility for elective mitral valve repair with severe MR. The referring TTE notes a possible cleft mitral valve. A repeat TTE is performed, and the cardiologist describes the anatomy as a congenitally corrected transposition of the great arteries.

**21.** Which of the following findings is *not* consistent with this anatomy?

a. situs solitus
b. AV discordance
c. AV concordance
d. ventriculoarterial discordance

**22.** What is the most likely explanation for the patient's MR?

a. a cleft mitral valve
b. Ebstein's anomaly of the tricuspid valve associated with the left-sided RV
c. Ebstein's anomaly of the mitral valve associated with the left-sided RV
d. mitral valve prolapse

## Case 9 (Questions 23 and 24)

A 30-year-old man is referred to a cardiology clinic for evaluation of a heart murmur. He had an uneventful childhood, except that on two separate occasions he fractured his arm and leg. He has also developed hearing loss over the past year. He has no shortness of breath or chest pain.

### Physical Examination

He is of normal stature. The vital signs are normal. The arm–span–height ratio is normal.
There is no pectus deformity. There is no scoliosis. There is no wrist sign.
The cardiac examination is notable for a decreased $S_1$ and normal $S_2$ with a III/IV diastolic decrescendo murmur. There are no gallops. The pulses are normal, and the extremities are hypermobile. There is no abnormality of the skin.
A TTE shows a dilated aortic root of 4.7 cm and severe aortic regurgitation with a dilated LV.

**23.** What other finding on the physical examination is most consistent with the patient's diagnosis?

a. ectopia lentis
b. blue sclerae
c. high-arched palate
d. thumb sign

**24.** What is the most likely diagnosis for this patient?

a. Ehlers-Danlos syndrome
b. Marfan syndrome
c. osteogenesis imperfecta
d. homocystinuria

## Case 10 (Questions 25–27)

A 65-year-old man presents to the ER with severe, tearing chest pain that started while he was shoveling snow. He has a history of HTN that is poorly regulated. He has a history of coronary disease, with a stent to the left anterior descending coronary artery 4 months ago.

### Physical Examination

BP is 190/110 mm Hg.
Pulse is 90 bpm.
The cardiac examination is notable for a normal $S_1$ and $S_2$, with an $S_4$ gallop and II/IV systolic ejection murmur at the left sternal border.
An ECG shows sinus rhythm and no ST changes. An initial set of cardiac enzymes is normal.

25. What is the most appropriate diagnostic test?
    a. cardiac catheterization
    b. TTE
    c. aortogram
    d. CT angiography of the aorta

26. A cardiologist in the ER seeing another patient offers to perform a TEE at the bedside. He sees an ascending aortic aneurysm measuring 6.2 cm, with a continuous crescentic area of wall thickening extending from the right coronary artery to the innominate artery. There are areas of echolucency within the walls. There is no intimal flap. There is intimal calcium that is displaced. What is the most appropriate management?
    a. medical therapy with beta-blockers and nitroprusside
    b. urgent aortic replacement surgery
    c. medical therapy with beta-blockers and nitroprusside and repeat TEE or CT in 24 hours
    d. MRI to confirm findings and assess branch vessels

27. Which of the following is a *false* statement about the aortic disease of this patient?
    a. The prognosis is similar to an aortic dissection with an intimal tear.
    b. Controversy exists regarding the management of patients with this condition occurring after iatrogenic procedures.
    c. Surgery is only indicated when a concomitant intimal tear is seen.
    d. Aortography may miss the diagnosis.

## Case 11 (Questions 28–30)

A 44-year-old man is admitted to the hospital because of a left hemisphere stroke with right arm and leg weakness. He has no known history of HTN or smoking, although his total cholesterol level is 314.

### Physical Examination

The ECG shows sinus rhythm. A carotid duplex ultrasound shows less than 20% obstruction bilaterally. A head CT demonstrates an area of left cortical echogenicity consistent with a middle cerebral artery territory embolism.

28. Which test is most likely to elucidate the etiology of the patient's stroke?
    a. TTE with contrast injection
    b. telemetry monitoring
    c. MRI/MRA
    d. TEE

29. The patient is maintained on telemetry, and sinus rhythm without atrial arrhythmias is present. A TTE shows normal LV function and no valvular abnormalities. A contrast study is negative for right-to-left shunt. A TEE shows extensive aortic arch atheroma. Which characteristic is *least* consistent with aortic atheroma resulting in the patient's stroke?

    a. size $\geq 4$ mm
    b. calcification of atheroma
    c. mobility of the atheroma
    d. absence of calcification of the atheroma

30. Which statement is *true* regarding performing CABG in a similar patient with aortic arch atheroma and focal areas of atheroma in the ascending aorta?

    a. Palpation of the aorta by the surgeon for calcified plaque correlates with findings of atheroma by TEE.
    b. Alternative sites of clamping or cannulation may reduce stroke risk.
    c. Aortic arch endarterectomy is recommended.
    d. Replacement of the ascending aorta is recommended because of increased likelihood of stroke.

## Case 12 (Questions 31 and 32)

A 24-year-old Asian man presents to his primary care doctor with the report of claudication and shortness of breath. He was diagnosed with a patent ductus arteriosus as a child but has had infrequent follow-up visits, because he has felt well until the past year.

### Physical Examination

He is normal in stature.
BP is 102/64 mm Hg in the right arm.
Pulse is 80 bpm.
There is no central cyanosis. Lung sounds are clear. The cardiac examination is notable for a normal $S_1$ and loud $S_2$ ($P_2$). The feet bilaterally are cyanotic.

31. Which additional physical examination finding is *not* consistent with the patient's abnormality?

    a. pink hands
    b. decreased BP in the lower extremities
    c. a diastolic heart murmur
    d. an RV heave

32. Which diagnosis best describes the patient's condition?

    a. Eisenmenger's physiology
    b. coarctation of the aorta
    c. patent ductus arteriosus without Eisenmenger's physiology
    d. Takayasu's arteritis

## Case 13 (Questions 33 and 34)

A 28-year-old man is referred to a cardiologist for exertional dyspnea and a cardiac murmur. As a child, he was evaluated by a pediatrician for congenital heart disease because of mild mental retardation. No specific diagnosis was made.

### Physical Examination

His vital signs are normal. The cardiac examination is notable for a III/IV systolic ejection murmur radiating to the neck. The left brachial pulse is diminished relative to the right brachial pulse.

NOTES

33. What diagnosis best explains the patient's disorder?
    a. patent ductus arteriosus
    b. coarctation of the aorta
    c. supravalvular pulmonary stenosis
    d. Williams syndrome

34. What additional finding on physical examination is *not* consistent with the patient's diagnosis?
    a. decreased BP in the left arm relative to the right arm
    b. decreased ($A_2$) component of $S_2$
    c. small chin and wide-spaced eyes

35. What abnormal protein is produced because of the genetic defect associated with Marfan syndrome?
    a. procollagen
    b. elastin
    c. fibrillin

36. A patient is rushed to the ER after a motor vehicle accident between two cars. The CXR shows widening of the mediastinum. What cardiac or aortic structure is *least* likely to be injured?
    a. aortic isthmus
    b. aortic cusp tear with aortic regurgitation
    c. right atrial rupture
    d. LV rupture

## Case 14 (Questions 37–39)

A 30-year-old man with a history of congenital heart disease is referred to you because of symptoms of dysphagia and an abnormal CXR. As a child he was told that his CXR was abnormal because of an "aortic anomaly" and that it was benign. He has a brother that has tetralogy of Fallot and has a similar finding on CXR. He was reassured that he does not have tetralogy of Fallot.

### Physical Examination

The vital signs are normal.

The cardiac examination is notable for normal intensity $S_1$ and $S_2$ heart sounds. There is an ejection click heard in the right upper sternal border (RUSB) though no murmur is audible. The upper and lower extremity pulses are equal.

37. The CXR shows what abnormality?
    a. bovine aortic arch
    b. cervical aortic arch
    c. right aortic arch
    d. aberrant right subclavian artery

38. The aortic anomaly seen in question 37 is not associated with which congenital heart disease?
    a. tetralogy of Fallot
    b. truncus arteriosus
    c. primum ASD
    d. transposition of the great vessels

39. The patient's dysphagia is likely caused by what abnormality associated with his aortic anomaly?
    a. aberrant left subclavian artery and diverticulum of Kommerell
    b. coarctation of the aorta
    c. isolated left subclavian artery
    d. interrupted aortic arch

## Case 15 (Question 40)

A 40-year-old man presents for follow-up after undergoing a surgical coarctation repair at age 9. He has no records and is uncertain of the type of repair. He has not had any testing done in the past 10 years. He has used antibiotic prophylaxis for dental procedures. He takes no other medications. He feels well, is active, and has no complaints.

### Physical Examination

BP right arm: 138/72; BP left arm: 126/70; P: 80 regular.

The heart sounds are normal intensity. There is an aortic ejection click in the RUSB. There is brief/short duration ejection murmur in the RUSB. There is no diastolic murmur. The upper and lower extremity pulses are equal. There is no radial femoral delay.

**40.** Which testing is least useful for this patient?

**a.** echocardiogram
**b.** CTA of the aorta
**c.** exercise stress echocardiogram
**d.** Holter monitor

## Case 16 (Questions 41 and 42)

A 34-year-old man has a routine CXR done prior to an elective inguinal hernia repair. He has no significant past medical history. He takes no medications. He has no cardiovascular-related symptoms. The vital signs are normal and the physical examination is unremarkable. The CXR is reviewed and shows a normal heart contour. There is a narrowing of the descending thoracic aorta. There is no "3-sign" or rib-notching.

**41.** What test would be most appropriate to determine if an aortic coarctation is present?

**a.** echocardiogram
**b.** aortogram with pull-back to determine gradient
**c.** MRI/MRA of the thoracic aorta
**d.** CTA of the thoracic aorta

**42.** What is the most likely diagnosis?

**a.** severe coarctation with significant collaterals
**b.** mild coarctation
**c.** aortic diverticulum
**d.** pseudo-coarctation

## Case 17 (Questions 43 and 44)

A 38-year-old man is referred for a cardiac surgical evaluation for bicuspid aortic regurgitation. He has known of an aortic valve disorder for 10 years. He is fully active with no limitations. He plays tennis on a regular basis. Vital signs are notable for a BP 120/40 mm Hg and a pulse of 68 bpm. A stress echocardiogram is performed and shows a bicuspid aortic valve with right-left fusion. There is holodiastolic flow reversal in the descending aorta. The aortic root measures 4.0 cm and the proximal ascending aorta is 3.9 cm with no ST junction effacement. The LV cavity dimensions are as follows: LVIDd 5.8 cm; LVIDs 3.9 cm. The LVEF is calculated at 58%. There is a reduction in LV cavity size with exercise and he performs 13 METs without symptoms.

NOTES

**43.** What is the most appropriate surgical recommendation?

    **a.** elective AVR and ascending aortic grafting

    **b.** elective AVR without ascending aortic grafting

    **c.** medical therapy/observation and add a beta-blocker

    **d.** AV repair and ascending aortic grafting

    **e.** observation only

**44.** Six months later the patient has developed dyspnea with moderate exertion and a significant reduction in exercise tolerance. A repeat echocardiogram shows similar LV cavity dimensions and LVEF calculated at 57%. The aortic root dimension is now 4.5 cm and the proximal ascending aorta is 3.9 cm. What is the appropriate recommendation at this time?

    **a.** AVR only

    **b.** composite AVR/aortic root/ascending aortic grafting (Bentall procedure)

    **c.** AVR and supra-coronary ascending aortic graft (root sparing procedure)

    **d.** stress echocardiogram to confirm change in exercise tolerance

## Case 18 (Questions 45 and 46)

A 66-year-old man is seen by his internist for an annual evaluation. Past medical history is notable for HTN and tobacco use. His BP is 136/80 mm Hg on monotherapy. His examination is unremarkable including an abdominal examination. He has a friend who was detected to have an AAA on routine screening and asks his physician whether it is indicated for him to be screened.

**45.** Which of the following recommendations regarding AAA screening is incorrect?

    **a.** Screening is indicated in males ≥65 years of age with a prior history of smoking.

    **b.** Screening is indicated in males ≥40 years of age with a family history of an aortic aneurysm.

    **c.** Screening for AAA in males ≥65 years of age has been shown in a randomized study to reduce aneurysm-related deaths compared to unscreened males of similar age.

    **d.** Screening abdominal ultrasound identifies an aortic aneurysm as a diameter of ≥3.0 cm.

**46.** A screening abdominal ultrasound shows an infrarenal AAA of 6.2 cm. The patient is advised repair though wishes to consider the option of a percutaneous aortic endovascular stent graft rather than an open repair. Which of the following statements regarding a comparison of open surgery for AAA versus percutaneous aortic endovascular stent grafting is incorrect?

    **a.** Greater than 30% of patients are not anatomically suitable for endovascular repair.

    **b.** Endovascular leaks occur in 30% of patients undergoing endovascular repair.

    **c.** The frequency of repeat aortic procedures is greater for endovascular repair compared to open surgery.

    **d.** Endovascular aortic repair is generally recommended for elderly patients and those with higher operative mortality for open repair.

## Case 19 (Questions 47 and 48)

A 38-year-old female is admitted to the internal medicine service for chest pain. She has experienced sharp chest pain unrelated to exertion and dyspnea for 2 days. Her family history is unknown since she was adopted. Past medical history is not well defined but notable for an uncharacterized connective tissue disorder. Admission ECG and cardiac enzymes are negative. She is unable to exercise because of her symptoms and therefore is sent for an adenosine cardiolite stress test. The test shows mild anteroseptal ischemia with no ECG changes. The cardiology service is consulted for a cardiac catheterization. On exam she is thin and in mild distress. Vital signs are stable. The cardiac examination reveals a normal $S_1$ and $S_2$ with a soft diastolic decrescendo murmur at the right sternal border. The general exam and skin exam are notable for joint hypermobility, hyperextensible skin, and bruises. There are no findings suggestive of Marfan syndrome.

**47.** What do you recommend?

    **a.** cardiac catheterization for coronary angiography

    **b.** cardiac catheterization for coronary angiography and an aortogram

    **c.** CT for PE protocol

    **d.** CT for "triple rule out" protocol

**48.** What should be done to better characterize the patient's connective tissue disorder?

    **a.** diagnosis based on clinical criteria

    **b.** laboratory markers

    **c.** gene testing

    **d.** skin biopsy

**49.** A 24-year-old man is referred to the cardiology clinic for consultation regarding an aortic aneurysm. He has a family history of ascending aortic aneurysms and therefore underwent an echocardiogram where an ascending aortic aneurysm of 4.6 cm was noted. There were widely set eyes. An examination of the oropharynx is performed (Fig. 6–3). There are no findings consistent with Marfan syndrome. The skin examination is normal. An ESR is normal. What is the diagnosis?

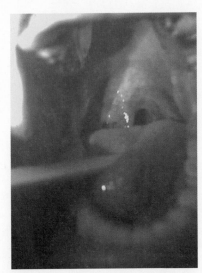

**FIGURE 6–3** Oropharynx image demonstrating a bifid uvula as seen in a patient with Loeys-Dietz syndrome.

    **a.** Cogan's syndrome

    **b.** Loeys-Dietz

    **c.** Ormond's disease

    **d.** Behçet's disease

**50.** An 80-year-old man with long-standing HTN and a dilated ascending aorta of 4.3 cm by echocardiography undergoes a routine surveillance CT of the aorta. He is asymptomatic and his BP is well controlled. CT aortography shows a dilated ascending aorta and arch with a maximal diameter of 4.4 cm. The descending thoracic aorta measures 6.0 cm and there is a 4-cm long dissection flap. He is admitted to the hospital despite his lack of symptoms. Which of the following statements is not accurate?

**NOTES**

a. The risk of paraplegia for descending aortic graft repair is ~5%.
b. The risk of death for descending aortic graft repair is ~5% to 15%.
c. The risk of aortic complications if the patient is treated medically is related to the patency of the false lumen.
d. An "elephant trunk" procedure should be considered for this patient.
e. Descending aortic aneurysms are generally repaired when the diameter is in the range of 6.0 to 6.5 cm.

# ANSWERS

1. **d.** Aortic dilation caused by aortic aneurysm. The clinical history, examination, and ECG do not suggest long-standing HTN as a contributing factor to valvular heart disease. There is no systolic ejection click to suggest a bicuspid valve, and the patient is older than most patients who present with aortic stenosis caused by a bicuspid valve. The murmur is not consistent with severe aortic stenosis because it is early peaking and $S_2$ ($A_2$) is audible. Therefore, the most likely etiology of the heart murmur is aortic dilation with associated aortic regurgitation. This type of murmur associated with an abnormality of the aorta is often heard along the right sternal border.

2. **b.** MRI of the aorta and MRA of the great vessels. The presence of aortic dilation, sinotubular effacement, a pericardial effusion, and an elevated erythrocyte sedimentation rate suggests an inflammatory etiology for aortic dilation. Aortic aneurysms can be classified as being a result of (a) arteriosclerosis, (b) connective tissue disorders, (c) trauma, (d) infectious diseases, (e) inflammatory diseases or "aortitis," and (f) annuloaortic ectasia. Inflammatory aortitis includes numerous systemic diseases that may involve the aorta, including systemic lupus erythematosus, rheumatoid and psoriatic arthritis, systemic sclerosis, relapsing polychondritis, the rheumatoid factor–negative spondyloarthropathies, and other primarily vascular disorders, such as Takayasu's and giant cell arteritis. MR of the aorta may distinguish characteristic thickening and tissue characteristics that are consistent with inflammatory aortitis.

3. **d.** Giant cell arteritis. The presence of systemic symptoms, such as headaches and myalgia, as well as pericardial effusion and an elevated sedimentation rate, is consistent with giant cell arteritis as the cause of the aortic aneurysm and secondary aortic regurgitation. Headaches suggest the associated problem of temporal arteritis. The disease affects women twice as often as it does men and is most commonly seen after age 55 years. The MRI showed sparing of the branch vessels and uniform thickening of the walls that is consistent with giant cell arteritis and not Takayasu's arteritis. Takayasu's arteritis generally involves younger patients with pulse differences and signs of arterial insufficiency. The MRI typically shows stenosis of branch vessels of the upper or lower extremity. Annuloaortic ectasia is a primary disease of the aorta that morphologically looks similar to Marfan syndrome and pathologically involves cystic medial necrosis, as in Marfan syndrome. However, there are no other noncardiovascular systems involved with annuloaortic ectasia.

4. **d.** No additional testing. The current diagnostic criteria revised by Gent require major criteria in one organ system and minor criteria in a different organ system for diagnosis of Marfan syndrome when a family history of the disease is present. If no family history is present, two major criteria are required in separate organ systems and one minor criterion in a third organ system. Organ involvement affects the skeletal, ocular, cardiovascular, pulmonary, neurologic, and dermatologic systems. The patient had a major criterion of ectopia lentis and multiple musculoskeletal criteria, including pectus carinatum, an arm-span–to–height ratio of $>1.05$, wrist and thumb sign, and high-arched palate. She also has mitral valve prolapse, which is a minor criterion.

5. **d.** Elective aortic replacement surgery. The most widely cited study of beta-blockade and Marfan syndrome was performed by Shores et al. This study was an open-label study of adult patients with mild or moderate aortic dilatation and Marfan syndrome who were randomized to propanolol or no treatment. Patients with asthma were excluded. The follow-up was near 10 years. Patients randomized to propanolol had less aortic dilatation and aortic complications, although the numbers were small for the latter end point. The timing of surgery

invasive procedure will add further risk of dissection, tamponade, or rupture. Therefore, most centers carefully select those patients who undergo coronary angiography, including those with known coronary disease, recent unstable coronary symptoms, and new regional wall-motion abnormalities. One study comparing outcomes of patients undergoing surgery for aortic dissection found that those not undergoing cardiac catheterization had similar mortality to those undergoing this procedure.

9. **c.** Cerebral aneurysm rupture. The history of HTN requiring therapy in a young man with a bicuspid valve suggests the possibility of an aortic coarctation. Given his recent well-being and well-controlled BP, aortic dissection, hypertensive crisis, and endocarditis are unlikely. A known association between aortic coarctation and cerebral aneurysms has been described. Screening for this abnormality with MRI or MRA is often performed for patients when any neurologic symptoms are present or before major surgery, such as cardiac surgery.

10. **c.** CT of the chest and abdomen. The patient's history is most suggestive of a distal aortic dissection. He has a known thoracic aortic aneurysm, atherosclerosis, and presents hypertensive, with back pain and diminished pulses. Although TEE may be accurate for diagnosis of aortic dissection above the diaphragm, CT scanning may extend imaging to the entire aorta, including the abdominal aorta, and provide information regarding the involvement of branch vessels. Therefore, if both tests were available with equal rapidity and expertise for interpretation, CT would be preferable. Aortography is invasive and could cause further injury to the aorta, although it could provide useful information along with angiography regarding the patency of the patient's bypass grafts and native circulation.

11. **d.** Transfer the patient to a nearby facility for CT of the aorta, including the chest and abdomen. The patient is experiencing ongoing pain, and the clinical history is still suggestive of an aortic dissection. Although aortography is accurate for diagnosis of an intimal flap with communication with the false lumen, it may not be accurate in detection of an intramural hematoma, because it provides information only about flow within the lumen. CT scanning may reveal a descending thoracic aortic intramural hematoma, and although management is generally medical therapy for distal involvement, the presence of ongoing pain requires diagnosis and could be a reason for surgical consideration. Therefore, immediate transfer and CT imaging should be undertaken.

12. **a.** Initiate a beta-blocker and repeat ultrasound in 6 months. A noninflammatory abdominal aortic aneurysm of <4 cm has a 0% to 2% risk of rupture over 2 years. Therefore, surgery or stenting is usually performed for asymptomatic patients when the size is larger than 5 cm, although consideration is given to surgery for high risk aneurysms or for women at smaller sizes. To determine the stability of an aortic aneurysm once it is detected, a follow-up ultrasound is usually performed in 6 months. The rate of change is also considered as a strong indicator of the risk of rupture with a growth rate of >0.5 cm/year considered to be rapid progression. Beta-blockers have been shown to delay the rate of aneurysm enlargement and would be indicated for this patient with HTN.

13. **a.** Cardiac catheterization is the least appropriate. The character of the pain that is different from a prior MI, the lack of relief with antianginal therapy, and the absence of ECG changes or positive enzymes suggest that an acute coronary syndrome is not the cause of the patient's discomfort. Other considerations include an aortic dissection. Less invasive imaging modalities are preferred to make this diagnosis. At most institutions, a TEE can be done with less time delay and with equal accuracy to an MRI.

14. **b.** Medical management and transfer to the operating room immediately; do intraoperative TEE. The finding on the aortogram is highly suggestive of a pseudoaneurysm of the aortic wall caused by inward rupture of atheroma into the aortic wall. This finding is an indication for immediate surgical correction

because of the potential for aortic rupture. Further confirmation of the diagnosis is not required. Two views of the TEE in this patient are shown in Figure 6–6, an aortogram in a patient with multiple penetrating aortic ulcers, seen as outpouching of the anterior surface of the ascending aortic wall. The arrows show three separate ulcers in the ascending aorta and in the aortic arch.

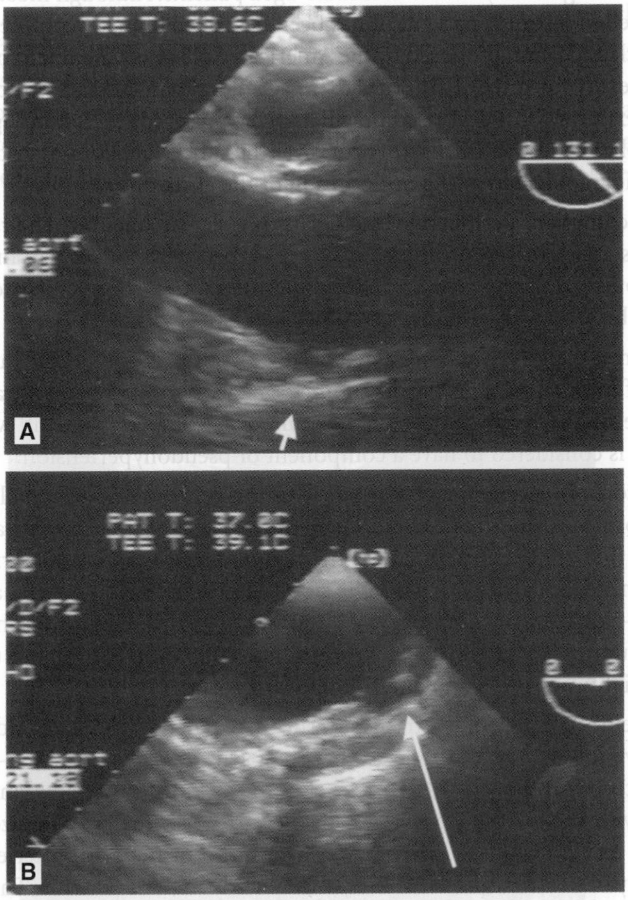

**FIGURE 6–6**  TEE (two views at different levels) in the same patient as in Figure 2. The images show extensive calcific aortic atheroma and two penetrating aortic ulcers. **A:** The arrow points to an ulcer in the ascending aorta. **B:** The arrow points to a second ulcer in the aortic arch. (Images compliments of Dr. Wael Jaber, Cleveland Clinic Foundation.)

**15. d.** Penetrating aortic ulcer. Aortic dissections can be broadly categorized into typical and variant forms. Svennson proposed a classification description as follows: (a) classic dissection or dual lumens, (b) intramural hematoma, (c) limited dissection, (d) penetrating aortic ulcer, and (e) iatrogenic or traumatic dissection. A penetrating aortic ulcer occurs when aortic atheroma ruptures into the aortic media through the internal elastic lamina. Subsequently, an aneurysm, pseudoaneurysm, localized dissection, hematoma, or aortic rupture may develop. Penetrating ulcers can be diagnosed by aortography, CT, MRI, or TEE. Typical findings include a focal outpouching and ulcer crater in the region of severe, calcified atheroma. A limited or a dissection flap may also be present. Localized flow can be seen by contrast opacification or color or pulsed Doppler. The presence of ongoing pain and the possibility of a pseudoaneurysm would be a definite indication for surgery in this patient.

**16. d.** Angiography. The patient presents with pulse deficits, bruits, or arterial insufficiency in multiple distributions, including the upper and lower extremity, suggesting a systemic disease. Angiography or aortography would most directly define the site and extent of arterial disease. The appearance of the lesions may also help with determining the etiology of the vascular disease (i.e., atherosclerotic vs. vasculitic).

**28. d.** TEE. With the absence of significant carotid artery disease and the location of the stroke in the middle cerebral artery territory, an embolic source is likely. Therefore, a TEE would be the more likely technique to reveal the etiology of the patient's event. It is possible that the patient has small-vessel intracranial disease that could be demonstrated by MRA, although, given his age and the absence of significant carotid artery disease, a cardioembolic source seems more likely.

**29. b.** Calcification of atheroma is least consistent with aortic atheroma resulting in the patient's stroke. Factors that are most highly associated with embolic risk include mobility, size ≥4 mm, and the absence of calcification. It is speculated that those plaques without calcification are more likely vulnerable plaques that may have superimposed thrombus. Some studies have also shown that ulcerated plaques are more often associated with embolic events.

**30. b.** Alternative sites of cross-clamping and cannulation, such as femoral or axillary arteries, may reduce the risk of stroke. Aortic arch endarterectomy has been found to increase the risk of perioperative stroke and is seldom recommended. Replacement of the ascending aorta in this patient would be unlikely to reduce the risk of stroke because of the presence of severe atheroma in the ascending aorta. Palpation of the aorta by the surgeon is usually not accurate in finding noncalcified atheroma that may be detected by TEE. Figure 6–8 shows aortic atheroma as seen by the TEE.

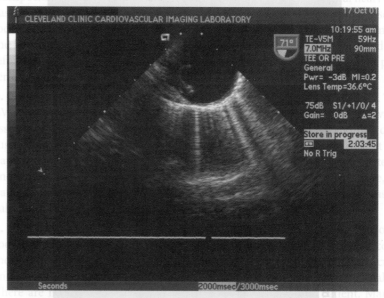

**FIGURE 6–8** TEE of a patient with severe protruding atheroma in the aorta.

**31. b.** Decreased BP in the lower extremities is not consistent with the patient's abnormality. The presence of cyanotic feet in a patient with a patent ductus arteriosus and pink upper extremities suggests the onset of pulmonary HTN and right-to-left shunting. Concomitant findings would include a loud $P_2$ and an RV heave. The classic machinery murmur of a patent ductus arteriosus will not be heard. Only a systolic component will be heard. The blood flow to the lower extremities will be deoxygenated blood, although the BP in the lower extremities would not necessarily be reduced.

**32. a.** Eisenmenger's physiology. The scenario described is most consistent with Eisenmenger's physiology with right-to-left shunting through a patent ductus arteriosus. The patient has severe pulmonary HTN, with pulmonary pressures greater than systemic pressures.

**33. d.** Williams syndrome. The patient has a clinical examination consistent with supravalvular aortic stenosis, with a systolic ejection murmur and associated decreased left brachial pulse. Patent ductus arteriosus and severe coarctation of the aorta more typically have continuous murmurs and would not have the pulse differences. Supravalvular pulmonary stenosis would also not have a pulse difference. The association of supravalvular aortic stenosis and mental retardation is found with Williams syndrome.

**34. b.** Decreased ($A_2$) component of $S_2$ is not consistent with the patient's diagnosis. Because the aortic stenosis is supravalvular, $S_2$ ($A_2$) is preserved and would not be diminished. Other findings consistent with Williams syndrome include a reduced BP or pulse in the left upper extremity caused by preferential deflection of flow to the right side of the body, a small chin and wide-spaced eyes, and hypercalcemia.

**35. c.** Fibrillin. A mutation in the fibrillin-1 protein is the defect associated with the autosomal-dominant inheritance of Marfan syndrome. Defects in procollagen are associated with osteogenesis imperfecta and Ehlers-Danlos syndrome.

**36. d.** LV rupture is least likely to occur. Common sites of injury of the heart and great vessels involve anterior structures, thin-walled structures, and those with some degree of tethering. The aortic isthmus is a common site of rupture, as are the innominate artery and subclavian artery. Cardiac structures most often injured include the right atrium and RV and, less commonly, the left-sided chambers.

**37. c.** The CXR (Fig. 6–9) shows a right aortic arch with the aortic knob on the right side and cardiac structures with normal sidedness. A bovine aortic arch describes the origin of the innominate artery arising from the left carotid artery. A cervical arch refers to a cranial take off of the aortic branch vessels above the sternum. It often presents as a pulsatile mass in the neck or supraclavicular region. It may be associated with compressive symptoms and other vascular anomalies.

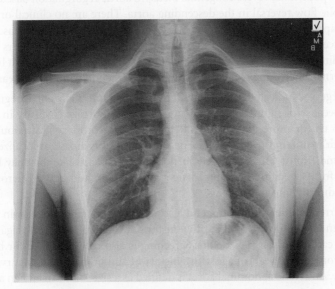

**FIGURE 6–9** CXR demonstrating right aortic arch.

**38. c.** A right aortic arch is associated with tetralogy of Fallot in ~25% of patients. It is also associated with other aortic anomalies, including truncus arteriosus and transposition of the great arteries. It is not associated with primum ASD.

**39. a.** Aortic arch anomalies may result in dysphagia, stridor, or wheezing associated with vascular rings that compress the esophagus or trachea. With a right aortic arch, the left subclavian may arise from the right side and cross posterior to the esophagus and trachea causing a vascular ring and compressive symptoms.

Often aberrant vascular vessels such as the left subclavian arise from aneurysmal segment called a diverticulum of Kommerell.

**40. d.** Arrhythmias are not a concern post-coarctation repair unless significant LVH or LV dysfunction has occurred. An echocardiogram should be performed since approximately 50% to 85% of patients with a coarctation have a bicuspid aortic valve. The patient's murmur is suggestive of a nonstenotic bicuspid aortic valve. Other associated cardiac abnormalities include a perimembranous VSD, PDA, or Shone's complex (multiple left heart obstructive lesions). Although the frequency of follow-up CTA of the aorta is not well defined, it is reasonable to do periodic surveillance of post-coarctation repair to establish the aortic anatomy and type of repair. Late complications include recoarctation, aneurysms in the region of the repair, and broncho-aortic fistulas. The types of coarctation repairs that have been performed surgically include end-end repair, a proximal to distal graft, a patch repair, and a left subclavian to distal aortic anastamosis. The patch repair is most often associated with aneurysms. An exercise stress echocardiogram is particularly useful to look for post-exercise gradients across the coarctation and to assess for exercise-induced HTN. Even in post-coarctation repair, there is an associated aortopathy that is associated with exercise induced HTN.

**41. b.** An aortogram is the best modality to assess both structural and hemodynamic effects of a coarctation. In adults, transthoracic echocardiogram may not adequately visualize the descending thoracic aorta, although gradients can be obtained to assess hemodynamic significance. CT or MRA are excellent modalities to assess the aorta but are not able to adequately determine hemodynamic effects.

**42. d.** In an asymptomatic individual without hypertension and an unremarkable physical examination the incidental finding on a CXR likely represents a pseudo-coarctation. A pseudo-coarctation is a kink in the aorta in the region of the ligamentum arteriosus that has no or minimal gradient.

**43. e.** The patient has severe congenital bicuspid aortic regurgitation based on holo-diastolic flow reversal in the descending aorta. There are no clinical or echocardiographic indications for surgery based on aortic valve or aortic disease. Current practice guidelines for valvular heart disease recommend beta-blockers for aortic root dimensions >4.0 cm only if moderate or severe AR is not present because of concern of increasing regurgitant volume and fraction with slower heart rate.

**44. b.** Surgery is indicated in this patient both for symptomatic aortic regurgitation and because of significant progression in aortic root size (increase in diameter of 0.5 cm or more per year). AVR plus a supra-coronary graft would isolate though maintain the enlarged aortic root that still is at risk of localized dissection and rupture. In specialized aortic centers, patients like this may be candidates for AV repair where the aortic sinuses are excised and a Dacron graft is sewn directly into the annulus.

**45. b.** Current guidelines recommend a screening ultrasound for AAA in men and women 60 to 65 years of age with a history of tobacco use (>100 cigarettes) or other cardiovascular risk factors. Screening is also recommended for both men and women >50 years of age with a history of abdominal aortic aneurysm in the family. An ectatic abdominal aorta is defined as a size ≥2.5 cm and an aneurysm ≥3.0 cm.

**46. b.** Two large trials of predominantly males showed that early elective AAA repair for aneurysms (4.0 to 5.5 cm) resulted in a similar mortality compared to surveillance. Therefore, repair is not generally indicated in asymptomatic patients with AAA <5.5 cm. However, the patient presented despite the lack of symptoms should undergo surgery. All the statements are correct except that endovascular leaks occur in 10% to 20% of cases. These are seen angiographically as persistent leak into the excluded aneurysmal sack and can lead to progressive aneurysm expansion and rupture.

**47. d.** The patient's skin examination has many features suggestive of Ehlers-Danlos syndrome. Since she has a low pretest probability and post-test probability of coronary ischemia, a cardiac catheterization is not advisable especially given the possibility of Ehlers-Danlos syndrome. The vascular type of Ehlers-Danlos syndrome is associated with spontaneous or idiopathic aortic complications including dissection and rupture, and therefore arterial puncture is generally contraindicated. A CTA for "triple rule out" would exclude multiple pathologies found in these patients including aortic aneurysm and dissection, pulmonary artery aneurysm and dissection, pericardial or pleural cysts, and pneumothorax.

**48. d.** Punch biopsy of the skin to obtain fibroblasts for culture is used to determine if there is defective production of type III collagen. If an abnormality is found, a specific gene mutation is then sought.

**49. b.** Loeys-Dietz is a recently described autosomal dominant genetic aortic aneurysm syndrome. It predominantly involves children and young adults with risk of rapid progression to aneurysms, arterial tortuosity and dissection. It is associated with a bifid uvula (shown in Fig. 6–3), cleft palate, and hyperteleorism. Cogan's syndrome is a rare large vessel vasculitis that involves the aorta and is associated with vestibular and ocular abnormalities, including uveitis and keratitis. Ormond's disease is an inflammatory form of aortitis associated with retroperitoneal fibrosis, and Behçet's disease is a medium-sized vessel arteritis associated with oral and genital ulcers and skin lesions.

**50. d.** An "elephant trunk" procedure is a staged procedure for patients requiring surgical repair of the ascending aorta or arch and descending aorta. The ascending aorta/arch are repaired first and a graft is sewn to the descending aorta distal to the left subclavian artery. The graft protrudes into the lumen of the native dilated descending aorta and can be used to clamp and form an anastomosis to the distal graft done through a left thoracotomy. The statements regarding timing of surgery, morbidity, and mortality are correct. A recent study showed that partial thrombosis of the false lumen in patients with a descending aortic dissection was associated with a higher mortality than if the false lumen were patent or completely thrombosed.

## Suggested Reading

Celermajer DS, Cullen S, Deanfield JE, et al. Congenitally corrected transposition and Ebstein's anomaly of the systemic atrioventricular valve: association with aortic arch obstruction. *J Am Coll Cardiol.* 1991;18:1056–1058.

Coady MA, Rizzo JA, Hammond GL, et al. What is the appropriate size criterion for resection of thoracic aortic aneurysms? *J Thorac Cardiovasc Surg.* 1997;113:476–491.

DePaepe A, Devereux RB, Dietz HC, et al. Revised diagnostic criteria for Marfan syndrome. *Am J Med Genet.* 1996;62:417–426.

Hagan PG, Nienaber CA, Isselbacher EM, et al. The International Registry of Acute Aortic Dissection (IRAD): new insights into an old disease. *JAMA.* 2000;283:897–903.

Isselbacher EM. Thoracic and abdominal aortic aneurysms. *Circulation.* 2005;111:816–828.

Isselbacher EM, Cigarroa JE, Eagle KA. Cardiac tamponade complicating proximal aortic dissection: is pericardiocentesis harmful? *Circulation.* 1994;90:2375–2378.

Januzzi JL, Isselbacher EM, Fattori R, et al. Characterizing the young patient with aortic dissection: results from the International Registry of Aortic Dissection (IRAD). *J Am Coll Cardiol.* 2004;43:665–669.

Loeys BL, Schwarze U, Holm T, et al. Aneurysm syndromes caused by mutations in the TGF-beta receptor. *N Engl J Med.* 2006; 355: 788–798.

Maraj R, Rerkpattanapipat P, Jacobs LE, et al. Meta-analysis of 143 reported cases of aortic intramural hematomas. *Am J Cardiol.* 2000;86:664–668.

McCready RA, Vincent AE, Schwartz RW, et al. Atherosclerosis in the young: a virulent disease. *Surgery.* 1984;96:863–869.

Nienaber CA, Von Kodolitsch Y, Nicolas V, et al. The diagnosis of thoracic aortic dissection by noninvasive imaging procedures. *N Engl J Med.* 1993;328:1–9.

**NOTES**

Penn MS, Smedira N, Lytle B, et al. Does coronary angiography before emergency aortic surgery affect in-hospital mortality? *J Am Coll Cardiol.* 2000;35:889–894.

Pretre R, Chilcott M. Blunt trauma to the heart and great vessels. *N Engl J Med.* 1997;336:626–632.

Schermerhorn ML, O'Malley AJ, Jhaveri A, et al. Endovascular vs. open repair of abdominal aortic aneurysms in the medicare population. *N Engl J Med.* 2008;358:464–474.

Shores J, Berger KR, Murphy EA, et al. Progression of aortic dilatation and the benefit of long-term beta-adrenergic blockage in Marfan's syndrome. *N Engl J Med.* 1994;330:1335–1341.

Song JK, Kim HS, Kang DH, et al. Different clinical features of aortic intramural hematoma versus dissection involving the ascending aorta. *J Am Coll Cardiol.* 2001;37:1604–1610.

Svennson LG, Labib SB, Eisenhauer AC, et al. Intimal tear without hematoma: an important variant of aortic dissection that can elude current imaging techniques. *Circulation.* 1999;99:1331–1336.

Tsai TT, Evangelista A, Nienaber CA, et al. Partial thrombosis of the false lumen in patients with acute type B aortic dissection. *N Engl J Med.* 2007;357:349–359.

Tsai TT, Nienaber CA, Eagle KA. Acute aortic syndromes. *Circulation.* 2005;112:3802–3813.

Tunick PA, Kronzon I. Atheromas of the thoracic aorta: clinical and therapeutic update. *J Am Coll Cardiol.* 2000;35:545–554.

Vilacosta I, San Roman JA, Aragoncillo P, et al. Penetrating atherosclerotic aortic ulcer: documentation by transesophageal echocardiography. *J Am Coll Cardiol.* 1998;32:82–89.

# chapter 7

# Peripheral Vascular Disease

DOUGLAS E. JOSEPH • OLUSEGUN OSINBOWALE • MARY C. DOWNING

## QUESTIONS

1. Based on epidemiological studies, which of the following risk factors has the lowest relative risk range for developing lower extremity peripheral arterial disease (PAD)?

   a. smoking
   b. diabetes
   c. hypertension
   d. hypercholesterolemia
   e. hyperhomocysteinemia

2. Among patients diagnosed with PAD, 50 years of age or older, whose presenting symptoms are consistent with critical limb ischemia, a fraction will require amputation while others will be alive with both limbs in 12 months. What is the reported 12-month rate of cardiovascular mortality among these patients?

   a. <5%
   b. 5% to 10%
   c. 15% to 20%
   d. 20% to 30%
   e. 50%

3. A 53-year-old male with a history of obesity, obstructive sleep apnea, hypertension, and hypercholesterolemia presents to the vascular medicine clinic complaining of a nonhealing ulcer on his left ankle present for the past month. His blood pressure is 160/78 mm Hg. His physical exam is remarkable for mild bilateral lower leg edema as well as lipodermatosclerosis and hyperpigmentation around the ankles. A mildly tender, superficial ulceration is observed with an irregular pink base above his medial malleolus. His feet and toes are warm, pink, and have 2-second capillary refill and intact sensation. Laboratory tests on this patient include a random blood sugar of 160 mg/dL, creatinine of 1.1 mg/dL, calcium of 10.4 mg/dL, phosphorus of 4.4 mg/dL, and serum intact parathyroid hormone level of 50 pg/mL. What is the most likely etiology of the ulceration?

   a. diabetes mellitus
   b. chronic venous insufficiency
   c. peripheral arterial disease
   d. calciphylaxis
   e. brown recluse spider bite

4. A 49-year-old female with a 60 pack per year history of smoking presents to the emergency department with complaints of constant, worsening right foot pain and tingling in the toes for several hours. She denies a history of trauma. On exam she is in moderate distress from pain and has a regular cardiac rhythm at a

rate of 104 bpm. Her right lower extremity has a palpable femoral pulse and cool, pale foot with nonpalpable pedal pulses. There is a faint dorsalis pedis arterial signal with continuous-wave handheld Doppler evaluation. Strength is intact in the foot and toes, but she reports pain during examination. What is the most appropriate next step?

**a.** Admit to the hospital; begin a heparin infusion and antiplatelet therapy. Obtain an urgent echocardiogram to identify the source of embolism.

**b.** Obtain urgent ankle-brachial indices and pulse volume recordings to determine the severity of disease and begin aggressive risk-factor-modifying medical therapy.

**c.** Admit to the hospital for an urgent diagnostic abdominal aortogram with runoff and potential endovascular revascularization.

**d.** Admit to the hospital for pain control and obtain a lumbar MRI to evaluate for lumbar canal stenosis and pseudoclaudication.

**e.** Obtain ankle brachial indices at rest and with exercise to assess for lower extremity peripheral arterial disease and a venous plethysmography of the lower extremities with exercise to evaluate for venous claudication.

**5.** A 65-year-old male presents with progressive, short-distance, intermittent claudication in his right leg and a declining ankle brachial index (ABI). He undergoes an abdominal aortic angiogram with runoff demonstrating a discrete 90% stenotic lesion of the superficial femoral artery. Percutaneous transluminal angioplasty followed by placement of a self-expanding nitinol mesh stent is performed with good post-procedural angiographic results. Which of the following is the most appropriate post-procedure surveillance program for this patient?

**a.** Regular visits with assessment for interval change in symptoms, vascular examination, and ABI measurement beginning in the immediate post-procedure period and at intervals for at least 2 years.

**b.** Regular visits with assessment for interval change in symptoms, vascular examination, and arterial duplex at 1 month, 3 months, and at month 12.

**c.** Regular visits with assessment for interval change in symptoms, vascular examination, and ABI measurement at 3 months, 6 months, 9 months, and at month 12.

**d.** Regular visits with assessment for interval change in symptoms, vascular examination, and arterial duplex at 3 months, 6 months, 12 months, and 2 years.

**e.** Annual visits with assessment for interval change in symptoms, vascular examination, ABI measurement, and arterial duplex.

**6.** A 38-year-old female presents to the vascular medicine clinic for a second opinion regarding renal artery stenosis. She has a 10-year history of hypertension treated with hydrochlorothiazide, metoprolol, and ramipril. Review of systems is negative for dysuria, hematuria, heart failure, or neurologic deficits. She admits to chronic back pain for which an MRI of the lumbar spine was obtained, demonstrating an atrophic left kidney. Subsequent computed tomographic angiography of the abdomen revealed hemodynamically significant bilateral renal artery stenosis (RAS). On physical exam her blood pressure is 125/70 mm Hg and tenderness is noted in her lumbar back. Laboratory studies include an unremarkable urinalysis and creatinine of 0.9 mg/dL. What is the most appropriate recommendation for the management of RAS in this patient?

**a.** Proceed with percutaneous revascularization.

**b.** Optimize medical therapy for cardiovascular risk factors.

**c.** Monitor closely for evidence of symptomatic RAS, including sudden unexplained pulmonary edema; accelerated, resistant, or malignant hypertension, despite adequate medical therapy; or declining renal function.

**d.** A and C are reasonable recommendations.

**e.** All of the above are reasonable recommendations.

## Case 1 (Questions 7 and 8)

A 59-year-old morbidly obese female is admitted for cholecystectomy and postoperatively is placed on deep venous thrombosis (DVT) prophylaxis with mini-dose subcutaneous heparin. On hospital day 2, a peripherally inserted central venous catheter is placed in the right arm. The patient is discharged to a rehabilitation facility on hospital day 5 after removal of the venous catheter. Two days later she presents to the emergency room with right upper extremity pain and swelling. She reports she has not felt well enough to participate with physical therapy since being discharged from the hospital. Venous duplex of the right arm demonstrates acute thrombosis of the right cephalic vein. CBC and chemistries are within normal range with a platelet count of 180 K/uL.

7. What is the most appropriate management of this patient?

   a. Admit to the hospital and start on intravenous anticoagulation with heparin or a direct thrombin inhibitor (DTI).
   b. Prescribe enoxaparin 1 mg/kg every 12 hours and coumadin. Admit for 4 to 5 days of overlap and discontinue enoxaparin once the INR is within therapeutic range for 2 consecutive days. Continue anticoagulant therapy for 3 months.
   c. Prescribe enoxaparin 1 mg/kg every 12 hours and coumadin. Discharge with instructions for 4 to 5 days of overlap and discontinue enoxaparin once the INR is within therapeutic range for 2 consecutive days. Continue anticoagulant therapy for 6 months.
   d. Prescribe enoxaparin 1 mg/kg every 12 hours and coumadin. Discharge with instructions for 4 to 5 days of overlap and discontinue enoxaparin once the INR is within therapeutic range for 2 consecutive days. Continue anticoagulant therapy for 12 months.
   e. None of the above.

8. What should the target activated partial thromboplastin time (aPTT) be to achieve optimal efficacy and safety if anticoagulation with a DTI were to be initiated in this patient?

   a. an aPTT of 3.0 to 4.0 times the baseline value
   b. an aPTT of 2.5 to 3.0 times the baseline value
   d. an aPTT of 2.0 to 3.0 times the baseline value
   e. an aPTT of 1.5 to 2.0 times the baseline value

## Case 2 (Questions 9–11)

A 15-year-old male presents to the vascular medicine clinic accompanied by his mother for evaluation of "red hands." He earned money last winter clearing sidewalks of snow and plans to do so again in the upcoming weeks. He reports developing red discoloration of his hands after returning home from the cold. The discoloration persisted for a few minutes until his hands were rewarmed. He denies weakness, paresthesia, pain, or skin lesions. He is otherwise healthy. At the time of consultation, inspection of his hands is unrevealing. Radial and ulnar pulses are 2+/2 bilaterally. The Allen's test and reverse Allen's test reveal return of color to the hands in 7 seconds bilaterally. His mother reports that she and her mother both have Raynaud's phenomenon. The patient's mother expresses concern that her son may have systemic lupus and she requests further testing.

9. What is the most likely diagnosis?

   a. Raynaud's disease
   b. Raynaud's phenomenon
   c. normal physiologic cold response
   d. acrocyanosis
   e. thermal injury

NOTES

**10.** Of the following, which is the most appropriate next step to objectively evaluate this patient?

    **a.** Obtain an upper extremity angiogram with selective imaging of the digital vessels and before and after administration of nitroglycerin.

    **b.** Obtain digital pulse volume recordings and transcutaneous partial pressure of oxygen measurements of the digits.

    **c.** Order a C-reactive protein level, erythrocyte sedimentation rate, and perform nailfold capillaroscopy.

    **d.** Order a C-reactive protein level, erythrocyte sedimentation rate, and plasma homocysteine level.

    **e.** Order antinuclear antibodies, erythrocyte sedimentation rate, and perform nailfold capillaroscopy.

**11.** When would be the most appropriate time to schedule a follow-up appointment?

    **a.** 5 years

    **b.** 3 years

    **c.** 2 years

    **d.** 1 year

    **e.** as needed

**12.** A 25-year-old man is referred to the vascular medicine clinic for complaints of his hands becoming painful and turning white, blue, and red with exposure to cold. As a consequence he avoids outside activities in cold weather. He is a nonsmoker and denies specific systemic symptoms suggestive of a connective tissue disorder or autoimmune disease. He has a normal antinuclear antibody and an elevated erythrocyte sedimentation rate of 30 mm per hour. Nailfold capillary microscopy reveals enlarged and distorted capillary loops. On examination his skin has normal turgor and there is no evidence of pitting, ulcers, or gangrene observed in his fingers or toes. His pulse exam is normal in all four extremities. You suspect he may have secondary Raynaud's phenomenon. He asks you if he is at risk for developing other medical conditions. Which of the following statements is least accurate?

    **a.** He is at risk for developing systemic lupus erythematosus.

    **b.** He is at risk for developing thromboangiitis obliterans.

    **c.** He is at risk for developing Sjogren's syndrome.

    **d.** He is at risk for developing scleroderma.

    **e.** He is at risk for developing mixed connective tissue disease.

## Case 3 (Questions 13 and 14)

A 49-year-old male presents to the vascular medicine clinic with complaints of progressive exertional dyspnea for several weeks. His speech is mildly breathless. Neck veins are distended bilaterally and there is moderate lower extremity edema. He denies chest pain. ECG shows sinus tachycardia without ST segment abnormality. Physical exam reveals a parasternal heave and systolic ejection murmur. Past medical history is significant for splenectomy after a car accident several years ago.

**13.** Which of the following will most accurately confirm the underlying cause of this patient's symptoms?

    **a.** chest computed tomography with intravenous contrast

    **b.** transthoracic echocardiogram

    **c.** transesophageal echocardiogram

    **d.** pulmonary arteriogram

    **e.** ventilation-perfusion scan

**14.** Which of the following statements is most accurate concerning this patient's underlying diagnosis?

a. Inflammatory mechanisms have not been implicated in the pathogenesis

b. Patients should be anticoagulated with a vitamin K antagonist and target INR of 2.5 to 3.5

c. Intravenous epoprostenol is an effective therapy in patients with advanced disease.

d. Inhaled iloprost has been demonstrated to improve exercise capacity.

e. Bosentan has been shown to improve exercise capacity in patients with mild to moderate liver disease.

15. A 67-year-old man with a history of low back pain presents to your office for evaluation of left leg swelling for several months. He has trouble walking long distances, and standing for too long causes his left leg to ache. On exam the left leg is swollen from the foot to the thigh. The right leg is not involved. Pulses are palpable in both feet and other than edema the skin of the lower leg appears normal. What is the next most appropriate step in the diagnostic workup and management for this patient?

    a. admit for evaluation of heart failure

    b. prescribe a course of diuretics

    c. prescribe compression stockings and follow-up in 3 months

    d. venous physiologic testing with outflow plethysmography

    e. none of the above

16. A 48-year-old male presents to the vascular medicine clinic for evaluation of bilateral lower leg swelling gradually worsening over the past year. His legs become swollen and are painful at the end of the day. He denies cough or dyspnea and reports the swelling is least in the morning and seems to become worse throughout the day. He has no other significant past medical history and states, "I haven't been sick a day in my life." He works full-time as a butcher at a local grocery store deli. His exam is remarkable for central obesity, tense edema of the lower legs, and pretibial brawny discoloration. He is normotensive with a regular cardiac rhythm, no murmur, and his lungs are clear. Jugular venous distension is not appreciated. Dorsalis pedis and posterior tibial pulses are 2+/2. What is the most appropriate next step for the management of this patient?

    a. admit for objective testing to evaluate for heart failure

    b. prescribe a course of diuretics

    c. prescribe graduated compression stockings and follow-up in 3 months

    d. order bilateral duplex ultrasound of the legs

    e. none of the above

17. You are consulted for recommendations regarding a deep vein thrombosis in a patient who is status post–aortic valve replacement with a bioprosthetic valve 4 days prior. Earlier on the day of consult he complained of pain and was diagnosed with a partially occlusive left femoral vein thrombosis. His postoperative course has been otherwise uncomplicated. On exam the patient is tender around the surgical site. There is moderate pitting edema in the legs bilaterally. He has palpable pulses in all extremities. What do you recommend?

    a. bolus subcutaneous low-molecular-weight heparin 80 mg/kg then dose at 1 mg/kg subcutaneously every 12 hours

    b. placement of a retrievable inferior vena cava filter

    c. catheter-directed thrombolysis

    d. begin a direct thrombin inhibitor

    e. begin a weight-based heparin infusion

18. A patient with a history of documented heparin-induced thrombocytopenia (HIT) 8 years before presents to your office for preoperative clearance for bioprosthetic aortic valve replacement and coronary artery bypass grafting. He requires

anticoagulation while on cardiopulmonary bypass pump during surgery. ELISA antiplatelet factor-4 antibody testing is currently negative (<0.400 optical density). He has had no subsequent heparin product exposures over the last 8 years. What is the most appropriate anticoagulation regimen you should recommend for this patient?

**a.** use of fondaparinux intraoperatively with daily monitoring of platelet counts

**b.** use of intraoperative low-molecular-weight heparin with daily monitoring of platelet counts

**c.** use of intraoperative argatroban with daily monitoring of platelet counts

**d.** use of intraoperative hirudin with daily monitoring of platelet counts

**e.** use of intraoperative unfractionated heparin with daily monitoring of platelet counts

19. A patient comes to your office 1 month after a hospital stay for gastric bypass surgery. She was diagnosed with a mesenteric vein thrombosis postoperatively. She denies a prior history of venous thromboembolism. She and her husband have questions about the duration of anticoagulation. They bring copies of laboratory results showing she was checked for a hypercoaguable condition. One laboratory test indicates she is heterozygous for a mutation of the methylenetetrahydrofolate reductase (MTHFR) enzyme. All other laboratory tests are within normal range. She asks you how these results impact duration and intensity of anticoagulation. The most accurate reply is

**a.** All first-episode deep venous thromboses are treated similarly; therefore, the discovery of this genetic mutation is of little clinical significance.

**b.** Given the clinical circumstances the laboratory finding is of doubtful clinical significance and you advise she should be anticoagulated with a vitamin K antagonist for 3 months with a target INR of 2.0 to 3.0.

**c.** She should be anticoagulated with a vitamin K antagonist for 3 months with an increased target INR of 2.5 to 3.5 because of increased thrombogenicity induced by the genetic mutation.

**d.** She should be anticoagulated with a vitamin K antagonist with a target INR of 2.0 to 3.0 for an extended duration of therapy to 6 months because of increased thrombogenicity induced by the genetic mutation.

**e.** She should be anticoagulated with a vitamin K antagonist with an INR target of 2.0 to 3.0 indefinitely because of the high rate of recurrent venous thromboembolism associated with the heterozygous form of this genetic mutation.

20. A 34-year-old female with a history of deep vein thrombosis who is chronically anticoagulated with warfarin discovers she is pregnant. Her due date is 34 weeks from now. Currently she is on warfarin and has an INR of 2.2. She presents to the vascular medicine clinic for recommendations regarding her anticoagulation management. Which of the following is true regarding venous thromboembolic disease, anticoagulation therapy, and pregnancy?

**a.** When deep vein thrombosis of the lower extremities complicates a pregnancy the right leg is affected significantly more often than the left, presumably because of exaggeration of the compressive effects of the left iliac artery compressing on the right iliac vein during pregnancy.

**b.** The incidence of teratogenic complications of pregnancy caused by warfarin, including nasal hypoplasia and stippled epiphyses, is greatest if warfarin exposure occurs during weeks 14 through 24.

**c.** Warfarin is contraindicated in the nursing mother because of a high incidence of inducing an anticoagulant effect in the infant fed with breast milk from a mother on warfarin therapy.

**d.** Fatal pulmonary embolism is a leading cause of maternal mortality in the Western world.

e. Low-molecular-weight heparins have been proven safe and efficacious in pregnant woman with prosthetic heart valves, and supplanted unfractionated heparin as the standard of care in this setting.

## Case 4 (Questions 21 and 22)

A 65-year-old-male presents to the vascular medicine clinic with complaints of episodic burning pain involving the soles of his feet and toes. He reports symptoms are most severe when the weather becomes hot and generally occurs when he is outside in the heat. His feet and toes turn red and feel hot to touch during episodes. When he returns to an air-conditioned area, symptoms begin to dissipate or some episodes may take hours for complete resolution. Elevating his legs relieves symptoms and walking barefoot on cold tile floors is also helpful. His past medical history includes hypertension, well controlled with atenolol, and he takes once daily low-dose aspirin for primary prevention.

### Physical Examination

Blood pressure is 120/70 and pulse is 84 bpm.
The cardiac and lung exams are normal.
The abdomen is soft and nontender with a normal-sized palpable aortic pulsation.
No bruit can be heard over the neck, abdomen, or either groin.
Radial, dorsalis pedis, and posterior tibial pulses are 2+/2 bilaterally.
A mild erythema and increased warmth are noted in toes and soles of the feet.

21. Which of the following is the most likely diagnosis?

    a. heat urticaria
    b. erythromelalgia
    c. chilblains (perniosis)
    d. Raynaud's phenomenon

22. What laboratory values should be followed serially in patients with this condition?

    a. electrolytes, blood urea nitrogen, and creatinine
    b. erythrocyte sedimentation rate
    c. ionic calcium
    d. complete blood count with differential

23. A young man presents to the emergency department (ED) after exposure to the freezing cold for 14 hours. His car had broken down during a winter storm and in his attempt to walk home he became lost. He was found the next morning by rescue workers, who immediately brought him to the ED. Luckily, he was wearing sufficient clothing and had enough experience outdoors to keep his core body temperature up; however, he did sustain severe frostbite to his feet bilaterally. Upon presentation his feet are edematous and have multiple small, dark colored blisters. Over the ensuing days the edema persists and the blisters are reabsorbed and replaced by black eschar. A week later the eschar is still present when he returns for follow-up. He complains of a throbbing pain in his feet, which he says began the day after he presented to the ED. His edema is unchanged. His vitals are normal and he has no other complaints. What should you do next?

    a. debride the black eschar
    b. give him a prescription for antibiotics
    c. admit him to the hospital for IV antibiotics and possible amputation
    d. follow-up in 1 week
    e. A and D
    f. B and D
    g. A, B, and D

**24.** A 17-year-old-male was involved in a motor vehicle accident, which resulted in multiple fractures as well as internal injuries that necessitated multiple abdominal surgeries over a 2-week period. He is expected to recover fully. An intraluminal filling defect was incidentally identified consistent with deep venous thrombosis of the right external iliac vein on a contrast-enhanced abdominal computed tomography scan. Anticoagulation was contraindicated because of a retroperitoneal hemorrhage. It was determined that placement of an inferior vena cava filter was necessary. Of the following types of filters, which filter is most appropriate in this case?

**a.** Bird's Nest vena cava filter
**b.** Gunther Tulip retrievable vena cava filter
**c.** TrapEase inferior vena cava filter
**d.** Greenfield vena cava filter
**e.** Simon Nitinol inferior vena cava filter

## Case 5 (Questions 25 and 26)

You are called to the bedside of a 68-year-old male in mild distress who underwent cardiac catheterization earlier in the day. He is complaining of increasing right groin pain. He complains of weakness and tingling in his foot and toes. He is presently on a heparin infusion because of atrial fibrillation. On inspection you note a large area of skin in his right groin and proximal thigh to be dark blue and there is a large, palpable, hard pulsatile mass. With ultrasound using color Doppler you note an irregular shaped area of flow measuring 4.0 $\times$ 3.3 cm near the common femoral artery, approximately 4.0-cm deep and connected to the artery by a 0.5-cm neck. There is surrounding hematoma observed. Spectral waveform analysis of the neck demonstrates a to-and-fro pattern.

**25.** What is the best treatment option for management of this patient's condition?

**a.** placement of a femoral compression device overnight and analgesics for pain
**b.** injection of thrombin by ultrasound guidance
**c.** ultrasound-guided compression for 30 minutes
**d.** surgical evacuation of the hematoma and suture repair of the artery
**e.** placement of a compression dressing with snugly applied bandages around the leg and serial duplex scans to monitor for resolution

**26.** Patients that undergo thrombin injection for repair of procedure-related pseudoaneurysms should be fully informed of potential complications. Which of the following is the least likely complication associated with this procedure?

**a.** acute intra-arterial thrombosis
**b.** anaphylactic reaction
**c.** deep vein thrombosis
**d.** infection
**e.** bleeding

**27.** A 74-year-old man is in the ICU recovering from coronary artery bypass surgery and has developed a hemorrhagic pericardial effusion. He is currently stable, but has noted swelling and pain in his left leg. An ultrasound is ordered and reveals acute thrombus in the left peroneal vein. Which of the following is the best management option?

**a.** observation
**b.** enoxaparin 1 mg/kg every 12 hours
**c.** enoxaparin 40 mg every 24 hours
**d.** pneumatic compression stockings
**e.** serial duplex ultrasound scans
**f.** continuous heparin infusion
**g.** inferior vena cava filter

## Case 6 (Questions 28 and 29)

A 25-year-old male presents to the vascular medicine clinic with complaints of pain in his feet with walking. He reports this has been going on for several months and has progressively worsened in the past few weeks. He is beginning to develop symptoms in his right calf and earlier this week noticed a black area on his great toe. He has no medical problems, takes no medications, and is in good health overall. He is a smoker and works as a computer salesman. He reports a family history of venous thromboembolism; his mother had a pulmonary embolism at the age of 50 and was diagnosed with the antiphospholipid antibody syndrome.

28. What is the most likely cause of his symptoms?

    a. elevated anticardiolipin antibodies
    b. thromboangiitis obliterans (Buerger's disease)
    c. Takayasu's arteritis
    d. premature atherosclerosis
    e. livedo vasculitis (atrophie blanche)

29. What is the most important aspect of therapy for this patient?

    a. anticoagulation with a vitamin K antagonist
    b. cessation of exposure to all forms of tobacco
    c. initiate immunosuppressive therapy with glucocorticoids
    d. antiplatelet therapy with aspirin
    e. admit to the hospital to begin tissue plasminogen activator therapy

## Case 7 (Questions 30 and 31)

A 24-year-old woman presents with complaints of a swollen, painful left leg. She has a history of two episodes of deep vein thrombosis in the past. She recalls that they were both on the left side, but is unsure of which veins were involved. She was on warfarin in the past but discontinued it when she began attempting to conceive. Venous duplex demonstrates an acute deep vein thrombosis of the left femoral vein. You initiate treatment with low-molecular-weight heparin monotherapy given she is actively attempting to become pregnant.

30. What is the most likely diagnosis?

    a. heterozygous prothrombin gene mutation
    b. heterozygous factor V Leiden mutation
    c. May-Thurner syndrome
    d. Klippel-Trenaunay syndrome
    e. Klippel-Trenaunay-Weber syndrome

31. Which of the following is the best management option?

    a. indefinite anticoagulant therapy with warfarin
    b. indefinite monotherapy with enoxaparin
    c. venography for thrombus removal and stent placement
    d. placement of an inferior vena cava filter and discontinue anticoagulants
    e. anticoagulate with either warfarin or enoxaparin for 6 months

32. A 68-year-old gentleman underwent coronary artery bypass surgery using the saphenous vein harvested from his left leg. He has done well postoperatively except for failure of the left leg incision to heal completely. Four months after surgery, his leg is still not fully healed and a peri-incisional ulcer is now present. He has significant edema in his leg, which was present prior to surgery. There are no symptoms or physical findings suggestive of infection. His ABI is 0.94 on the right and 0.89 on the left. You order an ultrasound, which is negative for acute thrombus but does reveal significant venous valvular reflux in the deep system. Which of the following is most likely to improve this patient's wound healing?

a. whirlpool therapy
b. antibiotics
c. topical steroids
d. compression stockings
e. plastic surgery consult
f. revascularization

33. You are providing postoperative care for a patient who is in the cardiovascular surgery postoperative intensive care unit, status post–coronary artery bypass surgery. A venous duplex ultrasound was performed to evaluate for new onset bilateral leg swelling. Results are reported as negative for deep venous thrombosis, but with monophasic flow noted within the bilateral common femoral veins. Which of the following is the next best step?

a. computed tomography venogram of the lower extremities
b. computed tomography venogram of the abdomen and pelvis
c. enoxaparin therapy 1 mg/kg subcutaneous injections every 12 hours
d. enoxaparin therapy 40 mg subcutaneous injections every 24 hours

## Case 8 (Questions 34 and 35)

A 39-year-old male presents to the emergency department (ED) with shortness of breath and tachycardia. He eventually develops hypotension with a systolic blood pressure of 80 mm Hg. A stat computed tomography scan of the chest reveals a saddle pulmonary embolism involving the main pulmonary artery trunk.

34. Which of the following is the next most appropriate step?

a. begin an intravenous heparin infusion at 18 U/kg/hour
b. begin alteplase 100 mg IV over 2 hours
c. begin enoxaparin subcutaneous injections 1 mg/kg every 12 hours
d. insert an inferior vena cava filter

35. Which of the following findings or laboratory values could be used to predict his prognosis?

a. C-reactive protein
b. atrial arrhythmia
c. left ventricular dysfunction
d. prolonged QT interval
e. elevated serum myoglobin

36. A 52-year-old man with metastatic prostate cancer has developed left lower extremity swelling. You order an ultrasound and a left acute external iliac deep vein thrombosis is visualized. You hospitalize the patient and his initial labs reveal hemoglobin 14.5 gm/dL and creatinine 1.0 mg/dL. Which of the following treatment options is most appropriate?

a. Begin a weight-based unfractionated heparin infusion and bridge to warfarin.
b. Begin enoxaparin 1 mg/kg subcutaneous injections every 12 hours.
c. Place an inferior vena cava filter.
d. Begin unfractionated heparin 5,000 units subcutaneous injections every 8 hours.

## Images (Questions 37–50)

Match the letter of the image to the most fitting corresponding description.

a. Refer to Figure 7–1
b. Refer to Figure 7–2
c. Refer to Figure 7–3
d. Refer to Figure 7–4
e. Refer to Figure 7–5
f. Refer to Figure 7–6

g. Refer to Figure 7–7
h. Refer to Figure 7–8
i. Refer to Figure 7–9
j. Refer to Figure 7–10
k. Refer to Figure 7–11
l. Refer to Figure 7–12
m. Refer to Figure 7–13
n. Refer to Figure 7–14

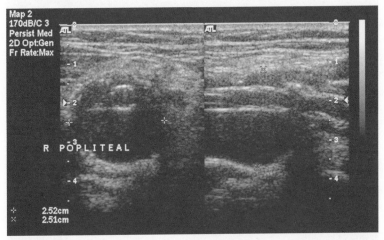

**FIGURE 7–1**

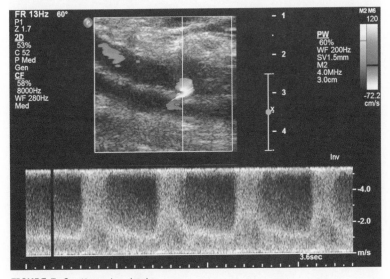

**FIGURE 7–2**   (See color plate)

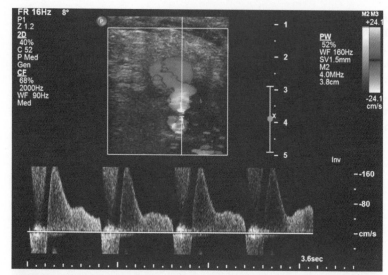

**FIGURE 7-3**    (See color plate)

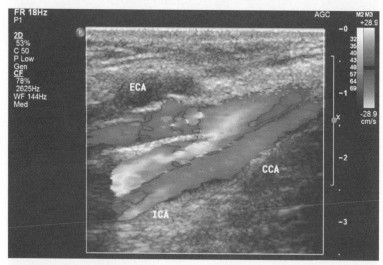

**FIGURE 7-4**    (See color plate)

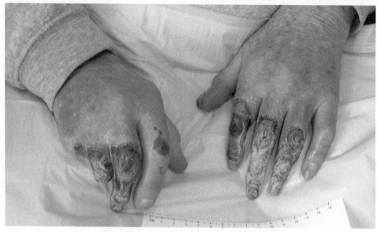

**FIGURE 7-5**

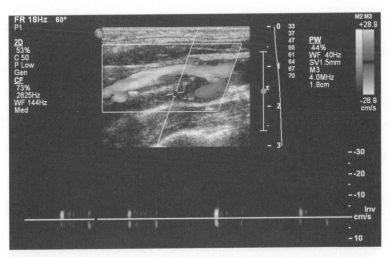

**FIGURE 7–6**  (See color plate)

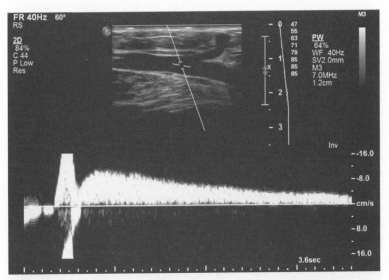

**FIGURE 7–7**

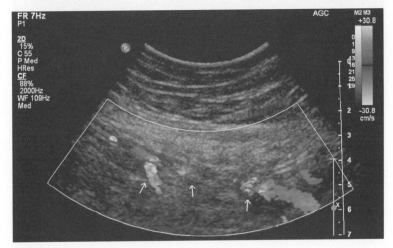

**FIGURE 7–8**  (See color plate)

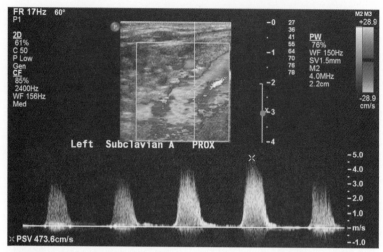

**FIGURE 7–9** (See color plate)

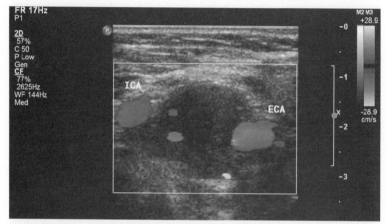

**FIGURE 7–10** (See color plate)

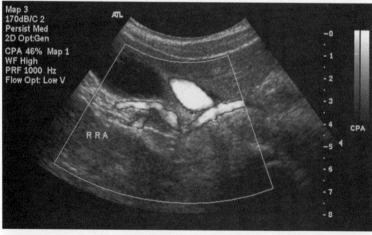

**FIGURE 7–11** (See color plate)

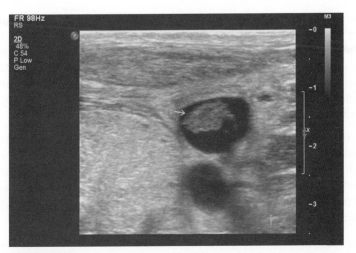

**FIGURE 7–12**

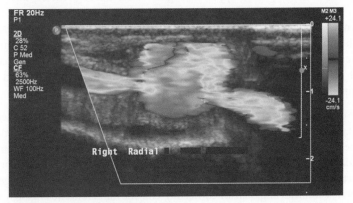

**FIGURE 7–13**   (See color plate)

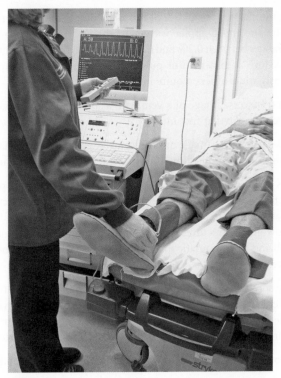

**FIGURE 7–14**

**37.** The condition illustrated is a significant cause of stroke in all age groups. This may develop following major or minor trauma, spontaneously, or, as in the patient presented, in association with Marfan syndrome or other connective tissue disorders. Patients may present with nonspecific head, neck, or face pain. Partial Horner's syndrome is often described as a presenting complaint. Management may be surgical, endovascular, or medical. Medical therapy usually consists of heparin and warfarin and, later, antiplatelet therapy.[1]

**38.** Pictured is the most common type of paraganglioma of the head and neck. It is most commonly discovered during the fifth decade of life. It may present with neck pain and swelling associated with hoarseness. Most often it is a benign neoplasm; however, 5% to 10% will exhibit malignant behavior. Treatment is dependent on the clinical circumstances, but may involve periodic clinical exam, palliative radiation therapy, or surgical excision.[2]

**39.** Patients presenting with this condition represent diagnostic and management dilemmas. Patients initially present with complaints of pain, cold intolerance, and ulceration. The diagnostic approach begins with a thorough history and examination including assessing for cardiovascular risk factors, claudication symptoms, Raynaud phenomenon, and connective tissue and autoimmune disorders. History pertaining to tobacco exposure and use of illicit drugs is especially important. Diagnostics should include noninvasive testing such as pulse volume recordings and diagnostic angiography. Treatment options include chemical and surgical sympathectomy as well as microvascular reconstruction.[3]

**40.** The image illustrates the classic vessel morphology of the disorder. It is often associated with hypertension, strokes, and arterial aneurysms and dissections. Females tend to be affected more than males. Patients may be asymptomatic or may complain of headaches. Examination may reveal hypertension, neurologic deficits, and bruits over affected arteries and diminished distal pulses. Treatment includes management of hypertension with angiotensin-converting-enzyme inhibitors and angiotensin receptor blockers, balloon angioplasty, and antiplatelet therapy. Surgical intervention may be required in some cases.[4]

**41.** Pictured is the classic appearance of this rare complication of percutaneous procedures. The spectral Doppler waveform shown is a classic to-and-fro signal. Incidence ranges between 0.2% and 0.5%. Patients typically present post–catheter-based procedure with a painful pulsatile mass. When small these may resolve spontaneously while others require intervention.[5]

**42.** Shown is a transverse image of a vein with a spectral Doppler waveform consistent with venous valvular incompetence.

**43.** Depicted is a transverse image of nonocclusive echogenic material within a vein. This is a common complication after placement of a central venous catheter.

**44.** Depicted is a rare complication of interventional percutaneous procedures. The classic spectral Doppler waveform consists of high velocity turbulent flow. Patients are often asymptomatic with a groin bruit discovered during physical exam. Avoiding low groin punctures may minimize the incidence of this complication. When small and asymptomatic these may be observed over time or surgical repair may be necessary.[6]

**45.** This image shows an artery with significant color aliasing, spectral broadening, and turbulent high velocity flow. Loss of the usual triphasic waveform is noted. High-grade stenosis of this vessel is important to detect prior to performing coronary artery bypass surgery using the internal mammary artery.

**46.** Shown is complete occlusion of an artery with collateralization and reconstitution.

**47.** The abnormality shown is rare. It may occur spontaneously but more often is iatrogenic. It may occur because of intrinsic abnormalities in the vessel wall, secondary to multiple punctures to obtain blood, or because of infection.[7]

**48.** Shown is a condition that is a cause of unilateral or bilateral leg swelling and pain. It is often associated with abdominal aortic and thoracic aortic aneurysm. Distal embolization, thrombosis, and compression of surrounding neurovascular structures are frequent complications. Risk factors include smoking, advanced age, hypertension, and family history.[8]

**49.** The test shown here is 95% sensitive and 99% specific for the detection of angiogram positive peripheral arterial disease.[9] This is a significant improvement compared to palpation of pedal pulses and using the Rose questionnaire of intermittent claudication.[10]

**50.** Shown is total occlusion of the internal carotid artery with lack of color filling and absence of a spectral Doppler waveform.

**NOTES**

# ANSWERS

1. **d.** Hypercholesterolemia. Among the risk factors listed, hypercholesterolemia has the lowest relative risk for the development of peripheral arterial disease with a relative risk of up to double that of nonsmokers. Smoking increases risk two- to sixfold, diabetes increases risk two- to fourfold, hypertension increases risk two and a half- to fourfold and hyperhomocysteinemia increases risk two- to threefold.[11]

2. **d.** 25%. 1% to 2% of patients with lower extremity PAD will present with clinical signs and symptoms of critical limb ischemia. One-year outcomes in this population was death caused by cardiovascular causes in 25%, amputation in 25%, and 50% were alive with two limbs.[11]

3. **b.** Chronic venous insufficiency. This patient has no history of neuropathy and has intact sensation, making a neurotrophic ulcer often associated with diabetes unlikely. While his glucose is elevated, inadequate information is provided to make the diagnosis of diabetes mellitus. Bilateral leg edema, hyperpigmentation of the ankles, and the location of the ulcer over the medial malleolus ("gaiter distribution") are findings consistent with a venous stasis wound. Ulcers secondary to arterial disease are usually painful, involve the toes, and are well circumscribed. The information provided suggests adequate arterial supply. Wounds associated with calciphylaxis may be anywhere. They are usually very painful, involve large areas of skin, and are associated with black eschar formation. These wounds are most often seen in patients with renal impairment and hyperparathyroidism, neither of which is true in this case. Nothing in the clinical vignette is suggestive of a brown recluse spider bite.[11]

4. **c.** Admit to the hospital for an urgent diagnostic abdominal aortogram with runoff and potential endovascular revascularization. The patient described is suffering from acute critical limb ischemia. The hallmarks of acute limb ischemia are the five "Ps", which are suggestive of impending tissue necrosis. They are pain, paralysis, paresthesia, pulseless, and pallor and some add poikilothermia (coldness) for a sixth "P." Our patient exhibits all but paralysis. Based on the Society for Vascular Surgery/International Society for Cardiovascular Surgery classification scheme for clinical categories of acute limb ischemia, her limb is marginally to intermediately threatened. Acute limb ischemia requires prompt diagnosis and intervention to avoid limb loss and life-threatening systemic illness resulting from tissue gangrene.[12]

5. **a.** Regular visits with assessment for interval change in symptoms, vascular examination, and ABI measurement beginning in the immediate post-procedure period and at intervals for at least 2 years. Unlike follow-up of autologous vein bypass grafts, well-established evidence-based guidelines for surveillance of post-endovascular revascularization patients do not exist. However, it is considered standard of care to evaluate these patients with interval history, examination, and measurement of the ABI regularly for at least 2 years after their percutaneous revascularization procedure.[13]

6. **e.** All of the above are reasonable recommendations. Endovascular intervention for asymptomatic RAS is controversial and there are no well-controlled prospective randomized trials evaluating the risk versus benefit of endovascular intervention in these patients. Recommendations to proceed with catheter-based interventions are based on expert opinion. It is not clear if treating asymptomatic RAS results in preservation of renal function, improved blood pressure control, or improved cardiovascular morbidity and mortality.[14]

7. **e.** None of the above. Empiric anticoagulation, including outpatient anticoagulation, for superficial vein thrombosis is not routinely recommended. The clinical

scenario may represent heparin-induced thrombocytopenia and she should have a follow-up platelet count in 2 days. Her prior platelet counts from her recent hospitalization should be evaluated for a drop in platelets of >50% from baseline.[15]

8. **e.** An aPTT prolongation of 1.5 to 2.0 times the baseline value. Although the recommended range for therapeutic anticoagulation for venous thromboembolism with a DTI is 1.5 to 2.5 times the baseline, which is not given as an option, published data indicate that anticoagulation with a DTI target aPTT of 1.5 to 2.0 times the baseline is just as efficacious and is associated with less bleeding risk.[16]

9. **c.** Normal physiologic cold response. This patient is exhibiting a normal response to prolonged exposure to cold. The diagnosis of Raynaud's phenomenon is clinical and includes the presence of pallor or acrocyanosis and pain with cold exposure. Redness of the hands with warming after prolonged cold exposure, without concomitant pain, may be a normal response in a healthy young individual. He should be counseled to wear gloves and report any change in his symptoms, as his family history does predispose him to development of Raynaud's phenomenon.[17]

10. **e.** Order antinuclear antibodies, erythrocyte sedimentation rate, and perform nailfold capillaroscopy. If all these tests are normal, it is very unlikely that this patient has Raynaud's phenomenon and no further testing is necessary.[18]

11. **e.** As needed. Although the patient does not have Raynaud's phenomenon, he should be encouraged to follow-up as needed because of his family history. Patients who have primary Raynaud's phenomenon should have clinical follow-up for a minimum of 2 years after diagnosis.[17]

12. **b.** He is at risk for developing thromboangiitis obliterans. Raynaud's phenomenon may precede the onset of many connective tissue diseases. All of the disorders listed can be associated with a secondary Raynaud phenomenon. However, the clinical history is not suggestive of thromboangiitis obliterans. Specifically, normal pulses in all extremities and the lack of tobacco exposure make this an unlikely diagnosis.[18]

13. **d.** Pulmonary arteriogram. An arteriogram is the test most likely to confirm pulmonary artery hypertension in this patient presenting with cor pulmonale, although a right heart catheterization is usually done first. This patient most likely has chronic thromboembolic pulmonary hypertension (CTEPH), a condition seen in otherwise healthy postsplenectomy patients. Other predisposing conditions include history of pulmonary embolism, myeloproliferative disorders, and chronic inflammatory conditions.[19]

14. **c.** Patients with CTEPH may be bridged to pulmonary endarterectomy with intravenous epoprostenol. The other answers are incorrect. Anticoagulation with a vitamin K antagonist is indicated; however, the INR target of 2.0 to 3.0 is recommended. The AIR study did not demonstrate improved exercise capacity with inhaled iloprost. Bosentan does improve exercise capacity and decreases pulmonary vascular resistance, but is not advocated for use in patients with moderate to severe hepatic dysfunction.[19]

15. **e.** None of the above. This patient has unilateral edema of uncertain etiology. The differential diagnosis of unilateral limb swelling includes, but is not limited to, cellulitis, lymphedema, venous thrombosis, pelvic mass causing external compression, and Charcot foot. An occult malignancy such as a pelvic tumor or soft tissue sarcoma is uncommon but should be a consideration. Initial workup should include venous duplex to rule out deep vein thrombosis. Venous outflow plethysmography can be used for screening patients for venous obstruction when the index of suspicion for acute DVT is low. Systemic conditions such as heart failure, renal insufficiency, hypoalbuminemia, and hypothyroidism are more associated with bilateral limb swelling.[20]

**16. c.** Prescribe compression stockings and follow-up in 3 months. The clinical history and exam are consistent with chronic venous insufficiency. Venous duplex to rule out an acute DVT in this setting is of low yield since his symptoms are chronic and have been progressing over at least the past year. Use of compression stockings is the mainstay for conservative treatment of chronic venous insufficiency. Daily use of compression stockings to control edema protects the skin from injury, reduces discomfort, and prevents the progressive inflammatory skin changes that lead to ulceration associated with venous stasis.[21]

**17. e.** Begin a weight-based heparin infusion. Although low-molecular-weight heparin may be appropriate as the initial anticoagulant of choice for the treatment of an acute DVT in the ambulatory as well as hospitalized patient, it does not require a bolus. In the setting of the postoperative state where rapid reversal of anticoagulation may be required, unfractionated heparin is favored. An inferior vena cava filter would be an appropriate recommendation if anticoagulation could not be administered at therapeutic levels. Thrombolytic therapy is contraindicated in the setting of recent open-heart surgery. Use of a direct thrombin inhibitor is not indicated for routine anticoagulation.[22]

**18. e.** Use of intraoperative unfractionated heparin with daily monitoring of platelet counts. The nature of immune response to heparin is anamnestic; this means a second exposure in the absence of positive antibodies is not associated with the development of a clinical hyperacute immune response. Perioperatively, heparin products should be avoided in patients with a history of HIT even with undetectable antiplatelet antibodies prior to cardiac surgery or vascular surgery. Nevertheless, heparin is favored over direct thrombin inhibitors in cardiac and vascular surgery because of its reversibility and relative ease of use. Acute HIT is unlikely to occur even in patients who have a remote history of HIT as long as there has been no heparin exposure within the previous 100 days. This recommendation is based on expert opinion (level 1C) and not on randomized controlled trials.[15]

**19. b.** Given the clinical circumstances the laboratory finding is of doubtful clinical significance and you advise she should be anticoagulated with a vitamin K antagonist for 3 months with a target INR of 2.0 to 3.0. While the site of thrombosis is somewhat out of the ordinary, it was in the setting of abdominal surgery and was her first episode; therefore, a routine course of 3 months of anticoagulation with a vitamin K antagonist and an INR target of 2.0 to 3.0 is appropriate. All first-episode venous thrombotic events are not treated the same. Patients with malignancy-related thrombosis, idiopathic events, and those with certain thrombophilic conditions such as the antiphospholipid antibody syndrome require a longer duration of therapy relative to patients with transient risk factors for venous thromboembolism (VTE). The MTHFR genetic mutation in the absence of hyperhomocysteinemia is not associated with increased risk of recurrence after discontinuation of anticoagulant therapy and has not been shown to increase thrombogenicity requiring a higher than usual INR target.[23]

**20. d.** Fatal pulmonary embolism is a leading cause of maternal mortality in the Western world. Thromboembolism is clearly the leading direct cause of maternal mortality according to the Seventh Report of the Confidential Enquiries into Maternal Deaths in the United Kingdom. The May-Thurner syndrome involves compression of the left iliac vein by the right iliac artery. The greatest teratogenicity of warfarin is seen during weeks 6 through 12. Use of low-molecular-weight heparin in pregnant women who have prosthetic heart valves is highly controversial and certainly not the standard of care.[24]

**21. b.** Erythromelalgia. The name of this condition is based on three Greek words: *erythro* meaning red, *melos* meaning extremity, and *algos* meaning pain. It is uncommon, affecting about 1 in 40,000. It may be primary or secondary. Primary erythromelalgia is usually bilateral, not associated with gangrene, and patients have normal pulses. Secondary erythromelalgia is often unilateral, can be associated with gangrene, and patients have variable pulses. Secondary erythromelalgia can be associated with medications including bromocriptine, nifedipine, nicardipine, and verapamil. It may also herald the onset of a myeloproliferative disease such as polycythemia vera or essential thrombocythemia.[24]

**22. d.** Complete blood count with differential (CBC with diff). Patients with this condition should have a CBC with diff checked periodically for at least 2 to 3 years. It is important for treating physicians to recognize that erythromelalgia can precede the laboratory manifestations of a myeloproliferative disorder by up to 2 to 3 years.[28]

**23. d.** Follow-up in 1 week. This question addresses a common mistake made with frostbite injury. The case of frostbite described is severe with development of hemorrhagic blisters similar in appearance to reperfusion bullae. The blisters are usually replaced by black eschar, which remains for several weeks. Generally, the eschar sloughs and reveals healing tissues. It is important to allow this eschar to slough on its own and not to debride unless there are signs or symptoms of infection. Early debridement may result in loss of otherwise viable tissue. Early amputation is also to be avoided for the same reason, unless infection is a concern, and, if possible, autoamputation should be permitted. Generally, a clear demarcation will develop between the healthy skin and the nonviable tissue. This may take weeks to fully declare. Ongoing pain is a common issue with frostbite. Severe pain usually accompanies the thawing process, and often narcotics are required for pain control. A throbbing pain caused by inflammation will often begin several days after thawing is complete. This may last for weeks. Patients may describe a prickly pain or a shooting electric pain that is more prevalent at night. This may represent an ischemic neuritis. Hyperhidrosis and a sensation of burning in the feet have been described and may reflect overactivity of the sympathetic nervous system. In the chronic state, sympathectomy has been shown to be helpful in this setting.[24]

**24. b.** Gunther Tulip retrievable vena cava filter. This patient is young and his deep vein thrombosis is situational. He is expected to recover fully with no sequelae, thus he does not require placement of a permanent inferior vena cava filter. Proximal iliac thrombus in the setting of a hospitalized trauma patient following multiple abdominal surgeries is a very high-risk scenario for development of serious, life-threatening venous thromboembolism (VTE). Anticoagulation is the treatment of choice when it can be safely administered; however, when contraindicated an inferior vena cava filter should be placed without delay. Patients with a temporary contraindication for anticoagulants should be reassessed at short intervals and, if circumstances permit, anticoagulants should be instituted for treatment of their VTE and to prevent recurrence. Of the filter types listed, only the Gunther Tulip is approved in the United States for retrieval. The OptEase is also approved for retrieval. The Bird's Nest filter is the only filter available for use in patients with a so-called megacava (vena cava greater than 28 mm). The Bird's Nest filter can be placed into an IVC of up to 42 mm in diameter. The TrapEase, Greenfield, and Simon Nitinol filters were not designed to have the option of retrieval.[25]

**25. d.** Surgical evacuation of the hematoma and suture repair of the artery. The patient complains of developing numbness in the setting of developing a large hematoma and pseudoaneurysm. To relieve the compressive affect of the hematoma, prevent irreversible injury, and relieve pain the most appropriate method of repair in this patient is to evacuate the hematoma. Most small to moderately sized pseudoaneurysms can be treated with either ultrasound-guided compression, thrombin injection, or when very small may be observed for spontaneous resolution. Placement of a femoral compression device (Fem-Stop) is not appropriate in this setting, and bandages should not be wrapped proximally around the thigh as this will cause worsening swelling and pain.[26]

26. **e.** Bleeding. All of the options have been reported as complications of ultrasound-guided thrombin injection of pseudoaneurysms except for bleeding.

27. **e.** Serial duplex ultrasound scans. The peroneal vein is a calf vein with less propensity for clinically significant sequelae. Anticoagulant therapy for calf vein deep venous thrombosis is controversial. However, in this setting there is a clear contraindication to anticoagulate. Even prophylactic doses of anticoagulants are not advisable in patients with hemorrhagic pericardial effusions status post–open heart surgery. Serial ultrasound scans have been studied as an alternative to anticoagulant therapy. If no propagation after several weeks, no anticoagulant therapy is necessary. If propagation occurs then anticoagulation versus placement of an inferior vena cava should be considered.[27]

28. **b.** Thromboangiitis obliterans. Thromboangiitis obliterans (TAO) classically manifests in young, male patients with a recent history of heavy tobacco use. The clinical presentation is consistent with ischemia, beginning distally and involving the small- and medium-sized arteries. Usually the lower extremities are involved, with ischemia or claudication of the feet or legs. Foot or arch claudication is typical. Occasionally, the hands are involved. If the disease progresses with continued exposure to tobacco, patients are at significant risk of progressive ischemia, ulceration, gangrene, and eventually amputation. Antiphospholipid antibody syndrome is certainly possible, but it is not a hereditary condition and most often manifests with venous thrombosis. Takayasu's arteritis does not usually present in this way. Nothing is suggestive of atrophie blanche, and premature atherosclerosis presenting in a 25-year-old male with claudication and ischemia would be highly unusual.[28]

29. **b.** Cessation of exposure to all forms of tobacco. The strong link between tobacco abuse and TAO is well recognized. There have been suggestions that some patients may demonstrate an abnormal sensitivity to a component of tobacco, which leads to small vessel occlusive disease. It has been shown that patients with TAO have higher tobacco consumption as well as higher carboxyhemoglobin levels than do patients with atherosclerosis.[28]

30. **c.** May-Thurner syndrome. Also known as iliac vein compression syndrome, Cockett syndrome, or iliocaval compression syndrome, May-Thurner syndrome is caused by compression of the left common iliac vein by the right common iliac artery. A history of chronic left lower extremity edema with or without the presence of DVT is suggestive of May-Thurner syndrome, especially in a female population. This phenomenon causes a partial obstruction caused by physical entrapment of the vein under the artery as well as by repetitive pulsatile force resulting in intimal hyperplasia of the vein. It has been estimated that this condition occurs in 2% to 5% of patients who are evaluated for lower extremity venous problems.[29]

31. **c.** Venography for thrombus removal and stent placement. May-Thurner syndrome is an anatomical anomaly that results in repeated venous trauma and often subsequent thrombus formation. Removal of thrombus followed by angioplasty, if needed, and placement of a stent is a potentially definitive treatment that could avoid the need for indefinite anticoagulant therapy in the young woman presented in this case.[29]

32. **d.** Compression stockings. The importance of edema control is often underestimated for wound healing. This patient has deep system venous reflux. He has no signs of infection complicating the healing of his incision, so antibiotics are unlikely to be helpful. Topical steroids offer no benefit in this case. His ABIs suggest adequate arterial inflow for wound healing. Whirlpool therapy is helpful in select cases, most often when multiple small wounds are present, which need cleansing and gentle debridement. Although the size of the wound is not clearly stated, these wounds are most often small and referral for skin grafting is not indicated.[30]

**33. b.** Computed tomography venogram of the abdomen and pelvis. Monophasic (loss of respiratory phasicity) flow is suggestive of proximal venous obstruction, especially in a patient with swollen limbs and under high-risk circumstances for venous thromboembolism. Monophasicity is not specific to thrombosis. Other potential causes include obesity, pregnancy, or a pelvic mass. Respiratory or cardiac dysfunction may also produce an abnormal venous flow pattern.[31]

**34. b.** Alteplase 100 mg IV over two hours. The patient presented has a clinically massive pulmonary embolism with hemodynamic compromise, thus thrombolytic therapy is indicated.[32]

**35. b.** Atrial arrhythmia. There have been many laboratory, electrocardiogram, and echocardiogram findings shown to be predictive of mortality and prognosis. Right ventricular dysfunction, particularly when accompanied by hypotension, is predictive of pulmonary embolism–related hospital mortality. Elevated serum troponin and elevated brain natriuretic peptide have also been shown to predict an increase risk of death. Additional findings associated with a poorer prognosis include atrial arrhythmia, right bundle branch block, inferior Q waves and precordial T wave inversions, and ST segment changes. The other distracters have not been shown to predict prognosis.

**36. b.** Begin enoxaparin 1 mg/kg subcutaneous injections every 12 hours. Cancer patients are at a sixfold increased risk of developing VTE. Patients with active cancer make up about 20% of all new VTE diagnosed in the community. The risk, however, varies somewhat with cancer type, and those that incur a higher risk include malignant brain tumors and adenocarcinoma of the ovary, pancreas, colon, stomach, lung, prostate, and kidney. Several studies have demonstrated a benefit to treatment with low-molecular-weight heparin (LMWH) as compared to coumadin in this patient population. One study, which compared dalteparin to coumadin, reported 27 of 336 patients in the LMWH group had recurrent VTE as compared to 53 of 336 in the coumadin group in a 6-month follow-up period. There was no increased risk of bleeding in the LMWH group.[33,34]

**37. d.**
**38. j.**
**39. e.**
**40. k.**
**41. c.**
**42. g.**
**43. l.**
**44. b.**
**45. i.**
**46. h.**
**47. m.**
**48. a.**
**49. n.**
**50. f.**

# References

1. Dziewas R, Konrad C, Drager B, et al. Cervical artery dissection. *J Neurol.* 2003;250(10): 1179–1184.
2. Mafee MF, Raofi B, Kumar A, et al. Glomus faciale, glomus jugulare, glomus tympanicum, glomus vagale, carotid body tumors, and simulating lesions. Role of MR imaging. *Radiol Clin North Am.* 2000;38(5):1059–1076.

**NOTES**

3. Wilgis EF. Evaluation and treatment of chronic digital ischemia. *Ann Surg.* 1981;193(6):693–698.

4. Slovut DP, Olin JW. Fibromuscular dysplasia. *N Engl J Med.* 2004;350(18):1862–1871.

5. Ferguson JD, Whatling PT, Martin V, et al. Ultrasound guided percutaneous thrombin injection of iatrogenic femoral artery pseudoaneurysms after coronary angiography and intervention. *Heart.* April;(85):e5.

6. Kelm M, Perings SM, Jax T, et al. Incidence and clinical outcome of iatrogenic femoral arteriovenous fistulas, implications for risk stratification and treatment. *J Am Coll Cardiol.* 2002;40(2):291–297.

7. McEllistrem RF, O'Toole DP, Keane P. Post cannulation radial artery aneurysm—a rare complication. *Can J Anaesth.* 1990;37: 907–909.

8. Podlaha J, Holub R, Konecny Z, et al. 20 year experience with operations for popliteal artery aneurysm. *BMJ/Bratisl Lek Listy.* 2005;106(12):421–422.

9. TASC Guidelines. Management of PAD. *J Vasc Surg.* 2000;(31):S1–S296.

10. Criqui MH, Fronek A, Klauber MR, et al. The sensitivity, specificity, and predictive value of traditional clinical evaluation of peripheral arterial disease: results from noninvasive testing in a defined population. *Circulation.* 1985;(71):516–522.

11. Hirsch AT, Haskal ZJ, Hertzer NR et al. ACC/AHA 2005 Practice Guidelines for the management of patients with peripheral arterial disease (lower extremity, renal, mesenteric, and abdominal aortic): a collaborative report from the American Association for Vascular Surgery/Society for Vascular Surgery, Society for Cardiovascular Angiography and Interventions, Society for Vascular Medicine and Biology, Society of Interventional Radiology, and the ACC/AHA Task Force on Practice Guidelines (Writing Committee to Develop Guidelines for the Management of Patients With Peripheral Arterial Disease). *Circulation.* 2006; 21;113:e471–e486.

12. Hirsch AT, Haskal ZJ, Hertzer NR, et al. ACC/AHA 2005 Practice Guidelines for the management of patients with peripheral arterial disease (lower extremity, renal, mesenteric, and abdominal aortic): a collaborative report from the American Association for Vascular Surgery/Society for Vascular Surgery, Society for Cardiovascular Angiography and Interventions, Society for Vascular Medicine and Biology, Society of Interventional Radiology, and the ACC/AHA Task Force on Practice Guidelines (Writing Committee to Develop Guidelines for the Management of Patients With Peripheral Arterial Disease). *Circulation.* 2006;21; 113: e525–e557.

13. Hirsch AT, Haskal ZJ, Hertzer NR, et al. ACC/AHA 2005 Practice Guidelines for the management of patients with peripheral arterial disease (lower extremity, renal, mesenteric, and abdominal aortic): a collaborative report from the American Association for Vascular Surgery/Society for Vascular Surgery, Society for Cardiovascular Angiography and Interventions, Society for Vascular Medicine and Biology, Society of Interventional Radiology, and the ACC/AHA Task Force on Practice Guidelines (Writing Committee to Develop Guidelines for the Management of Patients With Peripheral Arterial Disease). *Circulation.* 2006; 21;e527–e533.

14. Hirsch AT, Haskal ZJ, Hertzer NR, et al. ACC/AHA 2005 Practice Guidelines for the management of patients with peripheral arterial disease (lower extremity, renal, mesenteric, and abdominal aortic): a collaborative report from the American Association for Vascular Surgery/Society for Vascular Surgery, Society for Cardiovascular Angiography and Interventions, Society for Vascular Medicine and Biology, Society of Interventional Radiology, and the ACC/AHA Task Force on Practice Guidelines (Writing Committee to Develop Guidelines for the Management of Patients With Peripheral Arterial Disease). *Circulation.* 2006;21; 113:e547–e557.

15. Warkentin TE, Greinacher A. Review heparin-induced thrombocytopenia: recognition, treatment, and prevention: the Seventh ACCP Conference on Antithrombotic and Thrombolytic Therapy. *Chest.* 2004;126;311S–317S.

16. Warkentin TE, Greinacher A. Heparin-induced thrombocytopenia: recognition, treatment, and prevention: the Seventh ACCP Conference on Antithrombotic and Thrombolytic Therapy. *Chest.* 2004;126;311–337.

17. Wigley FM. Raynaud's phenomenon. *N Engl J Med.* 2002;347:1001–1008.

18. Creager MA, Dzau VJ, Loscalzo J. *Vascular Medicine: A Companion to Braunwald's Heart Disease.* Elsevier Health Sciences; Philadelphia, PA. 2006:689–706.

19. Hoeper MM, Mayer E, Simonneau G, et al. Chronic thromboembolic pulmonary hypertension. *Circulation.* 2006;113:2011–2020.

20. Ely JW, Osheroff JA, Chambliss ML, et al. Approach to leg edema of uncertain etiology. *J Am Board Fam Med.* 2006;19:148–160.

21. Eberhardt RT, Raffetto JD. Chronic venous insufficiency. *Circulation.* 2005;111:2398–2409.

22. Buller HR, Agnelli G, Hull RD, et al. Antithrombotic therapy for venous thromboembolic disease: the Seventh ACCP Conference on Antithrombotic and Thrombolytic Therapy. *Chest.* 2004;126:401S–428S.

23. Bates SM, Greer IA, Hirsh J, et al. See use of antithrombotic agents during pregnancy: the Seventh ACCP Conference on Antithrombotic and Thrombolytic Therapy, Section 5.0. *Chest.* 2004;126:627S–644S.

24. Young JR, Olin JW, Bartholomew JR, eds. *Peripheral Vascular Diseases,* 2nd ed. St. Louis, Mosby; 1996:614–617.

25. Hann CH, Streiff MB. The role of vena cava filters in the management of venous thromboembolism. *Blood Rev.* 2005;19:179–202.

26. Creager MA, Dzau VJ, Loscalzo J, eds. *Vascular Medicine: A Companion to Brunwald's Heart Disease.* Philadelphia, PA: Saunders; 2006:159160.

27. The Sixth ACCP Conference on Antithrombotic and Thrombolytic Therapy: evidence-based guidelines. *Chest Suppl.* 2001;119:176S–193S.

28. Creager MA, Dzau VJ, Loscalzo J, eds. *Vascular Medicine: A Companion to Brunwald's Heart Disease.* Philadelphia, PA: Saunders; 2006:641–654.

29. Cil BE, Akpinar E, Karcaaltincaba M, et al. Case 76: May-Thurner syndrome. *Radiology.* 2004;233:361–365.

30. Takahaski PY, Kiemele LJ, Jones JP. Wound care for elderly patients: advances and clinical applications for practicing physicians. *Mayo Clin Proc.* 2004;79:260–267.

31. Dewald CL, Jensen CC, Park YH, et al. Vena cavography with $CO_2$ versus iodinated contrast material for IVC filter placement: a prospective evaluation. *Radiology.* 2000;216:752–756.

32. The Seventh ACCP Conference on Antithrombotic and Thrombolytic Therapy: evidence-based guidelines. *Chest Suppl.* 2004;(126):413S.

33. Lee AYY, Levine MN, Baker RI, et al. Low-molecular-weight heparin versus coumadin for the prevention of recurrent venous thromboembolism in patients with cancer. *N Engl J Med.* 2003;349:146–153.

34. The Seventh ACCP Conference on Antithrombotic and Thrombolytic Therapy: evidence-based guidelines. *Chest Suppl.* 2004;(126):371S.

**NOTES**

# chapter 8

# Congestive Heart Failure

GARY S. FRANCIS · LESLIE CHO

## QUESTIONS

1. Which of the following characterizes heart failure?
   a. downregulation of $\beta_1$- and $\beta_2$-receptors
   b. downregulation primarily of $\beta_1$-receptors with little change in $\beta_2$-receptors
   c. downregulation of G proteins and $\beta_1$- and $\beta_2$-receptors
   d. increase in myocardial norepinephrine stores
   e. intact baroreceptor function

2. Which of the following treatments most consistently improves EF in patients who have systolic heart failure?
   a. diuretics
   b. beta-blockers
   c. ACE inhibitors
   d. vasodilators
   e. all of the above

3. When used chronically, all of the following drugs increase mortality *except*
   a. milrinone
   b. dobutamine
   c. vesnarinone
   d. xamoterol
   e. amlodipine

4. In the Veterans Administration Heart Failure Trial II (V-HeFT II), which combination of medications improved LV function and exercise tolerance?
   a. ACE inhibitors
   b. hydralazine plus nitrates
   c. ACE inhibitor plus hydralazine plus nitrates
   d. ACE inhibitor plus nitrates

5. A 56-year-old man presents to your clinic for follow-up after being discharged from the hospital 6 weeks ago. He underwent a successful primary angioplasty for acute anterior MI; however, his EF is now 40%. He is currently taking simvastatin (Zocor), acetylsalicylic aspirin, clopidogrel bisulfate (Plavix), metoprolol tartrate (Lopressor), and losartan (Cozaar). He states that he cannot afford all of these medications. He would like to know which medications are essential for a longer life. Which medications should you tell him are essential?
   a. all of them
   b. all of them except clopidogrel bisulfate
   c. all of them except losartan
   d. all except clopidogrel bisulfate and losartan

6. A 23-year-old woman presents to your clinic 8 weeks after delivery for a second opinion. She was diagnosed with peripartum cardiomyopathy, and her EF is 25%. She has been doing well and wants to know her prognosis. She is currently on an ACE inhibitor and a beta-blocker. She is not breast-feeding. What advice should you give her?

   a. Her EF will be 25%. She will need lifelong ACE inhibitors and beta-blockers.
   b. She is likely to make a full recovery and will not need any intervention.
   c. She has a 50% chance of recovery. If a TTE in 8 weeks shows abnormal EF, then she most likely will not recover.
   d. None of the above is your advice.

7. A 78-year-old woman with CHF (EF, 25%), chronic AFib, gastroesophageal reflux disease, hypertension (HTN), hyperlipidemia, diabetes, and osteoporosis takes 12 different pills. At the recent senior citizen day at the local church, a nurse told her that she does not need to take digoxin because she is on amiodarone. She wants to eliminate digoxin from her medication regimen, and she wants to know why you put her on it in the first place. What is your answer?

   a. Digoxin improves survival.
   b. Digoxin reduces hospitalization.
   c. Digoxin improves contractility.
   d. Digoxin decreases the volume of distribution of amiodarone.
   e. Digoxin reduces sympathetic nervous system activity.

8. Recently, a 43-year-old lawyer received heart transplantation. His hospital course was unremarkable, and he was discharged. He found out from the heart failure nurses that allograft vasculopathy is the leading cause of long-term morbidity and mortality in transplant patients. He wants to know what proven treatments prevent allograft vasculopathy. Which of the following treatments should you recommend?

   a. annual cardiac catheterization, intravascular ultrasound, and percutaneous coronary intervention (PCI), as needed
   b. annual stress test
   c. biannual stress test
   d. statins
   e. no known treatment

9. The following neurohormones are associated with vasoconstriction, cell growth, hypertrophy, and sodium retention *except*

   a. angiotensin II
   b. norepinephrine
   c. brain natriuretic peptide (BNP)
   d. endothelin
   e. arginine vasopressin

10. BNP has which of the following properties?

    a. Urine volume increases.
    b. Sodium excretion is enhanced.
    c. More BNP is secreted.
    d. A decrease in plasma aldosterone concentration occurs.
    e. All of the above occur.
    f. None of the above occurs.

11. A 34-year-old woman with dilated cardiomyopathy is admitted to the coronary care unit (CCU) for heart failure exacerbation. On examination, her respiratory rate is 25 with distended neck vein and prominent $S_3$. In addition to aggressive diuresis, a decision was made to start nesiritide (Natrecor). After the infusion, you notice hemodynamic changes. Which of the following changes is not related to the effects of nesiritide?

**a.** decrease in heart rate (HR)

**b.** decrease in BP

**c.** reduction in pulmonary capillary wedge pressure (PCWP)

**d.** no change in stroke volume index

**e.** all of the above

**f.** none of the above

**12.** A 72-year-old woman is transferred from another hospital. She was initially admitted with palpitation, diagnosed with AFib, and treated with amiodarone. A TTE showed an EF of 10% with a regional wall motion abnormality. She underwent cardiac catheterization and was found to have a heavily calcified 80% lesion in the mid–left anterior descending artery (LAD), a 40% lesion in a nondominant circumflex, and an 80% lesion in the posterior descending artery. Her children want to know what you plan to do for her. What should you recommend?

**a.** She has terrible EF and should be on medication only because coronary artery bypass graft (CABG) would be too high risk.

**b.** She should undergo PCI because she is too high risk for CABG.

**c.** She should undergo CABG because this is the definitive treatment.

**d.** She should have a positron emission tomography (PET) scan to assess the area of viability before proceeding with CABG or PCI.

**13.** A 53-year-old woman with a history of CHF presents to the emergency room (ER). She is cool and clammy. She reports being short of breath. Her BP is 71/40 mm Hg, her HR is 110 bpm, and her respiratory rate is 30. She has elevated neck veins and a prominent $S_3$. Her ECG shows sinus tachycardia. She is admitted to the CCU with heart failure. A PA catheterization is performed, and her hemodynamics are as follows: right atrial pressure, 12 mm Hg; PA pressure, 62/30 mm Hg; cardiac output, 1.9 L/minute/m²; PCWP, 36 mm Hg; and systemic vascular resistance (SVR), 2,000 dyne/second/cm⁵. Which of the following is your next step?

**a.** Start furosemide (Lasix).

**b.** Start dopamine.

**c.** Insert IABP.

**d.** Begin dobutamine.

**e.** Start nesiritide.

**14.** This patient continues to deteriorate after your initial treatment. Her BP is 64/32 mm Hg, and her HR is 132 bpm. She is now intubated on maximal pressor support and has an IABP in place. Which of the following should be your next therapeutic option?

**a.** There is no option. She is on maximal therapy.

**b.** Consider emergent cardiac transplant.

**c.** Consider LV assist device.

**d.** Consider cardiopulmonary bypass.

**15.** A 35-year-old man with a history of HTN presents to the ER in respiratory distress. He is intubated in the ER for respiratory distress. His BP is 73/48 mm Hg, his HR is 130 bpm, and his respiratory rate is 20. He is taken to the medical ICU, and a PA catheterization is performed. His hemodynamics are as follows: RA pressure, 22 mm Hg; PA pressure, 20/10 mm Hg; cardiac output, 3.5 L/minute/m²; PCWP, 12 mm Hg; and SVR, 1,690 dyne/second/cm⁵. What is your diagnosis?

**a.** pulmonary embolism

**b.** cardiogenic shock

**c.** acute RV failure

**d.** decompensated heart failure

**e.** hypovolemic shock

**16.** You receive a call from a cardiologist in a small community hospital regarding a patient in heart failure. She states that the patient was admitted last night with heart failure and was started on IV nitroglycerin; IV furosemide infusion;

captopril, 12.5 mg t.i.d.; and digoxin. There has been no improvement; therefore, the cardiologist placed a Swan-Ganz catheter this morning. The patient's hemodynamics are as follows: BP, 120/89 mm Hg; HR, 89 bpm; cardiac output, 2.0 L/minute/$m^2$; PCWP, 29 mm Hg; and SVR, 1,766 dyne/second/$cm^5$. The cardiologist also added dobutamine. Which of the following additional therapies should you recommend to the cardiologist for this patient?

a. Begin patient transfer arrangement.

b. Suggest nitroprusside.

c. Suggest nesiritide.

d. Suggest dopamine.

e. Suggest IABP.

17. A 57-year-old woman, who experienced inferior wall MI in 1992, has an EF of 30% and was diagnosed with nonsustained VT (four beats of VT) at another hospital on a routine ECG that she needed before cataract surgery. She has been in excellent health and has never been hospitalized for CHF. She has never had palpitation or syncopal episodes. Her doctors advised her that she would need an implantable defibrillator. She does not agree and wants a second opinion. She wants to know if there is any evidence to support the implantable defibrillators. What is your advice?

a. Place an implantable defibrillator.

b. Do not place an implantable defibrillator: A single episode is probably insignificant.

c. Perform an EP study.

d. Begin beta-blockers with amiodarone.

18. A 49-year-old man is admitted with new-onset heart failure. He is diagnosed with dilated cardiomyopathy with an EF of 20%. On hospital day 1, he is diuresed and started on a regimen of furosemide, digoxin, acetylsalicylic aspirin, captopril, and simvastatin. A medical student wants to know why you did not start him on a beta-blocker. What is your explanation?

a. Beta-blockers have not been shown to decrease mortality in dilated cardiomyopathy patients. Only ischemic cardiomyopathy patients have derived benefit.

b. There have been several conflicting results from randomized trials; therefore, beta-blockers are not recommended as the first line of therapy.

c. Beta-blockers have been shown to improve survival but should only be used in patients with an EF greater than 25%.

d. Beta-blockers should be started in stable CHF patients.

19. The same medical student wants to know whether the patient should also be started on calcium channel blockers. What is your answer?

a. There has never been a study to demonstrate the benefit of calcium channel blockers.

b. Diltiazem has proved to be of small but significant benefit in nonischemic cardiomyopathy patients and should be started.

c. Calcium channel blockers should be started after discharge once the patient has stabilized.

d. Felodipine has proved to be of small benefit only in ischemic cardiomyopathy patients. This patient does not fit this criterion.

e. Amlodipine proved to be of small benefit in a New York Heart Association (NYHA) class III or IV patient with an EF <30%. This benefit was seen more in dilated cardiomyopathy patients.

20. A 24-year-old female medical student presents to urgent care with 5 days of fever and shortness of breath. She is diagnosed with a viral infection and sent home. Five months later during her physical examination class, she is found to have an $S_3$ by her fellow students. She presents to your office for a second opinion. On examination, she appears healthy and in no distress. Her BP is 96/50 mm Hg, with an HR of 71 bpm and a respiratory rate of 12. Her neck veins are not distended, and

her examination is unremarkable except for an enlarged heart. You do not appreciate an $S_3$. You order a TTE, which shows an EF of 20% with a dilated heart. There is no valvular abnormality. Which of the following is your recommendation?

a. Begin ACE inhibitor, beta-blockers, and steroid.

b. Begin ACE inhibitor and beta-blockers.

c. Begin ACE inhibitor, beta-blockers, diuretics, and digoxin.

d. Begin ACE inhibitor, beta-blockers, diuretics, and spironolactone.

e. She is well compensated; nothing needs to be done.

21. A 79-year-old man with diabetes, HTN, chronic renal insufficiency, and ischemic cardiomyopathy was recently admitted with CHF exacerbation. At home, he takes captopril, 75 mg t.i.d.; digoxin, 0.125 mg per day; furosemide, 60 mg b.i.d.; aspirin; and atorvastatin calcium (Lipitor). When admitted, he was in heart failure with elevated neck veins and $S_3$. During his admission, he was diuresed with IV furosemide and metolazone. His baseline creatinine was 1.7 and now is 2.5, with a BUN of 100. What is your next step?

a. Stop captopril.

b. Stop diuretics.

c. Rule out renal artery stenosis.

d. Stop aspirin and ACE.

22. The severity of symptomatic exercise limitation in heart failure

a. is caused by elevated PCWP

b. is caused by reduced blood flow to skeletal muscles

c. bears little relation to the severity of LV dysfunction

d. can be reversed by inotropic therapy

e. is related to markers of central hemodynamic disturbance

23. A 59-year-old woman with CHF and an EF of 30% comes to your office for follow-up. She is on carvedilol (Coreg), enalapril, aspirin, atorvastatin calcium, digoxin, and furosemide. She has been doing well without any rehospitalization. However, she wants to improve her exercise tolerance. What should you recommend?

a. cardiac transplantation

b. IV dobutamine

c. higher doses of ACE inhibitor

d. adding spironolactone

e. enrolling her in an exercise training program

24. Prognosis in heart failure correlates best with which of the following?

a. peak $\dot{V}O_2$ during exercise

b. $\dot{V}E/\dot{V}O_2$ slope during exercise

c. EF at rest

d. blood gases during exercise

e. myocardial contractility measurements

25. An 86-year-old woman is transferred from a nursing home in respiratory distress. She was found to be short of breath. On examination, she has labored breathing, and her BP is 62/34 mm Hg with an HR of 60 bpm. She is intubated in the ER and admitted to the CCU. She is started on norepinephrine and dopamine at high doses without significant effect. Her ECG shows sinus bradycardia but is otherwise unremarkable. Her CXR shows pulmonary edema. The nursing home calls and says that she has mistakenly received 100 mg IV metoprolol tartrate. Which of the following should be your next step?

a. glucagon and milrinone

b. glucagon and dobutamine

c. IABP

d. fluid resuscitation

e. transvenous pacemaker

**26.** A 62-year-old man with an EF of 20% and chronic renal insufficiency presents to your office for follow-up. He has non–insulin-dependent diabetes mellitus and has developed worsening renal failure caused by diabetes. His medication regimen includes a beta-blocker that is significantly affected by reduced renal function. Which of the following beta-blockers is he taking?

  **a.** propanolol
  **b.** atenolol
  **c.** carvedilol
  **d.** metoprolol
  **e.** sotalol

**27.** A 38-year-old patient with CHF is transferred from another hospital. You are doing rounds in the CCU while the clinicians are performing a TTE. They ask you to assess his LV function. You notice the E:A wave ratio is greater than 1.5, with an E-wave deceleration time of 120 milliseconds. Which of the following do you guess is his PCWP?

  **a.** PCWP is 12 mm Hg.
  **b.** PCWP is 18 mm Hg.
  **c.** PCWP is 26 mm Hg.
  **d.** You cannot tell from the E:A wave ratio and deceleration time.

**28.** For the patient in the previous question, the E:A wave ratio and the E-wave deceleration time indicate which of the following?

  **a.** low filling pressure and reduced LV compliance
  **b.** high filling pressure and increased LV compliance
  **c.** low filling pressure and increased LV compliance
  **d.** high filling pressure and reduced LV compliance

**29.** A 67-year-old patient with HTN, hyperlipidemia, and an EF of 45% comes to your office for a second opinion. He had an exercise test and was told that his HR recovery was abnormal. His physician told him not to worry *unless* his heart function deteriorates. He is not convinced and wants your opinion and treatment. What should you recommend?

  **a.** Abnormal HR recovery does not predict mortality in patients with an EF greater than 35%; therefore, no treatment is needed.
  **b.** Abnormal HR recovery predicts mortality only in patients after MI; therefore, no treatment is needed.
  **c.** Abnormal HR recovery predicts mortality in all patients; however, there is no treatment.
  **d.** Abnormal HR recovery predicts mortality in all patients, and exercise training is the treatment of choice.

**30.** All of the following are indications for heart transplantation *except*

  **a.** dilated cardiomyopathy
  **b.** diabetes
  **c.** hypertrophic cardiomyopathy
  **d.** age
  **e.** amyloid heart disease

**31.** A 41-year-old man presents to the CCU with CHF symptoms. On examination, he has elevated neck veins, severe peripheral edema, and $S_3$ gallop. He is started on medication and has improvement in all of his symptoms. He has a PET scan, which shows a large area of hibernating myocardium. His cardiac catheterization reveals mild disease in the right coronary artery, a focal 80% lesion in the circumflex, and a focal 70% lesion in the LAD. All of his lesions are type A American College of Cardiologists/American Heart Association score. His EF is 15%. According to randomized clinical trials, which of the following is the best treatment for this patient?

a. percutaneous transluminal coronary angioplasty (PTCA)/stent with abciximab and clopidogrel bisulfate

b. PTCA/stent with cardiothoracic surgery backup

c. CABG

d. PTCA/stent with abciximab and IABP

**32.** A 28-year-old woman comes to your office for a second opinion. She had peripartum cardiomyopathy and wants to get pregnant again. You obtain a TTE, which shows a normal LV. What should you recommend?

a. She should not have another pregnancy because she is likely to have recurrent cardiomyopathy.

b. She may conceive again because her LV is normal. Her chance of having recurrent cardiomyopathy is less than 5%.

c. She may conceive again because her LV is normal. However, her chance of having recurrent cardiomyopathy is 30% to 50%.

d. She should undergo exercise testing for better assessment.

**33.** Primary causes of diastolic heart failure include all of the following *except*

a. hypertrophic cardiomyopathy

b. dilated cardiomyopathy

c. HTN

d. MI

e. infiltrative cardiomyopathy

**34.** A 78-year-old retired federal judge comes to your office for follow-up. He has long-standing HTN and has undergone PTCA/stent for a mid-LAD lesion. He has normal LV function and is active and healthy. Currently, he is on ramipril (Altace), atorvastatin, and aspirin. He heard on television that the combination of aspirin and ramipril increases mortality. He wants your opinion. What is your answer?

a. These are only observational studies, and they have not been proven. Continue the current regimen.

b. There are randomized studies to support this; however, the sample size was too small to make any conclusive recommendations. Continue the current regimen.

c. This has been shown in large trials; we should change aspirin to clopidogrel bisulfate or ramipril to metoprolol tartrate.

d. Although this has been seen in retrospective trials, it has not been validated in a randomized trial; therefore, continue the current regimen.

**35.** A 56-year-old man with dilated cardiomyopathy with an EF of 15% comes to your office for an opinion regarding medication. He is in NYHA class II and wants to know about biventricular pacing. He heard on television news that this may save lives. His ECG shows a sinus rate of 71, a PR interval of 210 milliseconds, a QRS duration of 188 milliseconds, and a QT/$QT_C$ of 364:427 milliseconds. What should you recommend?

a. Refer the patient for biventricular pacing based on PR interval.

b. Refer the patient for biventricular pacing based on QRS duration.

c. Refer the patient for biventricular pacing based on QT/$QT_C$ interval.

d. Refer the patient for exercise test to further assess.

**36.** A 31-year-old woman with hypertrophic cardiomyopathy presents to your office for follow-up. She has been doing well. She denies any palpitation or syncope. She has researched her disease on the Web and found out that most people die of arrhythmia. She would like to have an EP study. Which of the following is the predictive value of the EP study for ventricular arrhythmia?

a. 20%

b. 40%

c. 50%

d. 80%

e. 100%

**37.** A 61-year-old woman with an EF of 50% is admitted with an AFib with rapid ventricular response. She is started on metoprolol tartrate with excellent rate control and heparin. Her daughter, who is a nurse, wants to know why you did not start her on dofetilide because this is the best new drug. What is your response?

   **a.** Dofetilide showed increased mortality when compared to amiodarone and would be a bad choice for her mother.
   **b.** Dofetilide had safety and efficacy comparable to those of beta-blockers.
   **c.** Dofetilide was used in patients with an EF less than 35%.
   **d.** Dofetilide has safety and efficacy comparable to those of calcium channel blockers.
   **e.** Dofetilide is reserved for patients with chronic renal insufficiency.

**38.** A 79-year-old woman with HTN and non–insulin-dependent diabetes mellitus comes to your office for a second opinion. She is doing well and is currently on enalapril, aspirin, simvastatin, glipizide, and metformin. She read in her monthly American Association of Retired Persons newsletter that losartan is better than enalapril. She wants you to change her prescription. Based on trial data, which of the following is your recommendation?

   **a.** Losartan did not show mortality benefit but did show reduced hospitalization; because she has no history of CHF, there is no reason to change her medication.
   **b.** Losartan showed neither mortality benefit nor reduced hospitalization.
   **c.** Losartan did not show mortality benefit but decreased the risk of MI; therefore, she should have her prescription changed.
   **d.** Losartan did show mortality benefit, but only in patients younger than 60 years.

**39.** A 77-year-old man presents to the ER with shortness of breath. He is found to have an HR of 90 with a respiratory rate of 26. His BP is 110/63 mm Hg. His examination is remarkable for distended neck vein, $S_3$ gallop, edema, and ascites. His CXR shows pulmonary congestion. His ECG shows sinus rhythm and an old anterior MI. He is diuresed; on hospital day 4, he has a TTE. His TTE shows abnormal LV and RV diastolic function. Also, there is thickened myocardium, which appears to sparkle. He is diagnosed with amyloidosis. Which of the following is the treatment of choice for this patient?

   **a.** melphalan, prednisone, and colchicine
   **b.** cardiac transplantation
   **c.** pacer
   **d.** calcium channel blockers
   **e.** no known treatment available

## Questions 40–42

In Table 8–1, interpret the echocardiographic diastolic filling pattern:

**TABLE 8–1   Echocardiographic Diastolic Filling Patterns**

| Question | 40 | 41 | 42 |
|---|---|---|---|
| E:A wave ratio | 1.3 | 2.7 | 1.7 |
| Mitral deceleration time (msec) | 200 | 110 | 167 |
| Systolic/diastolic ratio | 1.6 | 0.5 | 0.9 |
| Isovolemic relaxation time (msec) | 80 | 40 | 82 |

   **a.** pseudonormal filling pattern
   **b.** restrictive filling pattern
   **c.** normal filling pattern

**43.** A 61-year-old woman with CHF and an EF of 25% is admitted with CHF exacerbation to your partner's service. On the day of discharge, your partner is sick, and you must explain her discharge medications. You explain to her the benefits of lisinopril, simvastatin, aspirin, digoxin, and furosemide. Finally, you want to explain the benefit of spironolactone (Aldactone) to her. What is your explanation?

   **a.** Spironolactone in addition to standard therapy (ACE inhibitor, diuretic) does not decrease mortality or morbidity.
   **b.** Spironolactone in addition to standard therapy only decreases rehospitalization— it does not improve NYHA functional class.
   **c.** Spironolactone in addition to standard therapy decreases mortality and rehospitalization.
   **d.** Spironolactone only benefits those not on standard therapy.

**44.** A 63-year-old man with non–insulin-dependent diabetes mellitus, HTN, hyperlipidemia, and chronic renal insufficiency is admitted with acute anterior wall MI 10 hours after symptom onset. He is taken emergently to the cardiac catheterization laboratory. He is noted to have proximal LAD occlusion, and he undergoes a successful PTCA/stent to the LAD with abciximab and heparin. His EF is noted to be 30% on a TTE performed 3 days later. On hospital day 4, he reports chest pain and is found to be in AFib with an HR of 121. His BP is 90/44 mm Hg, and he is short of breath and anxious. Which of the following should you administer next?

   **a.** procainamide
   **b.** lidocaine
   **c.** amiodarone
   **d.** metoprolol tartrate
   **e.** cardioversion

**45.** Common precipitating causes of acute decompensated heart failure include all of the following *except*

   **a.** exercise
   **b.** nonsteroidal anti-inflammatory drug use
   **c.** noncompliance with diet and medication
   **d.** infection
   **e.** trastuzumab (Herceptin)

**46.** An LV pressure volume loop is shown in Figure 8–1. Label A, B, C, and D.

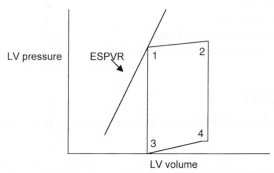

**FIGURE 8–1**  ESPVR, end-systolic pressure-volume relation. (From Little WC, Braunwald E. Assessment of cardiac function. In: Braunwald E, ed. *Heart Disease: A Textbook of Cardiovascular Medicine*, 5th ed. Philadelphia: WB Saunders; 1997, with permission.)

   **a.** mitral valve opening
   **b.** end-diastole
   **c.** aortic valve opening
   **d.** end-systole

**47.** A 57-year-old man with a history of CHF presents with acute pulmonary edema. His BP is 110/60 mm Hg with an HR of 92 bpm. His examination is consistent with heart failure. His hemodynamics are as follows: PA pressure, 62/27 mm Hg; PCWP, 12 mm Hg; cardiac output, 1.8 L/minute/m²; and SVR, 1,968 dyne/second/cm⁵. Which way should the LV pressure volume loop be shifted?

   **a.** to the right
   **b.** to the left
   **c.** up
   **d.** down

## Questions 48–52

In Figure 8–2, identify which drugs would have this effect on the same patient during hospitalization.

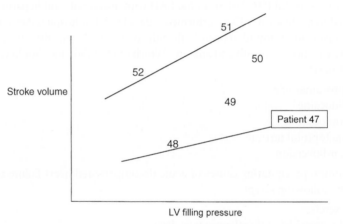

**FIGURE 8–2**   (From Smith TW, Kelly RA, Stevenson LW, et al. Management of heart failure. In: Braunwald E, ed. *Heart Disease: a Textbook of Cardiovascular Medicine*, 5th ed. Philadelphia: WB Saunders; 1997, with permission.)

   **a.** diuretic only
   **b.** vasodilator only
   **c.** inotropic agent only
   **d.** inotropic agent with vasodilator
   **e.** inotropic agent, vasodilator, and diuretic

## Questions 53–57

Figures 8–3 to 8–7 are schematic illustrations of the carotid pulse. Match the diagnosis with the pulse.

   **a.** normal
   **b.** aortic stenosis
   **c.** aortic regurgitation
   **d.** hypertrophic cardiomyopathy
   **e.** severe CHF decompensation

**53.**

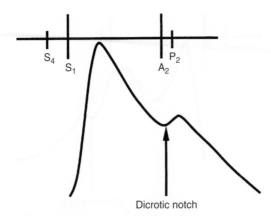

Dicrotic notch

**FIGURE 8–3**  (From Chatterjee K. Physical examination. In: Topol EJ, ed. *Textbook of Cardiovascular Medicine*, 2nd ed. Philadelphia: Lippincott Williams & Wilkins; 2002: Fig. 15.2, with permission.)

**54.**

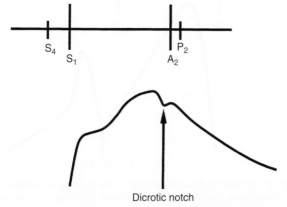

Dicrotic notch

**FIGURE 8–4**  (From Chatterjee K. Physical examination. In: Topol EJ, ed. *Textbook of Cardiovascular Medicine*, 2nd ed. Philadelphia: Lippincott Williams & Wilkins; 2002: Fig. 15.2, with permission.)

**55.**

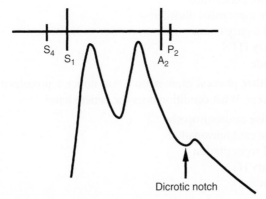

Dicrotic notch

**FIGURE 8–5**  (From Chatterjee K. Physical examination. In: Topol EJ, ed. *Textbook of Cardiovascular Medicine*, 2nd ed. Philadelphia: Lippincott Williams & Wilkins; 2002: Fig. 15.2, with permission.)

**56.**

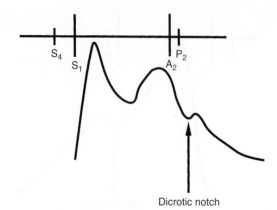

Dicrotic notch

**FIGURE 8–6**   (From Chatterjee K. Physical examination. In: Topol EJ, ed. *Textbook of Cardiovascular Medicine*, 2nd ed. Philadelphia: Lippincott Williams & Wilkins; 2002: Fig. 15.2, with permission.)

**57.**

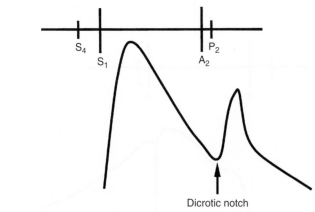

Dicrotic notch

**FIGURE 8–7**   (From Chatterjee K. Physical examination. In: Topol EJ, ed. *Textbook of Cardiovascular Medicine*, 2nd ed. Philadelphia: Lippincott Williams & Wilkins; 2002: Fig. 15.2, with permission.)

**58.** During physical examination, you notice an elevated systemic *venous* pressure with sharp *y* descent Kussmaul's sign and quiet pericardium. What might the patient have?

  **a.** constrictive pericarditis
  **b.** restrictive myocardial disorder
  **c.** tricuspid regurgitation
  **d.** pulmonary HTN
  **e.** tamponade

**59.** During another physical examination, you notice a prominent *v* wave with a sharp *y* descent. What condition does the patient have?

  **a.** constrictive cardiomyopathy
  **b.** restrictive cardiomyopathy
  **c.** tricuspid regurgitation
  **d.** pulmonary HTN
  **e.** tamponade

**60.** Again you notice an elevated systemic *venous* pressure without obvious *x* or *y* descent and quiet precordium and pulsus paradoxus. What does the patient have?

  **a.** constrictive cardiomyopathy
  **b.** restrictive cardiomyopathy
  **c.** tricuspid regurgitation
  **d.** pulmonary HTN
  **e.** tamponade

# ANSWERS

1. **b.** Downregulation primarily of $\beta_1$-receptors with little change in $\beta_2$-receptors.

2. **b.** Beta-blockers. Although ACE inhibitors have been shown to improve survival, they have not consistently been shown to improve EF in patients with systolic heart failure. Vasodilators and diuretics have not been shown to improve EF.

3. **e.** Amlodipine. Vasopressors have been found to increase mortality when taken chronically. Amlodipine did not increase mortality in the Prospective Randomized Amlodipine Survival Evaluation trial.

4. **b.** Hydralazine plus nitrates. In the V-HeFT II, although ACE inhibitors improved survival, it was hydralazine in combination with nitrates that had greater improvement in LV function and exercise tolerance.

5. **c.** All of them except losartan. There is no trial evidence that angiotensin II-receptor blocker improved mortality in post-MI patients. The Studies of Left Ventricular Dysfunction (SOLVD) prevention used ACE inhibitors in patients with an EF less than 35%.

6. **d.** None of the above is your advice. Approximately 50% of patients spontaneously recover in 6 months. Improvement after that time is unlikely. While the patient is waiting, she should be placed on the usual CHF medications, including ACE inhibitors and beta-blockers, and discouraged from breast-feeding.

7. **b.** Digoxin reduces hospitalization. In the large Digitalis Investigation Group study, digitalis only improved hospitalization. It had no effect on survival.

8. **e.** No known treatment. Allograft vasculopathy is the leading cause of long-term morbidity and mortality for cardiac transplant patients. Routine cardiac catheterization has been advocated for these patients but has not shown survival benefit with revascularization. Statin therapy appears to improve long-term survival in these patients and should be used for all heart transplant patients. However, its effect on allograft vasculopathy is unknown.

9. **c.** BNP. The release of BNP is a result of increased myocardial stretch in the ventricle. Plasma levels of BNP mainly reflect the degree of LV overload. Like atrial natriuretic factor, both C-type natriuretic peptide and BNP can elicit vasorelaxant activity.

10. **e.** All of the above occur. BNP has all of the above characteristics in addition to being a vasorelaxant.

11. **a.** Decrease in HR. BNP increases HR. All of the others are effects of BNP on hemodynamic parameters.

12. **d.** She should have a PET scan to assess the area of viability before proceeding with CABG or PCI. This patient is at high risk for any type of intervention because of her low EF. However, if there are areas of viability on the PET scan, her EF might improve with complete revascularization. Studies have consistently shown that patients with low EF do better with CABG than with PCI.

13. **b.** Start dopamine. This patient is in cardiogenic shock. She needs BP support before all else. In these patients, dopamine is the first line of choice, followed by norepinephrine. If there is no change with dopamine and norepinephrine, then dobutamine may be added while the patient is being prepared for IABP placement.

14. **c.** Consider LV assist device. This is a relatively young patient with no contraindication to cardiac transplant. However, in the current state, she is not eligible for transplantation. LV assist device as a bridge to transplant has been performed with success.

15. **c.** Acute RV failure. His hemodynamic pressures are characteristic of acute RV failure. He needs aggressive fluid resuscitation.

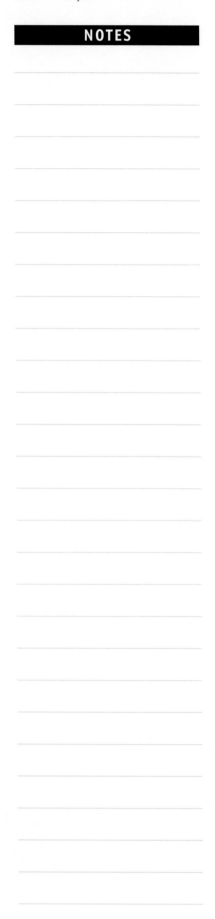

16. **b.** Suggest nitroprusside. This patient is in heart failure and needs to have her BP and SVR lowered. BP is adequate and does not need vasopressor or IABP support. Although nesiritide has been approved for use in acute heart failure, it only mildly lowers the BP.

17. **a.** Place an implantable defibrillator. She fits the criteria of the initial Multicenter Automatic Defibrillator Trial (MADIT). Therefore, based on randomized clinical trial data, she would benefit from an implantable defibrillator. Also, secondary prevention trials such as the Antiarrhythmics Versus Implantable Defibrillators Trial, the Canadian Implantable Defibrillator Study, and the Cardiac Arrest Study Hamburg trial also support an implantable defibrillator in this patient.

18. **d.** Beta-blockers should be started in stable CHF patients. They should not be started when the patient is congested. Although nonselective agents with vasodilating effects may be preferred, this is not clear at this time.

19. **e.** In the Prospective Randomized Amlodipine Survival Evaluation Trial, in which NYHA class III or IV patients with an EF less than 30% were enrolled, there was a statistically insignificant reduction in the combined mortality and morbidity in the amlodipine group. However, the benefit appeared to be greater in patients with nonischemic cardiomyopathy.

20. **b.** Begin ACE inhibitor and beta-blockers. She has well-compensated cardiomyopathy. Only medication that prolongs her life needs to be started. She does not need medication for symptom relief; therefore, ACE inhibitor and beta-blockers should be started.

21. **b.** Stop diuretics. This patient has prerenal azotemia caused by aggressive diuresis. His renal function should recover.

22. **c.** Bears little relation to the severity of LV dysfunction. Short-term administration of positive inotropic agents and vasodilators does not improve maximal exercise capacity in patients with CHF. Moreover, ACE inhibitors have failed to show consistent improvement in exercise tolerance. Numerous studies have not shown a correlation between LV function and exercise tolerance.

23. **e.** Enrolling her in an exercise training program. As stated, there is no medication that has consistently shown improvement in exercise tolerance; exercise training is the only method that has shown consistent improvement in these patients.

24. **b.** $\dot{V}E/\dot{V}O_2$ slope during exercise. This is the best correlate of prognosis. There is a higher ventilation for any given $CO_2$ production ($\dot{V}E/\dot{V}O_2$ slope), which reflects the severity of heart failure and prognosis.

25. **a.** Glucagon and milrinone. Milrinone is a second-generation phosphodiesterase inhibitor. It has no beta effect; therefore, it is an ideal vasopressor in the setting of beta-blocker overdose. Although a pacer is a good idea and should be placed, giving medication is faster and should be instituted first.

26. **b.** Atenolol. Atenolol is most affected by reduced renal function. Depending on how severe his creatinine clearance is, he should have his medication dose or frequency adjusted.

27. **c.** PCWP is 26 mm Hg. Restrictive mitral inflow pattern in the presence of a short E-wave deceleration time has been shown to correlate with high pulmonary capillary pressure, impaired functional class, and bad prognosis in postinfarction patients.

28. **d.** High filling pressure and reduced LV compliance. These conditions are indicated by a restrictive mitral inflow pattern with short E-wave deceleration time.

29. **c.** Abnormal HR recovery predicts mortality in all patients; however, there is no treatment. A delayed decrease in HR after exercise or an abnormal HR recovery predicts all-cause mortality in healthy adults and in patients referred for exercise testing—independent of ischemia. However, at this time, there is no treatment to improve abnormal HR recovery.

**30. e.** Amyloid heart disease. Although severe diabetes and age older than 70 years are exclusion criteria for transplantation, diabetes without end-organ damage and age from 60 to 70 years are not.

**31. c.** CABG. This patient has left main trunk equivalent with low EF. He is a candidate for CABG with left internal mammary artery to the LAD. CABG will prolong his long-term survival compared to PTCA/stent.

**32. d.** She should undergo exercise testing for better assessment. Recurrent peripartum cardiomyopathy occurs in 20% of patients with normal resting LV function but abnormal stress ventricular response. Recurrent peripartum cardiomyopathy with decompensation occurred in 41% of patients with abnormal resting LV function.

**33. b.** Dilated cardiomyopathy. All of the others may cause diastolic heart failure, whereas dilated cardiomyopathy causes systolic heart failure.

**34. d.** Although this has been seen in retrospective trials, it has not been validated in a randomized trial; therefore, continue the current regimen. In a substudy done by the Gruppo Italiano per lo Studio della Sopravvivenza nell'Infarto Miocardico, aspirin did not decrease the mortality benefit of lisinopril after MI or increase the risk of adverse clinical events. There have been some retrospective studies to assess this question that have had conflicting results; therefore, it is best to stay with the current regimen.

**35. b.** Refer the patient for biventricular pacing based on QRS duration. Patients with QRS duration greater than 150 to 160 milliseconds derived the greatest benefit from biventricular pacing.

**36. a.** 20%. There is no role for routine EP study in the asymptomatic hypertrophic cardiomyopathy patient.

**37. c.** Dofetilide was used in patients with an EF less than 35%. The study compared dofetilide to amiodarone. Dofetilide did not increase mortality. It has not been studied against beta-blockers or calcium channel blockers in patients with normal EF.

**38. b.** In the large Evaluation of Losartan in the Elderly II study, losartan did not show mortality benefit or reduced hospitalization. Losartan was better tolerated than captopril. Because the patient has no side effects with enalapril, her prescription should not be changed.

**39. e.** No known treatment available. There have been two randomized trials of chemotherapy showing benefit in amyloid patients with melphalan, prednisone, and colchicine when the major features were not cardiac or renal. For patients with cardiac manifestation, no treatment has shown clear benefit.

**40. c.** Normal filling pattern.

**41. b.** Restrictive filling pattern.

**42. a.** Pseudonormal filling pattern.

**43. c.** Spironolactone in addition to standard therapy decreases mortality and rehospitalization. In the Randomized Aldactone Evaluation Study, patients with NYHA class III or IV with an EF less than 35% had improvement in mortality, reduction in hospitalization, and improvement in functional class when spironolactone was taken in addition to standard therapy (ACE inhibitor and diuretic).

**44. e.** Cardioversion. This patient has post-MI AFib. He has LV dysfunction and renal insufficiency. Procainamide should be used in patients with normal LV and renal clearance. Amiodarone would take too long to work, and he is already in distress. Lidocaine is not used in AFib. Metoprolol tartrate would exacerbate his heart failure; therefore, cardioversion is the only choice.

**45. a.** Exercise. Exercise is recommended in patients with stable heart failure. Nonsteroidal anti-inflammatory drugs, trastuzumab (Herceptin), infection, and noncompliance are well-known causes of acute decompensated heart failure.

**NOTES**

**46.** An LV pressure volume loop.
   **a.** = 1. mitral valve opening
   **b.** = 2. end-diastole
   **c.** = 3. aortic valve opening
   **d.** = 4. end-systole

**47. c.** Up. The response of the LV to increased afterload is to shift the loop up. Increased preload would shift the loop to the right.

**48. a.** Diuretic only. This loop represents a Frank-Starling ventricular function curve in a heart failure patient because of systolic dysfunction.

**49. b.** Vasodilator only.

**50. c.** Inotropic agent only.

**51. d.** Inotropic agent with vasodilator.

**52. e.** Inotropic agent, vasodilator, and diuretic.

**53. a.** Normal.

**54. b.** Aortic stenosis.

**55. c.** Aortic regurgitation.

**56. d.** Hypertrophic cardiomyopathy.

**57. e.** Severe CHF decompensation.

**58. a.** Constrictive pericarditis.

**59. c.** Tricuspid regurgitation.

**60. e.** Tamponade.

## Suggested Reading

Braunwald E, Coluccci WS, Grossman W. Clinical aspects of heart failure: high output heart failure: pulmonary edema. In: Braunwald E, ed. *Heart Disease: A Textbook of Cardiovascular Medicine*, 5th ed. Philadelphia: WB Saunders; 1997.

Chatterjee K. Physical examination. In: Topol EJ, ed. *Textbook of Cardiovascular Medicine*, 2nd ed. Philadelphia: Lippincott Williams & Wilkins; 2002.

Francis G. Pathophysiology of the heart failure clinical syndrome. In: Topol EJ, ed. *Textbook of Cardiovascular Medicine*, 2nd ed. Philadelphia: Lippincott Williams & Wilkins; 2002.

Haas GJ, Young JB. Acute heart failure management. In: Topol EJ, ed. *Textbook of Cardiovascular Medicine*, 2nd ed. Philadelphia: Lippincott Williams & Wilkins; 2002.

Smith TW, Kelly RA, Stevenson LW, et al. Management of heart failure. In: Braunwald E, ed. *Heart Disease: A Textbook of Cardiovascular Medicine*, 5th ed. Philadelphia: WB Saunders; 1997.

Young JB. Chronic heart failure management. In: Topol EJ, ed. *Textbook of Cardiovascular Medicine*, 2nd ed. Philadelphia: Lippincott Williams & Wilkins; 2002.

# Adult Congenital Heart Disease

## Part A

SASAN GHAFFARI · RAYMOND Q. MIGRINO

## QUESTIONS

1. What is the most common coexisting congenital anomaly in patients with coarctation of the aorta?

   a. cleft mitral valve
   b. bicuspid aortic valve
   c. Ebstein's anomaly
   d. VSD
   e. patent ductus arteriosus (PDA)

2. All of the following are characteristic findings of ostium primum atrial septal defect (ASD) *except*

   a. precordial heave
   b. fixed split $S_2$
   c. right-axis deviation
   d. systolic ejection murmur
   e. prominent pulmonary vascular markings on CXR

3. All of the following are complications of unrecognized coarctation of the aorta *except*

   a. aortic dissection
   b. cerebrovascular aneurysms
   c. CHF
   d. LV hypertrophy
   e. SVT

4. All of the following statements are true regarding bicuspid aortic valve *except*

   a. In approximately 20% of cases, there are associated congenital conditions, such as coarctation of the aorta.
   b. A coexisting abnormality in the medial layer of the aorta causes dilatation of the aortic root.
   c. It is associated with diminished life expectancy.
   d. It is more common in males than females.
   e. With aortic valve stenosis, percutaneous balloon valvotomy has good short-term results in children but not in adults.

5. All of the following statements regarding pulmonary stenosis are true *except*

   a. Balloon valvuloplasty is the procedure of choice and has good long-term results.
   b. The majority of cases are subvalvular or supravalvular in location.
   c. Valve replacement is usually reserved for dysplastic and calcified leaflets or for cases with significant regurgitation.

**NOTES**

**d.** Among patients with valvular stenosis, only approximately 10% to 15% of cases have dysplastic leaflets.

**e.** Adults are usually asymptomatic when first diagnosed.

6. A 19-year-old man seeks your advice regarding profound dyspnea on exertion. He was born cyanotic, and he has not had regular follow-up. On examination, there is significant clubbing and cyanosis of all digits. There is RV lift, with a loud systolic ejection murmur in the left upper sternal border with a thrill. $P_2$ is absent. CXR demonstrates RV enlargement and pulmonary oligemia. His ECG reveals sinus rhythm with RV hypertrophy. Which of the following two-dimensional TTE findings will *not* be seen in this condition?

    **a.** pulmonary stenosis
    **b.** apical displacement of tricuspid leaflets
    **c.** RV hypertrophy
    **d.** overriding aorta
    **e.** VSD

7. The above patient undergoes surgical repair. Which of the following statements regarding long-term post-repair follow-up is *false*?

    **a.** The survival rate is 86% 32 years after surgery.
    **b.** Ventricular arrhythmias and sudden death pose long-term health hazards.
    **c.** On 12-lead ECG, a QRS duration of longer than 180 milliseconds is associated with VT.
    **d.** A palliative shunt is the preferred surgical strategy.
    **e.** He is at increased risk of infective endocarditis.

8. All of the following statements regarding PDA are true *except*

    **a.** The majority of cases close spontaneously after infancy.
    **b.** There is a higher incidence in mothers who acquired rubella during pregnancy.
    **c.** A decrease in the duration and intensity of the murmur has a poor prognostic implication.
    **d.** LV hypertrophy precedes RV hypertrophy.
    **e.** If it is uncorrected, approximately one third of patients die by the age of 40 years.

9. All of the following are found in cor triatriatum *except*

    **a.** pulmonary hypertension
    **b.** increased mitral orifice inflow velocity by pulsed-wave Doppler
    **c.** a double-chamber left atrium
    **d.** diastolic fluttering of the mitral leaflet
    **e.** a fibromuscular diaphragm inferior to the left atrial appendage

10. A 20-year-old asymptomatic man is referred for further evaluation of uncontrolled hypertension. He has a strong family history of premature hypertension. His vital signs reveal a left upper extremity BP of 150/100 mm Hg and a right lower extremity BP of 130/94 mm Hg. Heart rate is 88 bpm. His cardiac examination is remarkable for a 2/6 systolic ejection murmur in the right upper sternal border and an $S_4$ gallop. There is brachial-femoral pulse delay. The rest of the physical and neurologic examinations are within normal limits. A TTE confirmed a diagnosis of coarctation of the aorta, with a maximum gradient of 26 mm Hg. He has a bicuspid aortic valve with peak/mean gradients of 12/6 mm Hg and trivial aortic insufficiency. Cardiac catheterization reaffirms the transcoarctation gradient and demonstrates a narrowed segment in the descending aorta distal to origin of the subclavian artery. What is the most appropriate management strategy?

    **a.** surgical repair with end-to-end anastomosis
    **b.** percutaneous balloon angioplasty
    **c.** BP control that includes a beta-blocker agent
    **d.** EP testing for risk stratification
    **e.** repeat cardiac catheterization in 6 months

**11.** Congenital MR is commonly encountered in all of the following conditions *except*

    **a.** cor triatriatum

    **b.** ostium primum ASD

    **c.** coarctation of the aorta

    **d.** congenitally corrected transposition of the great arteries

    **e.** subaortic stenosis

**12.** Which of the following is the most common coronary artery anomaly?

    **a.** Bland-Garland-White syndrome (left main coronary artery arising from the PA)

    **b.** coronary arteriovenous fistula

    **c.** left circumflex artery arising from the right coronary artery

    **d.** left coronary artery arising from the right sinus of Valsalva

    **e.** coronary cameral fistula

**13.** Which of the following differentiates valvular aortic stenosis from subvalvular aortic stenosis?

    **a.** male preponderance

    **b.** surgical risk of repair

    **c.** dilatation of the ascending aorta

    **d.** aortic regurgitation

    **e.** valvular calcification

**14.** Besides pulmonary valve stenosis, which of the following is the most common associated cardiac defect present in patients with PA stenosis?

    **a.** VSD

    **b.** ASD

    **c.** coarctation of the aorta

    **d.** PDA

    **e.** bicuspid aortic valve

**15.** The following cardiovascular malformations are all associated with congenital rubella *except*

    **a.** PDA

    **b.** PA stenosis

    **c.** Ebstein's anomaly

    **d.** tetralogy of Fallot

    **e.** coarctation of the aorta

**16.** Which of the following statements about coronary arteriovenous fistula is *true*?

    **a.** The left coronary artery is most commonly involved.

    **b.** The fistula most commonly empties into the LV.

    **c.** Despite the success of surgical closure, the prognosis is still poor.

    **d.** Spontaneous closure rarely occurs.

    **e.** A large right-to-left shunt may cause CHF.

**17.** A 20-year-old asymptomatic man was diagnosed to have a subaortic membrane. The peak gradient across the membrane is 20 mm Hg. The aortic valve remains mobile, but there is associated moderate aortic valve insufficiency. What should you advise this patient?

    **a.** Elective surgical resection should be considered.

    **b.** TTE should be performed twice per year, and surgical correction is performed when the peak gradient across the membrane becomes >40 mm Hg.

    **c.** Transluminal balloon dilatation should be performed, because the long-term results are superior to surgical treatment.

    **d.** Endocarditis prophylaxis is not necessary.

    **e.** Surgical resection is rarely curative.

**18.** Which of the following syndromes is associated with pulmonary arteriovenous fistula?

  **a.** Williams syndrome
  **b.** Weber-Osler-Rendu syndrome
  **c.** Bland-Garland-White syndrome
  **d.** Kartagener's syndrome
  **e.** Crouzon's syndrome

**19.** In which of the following cases is surgical correction recommended?

  **a.** asymptomatic small VSD to decrease risk of endocarditis
  **b.** PDA with severe pulmonary hypertension
  **c.** asymptomatic subaortic stenosis with severe aortic valve insufficiency
  **d.** coarctation of the aorta with a transcoarctation gradient of 20 mm Hg
  **e.** small ASD to prevent paradoxical embolization

**20.** All of the following statements regarding anomalous pulmonary venous drainage are true *except*

  **a.** It is frequently associated with the secundum-type ASD.
  **b.** The degree of pulmonary hypertension depends on the number of anomalous veins involved.
  **c.** Oximetry is of limited value if the pulmonary vein drains into the inferior vena cava.
  **d.** It may be associated with VSD.
  **e.** TTE frequently misses this finding.

**21.** Which of the following is an indication for aortic surgical repair in patients with coarctation of the aorta?

  **a.** 50-mm Hg transcoarctation pressure gradient
  **b.** headaches
  **c.** chest pain
  **d.** presyncope
  **e.** right upper extremity claudication

**22.** All of the following statements regarding Ebstein's anomaly are true *except*

  **a.** The majority of patients have interatrial communication with potential for right-to-left shunting.
  **b.** There may be widely split $S_1$ and $S_2$ with triple or quadruple rhythm and a holosystolic murmur at the left lower sternal border.
  **c.** Approximately 20% of patients have ventricular pre-excitation or other forms of tachyarrhythmias.
  **d.** There is displacement of mitral leaflets into the LV.
  **e.** With valve replacement, bioprosthetic durability compares favorably with other cardiac valve positions.

**23.** A patient with congenitally corrected transposition may present with all of the following clinical features *except*

  **a.** CHB
  **b.** platypnea-orthodeoxia
  **c.** heart failure
  **d.** AV valve regurgitation
  **e.** supraventricular arrhythmias

**24.** Patients with Eisenmenger's syndrome should avoid all of the following *except*

  **a.** dehydration
  **b.** high altitude
  **c.** heavy exertion
  **d.** vasodilators
  **e.** phlebotomy

**25.** With which of the following adult congenital heart conditions can the following ECG tracing be seen (Fig. 9A–1)?

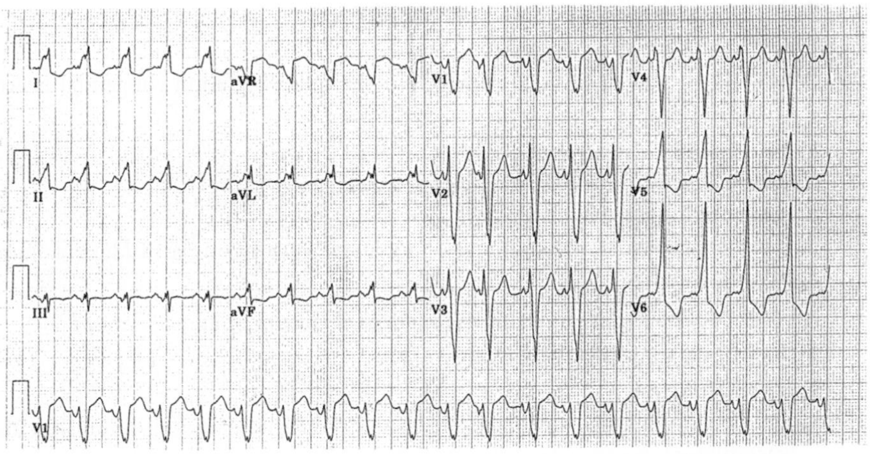

**FIGURE 9A–1**

    **a.** primum ASD
    **b.** congenitally corrected transposition
    **c.** Ebstein's anomaly
    **d.** VSD
    **e.** coarctation of the aorta

**26.** A 25-year-old man is referred to you for an abnormal heart sound. The patient is asymptomatic and very active. He has a continuous murmur at the left upper sternal border. A TTE reveals a small PDA with normal LV and RV and normal pulmonary pressures. How would the patient be best managed?

    **a.** ligation or closure of the PDA
    **b.** repeat TTE in 1 year
    **c.** stress TTE to determine LV enlargement or dysfunction postexercise
    **d.** endocarditis prophylaxis
    **e.** TEE

**27.** All of the following statements are consistent with the natural history of ASD *except*

    **a.** In the sixth decade, the mortality rate can approach 10%.
    **b.** Most patients are minimally symptomatic in the first three decades.
    **c.** LV dysfunction is unusual (<5%) in patients older than 50 years.
    **d.** The majority of patients are symptomatic by the fifth decade.
    **e.** Approximately one half of patients older than 40 years develop pulmonary hypertension.

**28.** A 30-year-old man with Eisenmenger's syndrome and irreversible pulmonary hypertension caused by untreated VSD is at risk for developing symptoms and signs of hyperviscosity. All of the following are associated with hyperviscosity syndrome *except*

    **a.** coronary artery ectasia
    **b.** erythrocytosis
    **c.** visual disturbances
    **d.** paresthesias
    **e.** iron-deficiency anemia

**29.** Bacterial endocarditis prophylaxis is indicated in all adults who have the following congenital heart diseases *except*

**NOTES**

a. VSD
b. coarctation of the aorta
c. secundum ASD
d. hypertrophic obstructive cardiomyopathy
e. PDA

30. Pregnancy should be avoided in which of the following adult congenital heart diseases?

a. Eisenmenger's syndrome
b. Marfan's syndrome with an enlarged aortic root
c. severe pulmonary hypertension
d. congenital aortic stenosis with New York Heart Association class III heart failure
e. all of the above

31. All of the following are indications for surgical closure of an ASD *except*

a. significant symptoms in a 65 year old
b. RV dysfunction
c. pulmonary vascular resistance >15 Wood units that does not diminish with vasodilators
d. an asymptomatic 20 year old with a Qp/Qs of 1.7 with no pulmonary hypertension
e. RV enlargement

32. All of the following statements regarding PDA are true *except*

a. The pulmonic bed is usually dilated.
b. The most common location is distal to the left subclavian artery.
c. Infectious endocarditis frequently occurs at the pulmonary end.
d. The risk of endocarditis is less in patients with inaudible PDA.
e. Transcatheter-device closure or coil occlusion is the procedure of choice for closure in adults.

33. All of the following physical examination findings are usually associated with ostium secundum ASD *except*

a. precordial heave
b. fixed split $S_2$
c. lateral and inferior displacement of the apex beat
d. soft systolic ejection murmur in the second left intercostal space
e. normal $S_1$

34. Which of the following is an absolute contraindication to pregnancy?

a. surgically corrected transposition of great arteries
b. congenitally corrected transposition of great arteries
c. Ebstein's anomaly
d. Eisenmenger's syndrome
e. status post Fontan operation

35. A 45-year-old man with known Ebstein's anomaly seeks your advice with regard to optimal management. He is asymptomatic and has an active lifestyle without any limitations. His physical examination is remarkable for the absence of cyanosis. He has a loud holosystolic murmur at the left lower sternal border that is accentuated with respiration. He has no organomegaly or peripheral edema. His TTE reveals moderately severe 3+ tricuspid regurgitation with an RV systolic pressure of 46 mm Hg and normal LV and RV systolic functions. There is no evidence of interatrial communication. Which of the following should you recommend?

a. furosemide and digoxin
b. tricuspid valve repair
c. tricuspid valve replacement
d. dual-chamber pacemaker
e. regular follow-up with repeat TTE in 6 months

## Questions 36–40

Match the following conditions with their corresponding surgical procedures. There may be more than one answer for each question.

    **a.** Ross
    **b.** Blalock-Taussig
    **c.** Senning or Mustard
    **d.** arterial switch
    **e.** Fontan
    **f.** Rashkind
    **g.** none of the above

**36.** Pulmonary atresia

**37.** Transposition of great vessels

**38.** Tricuspid atresia

**39.** Congenitally corrected transposition

**40.** Aortic stenosis

## Questions 41–45

Match the following disease conditions with their gender preponderance.

    **a.** predominantly male
    **b.** predominantly female
    **c.** equal preponderance

**41.** VSD

**42.** ASD

**43.** Bicuspid aortic valve

**44.** Coarctation of the aorta

**45.** Pulmonary atresia with an intact ventricular septum

## Questions 46–50

Match the following cardiac catheterization still-frame slides (Figs. 9A–2 through 9A–6) to their respective diagnoses.

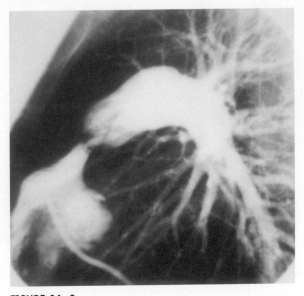

**FIGURE 9A–2**

NOTES

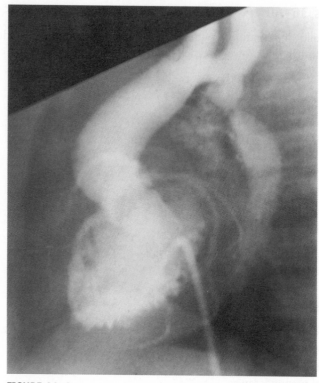

**FIGURE 9A–3**

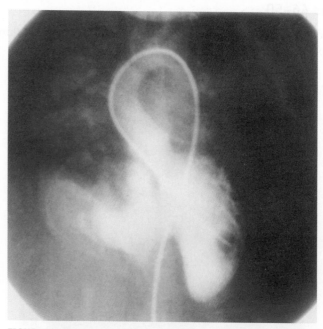

**FIGURE 9A–4**

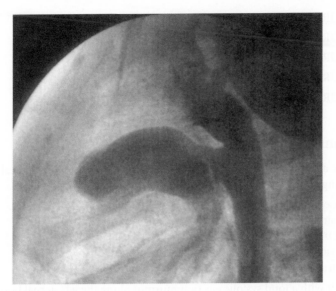

**FIGURE 9A–5**

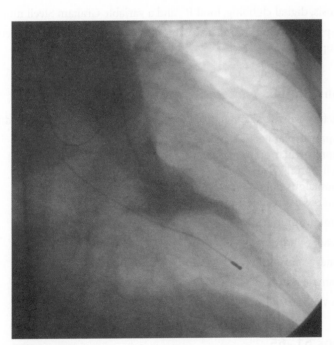

**FIGURE 9A–6**

**a.** coarctation of the aorta
**b.** PDA
**c.** hypertrophic cardiomyopathy
**d.** pulmonic stenosis
**e.** VSD

**NOTES**

46. FIGURE 9A–2
47. FIGURE 9A–3
48. FIGURE 9A–4
49. FIGURE 9A–5
50. FIGURE 9A–6

## Questions 51–55

Match the adult congenital heart disorder with the corresponding physical examination findings.

   **a.** Eisenmenger's syndrome
   **b.** coarctation of the aorta
   **c.** PDA
   **d.** Ebstein's anomaly
   **e.** tetralogy of Fallot

51. RV lift with a loud systolic ejection murmur along the left sternal border, with a single $S_2$

52. Loud $S_1$, holosystolic murmur in left lower sternal border, systolic ejection click, and hepatomegaly

53. Weak or delayed femoral arterial pulses, harsh systolic ejection murmur in the back, and a systolic ejection click in the aortic area

54. Cyanosis, digital clubbing, loud $P_2$, and a variable Graham Steell murmur

55. Wide pulse pressure, prominent LV impulse, and a continuous machinery murmur enveloping $S_2$

## Questions 56–60

Match the following congenital defects with their associated disease conditions.

   **a.** supravalvular aortic stenosis
   **b.** supravalvular pulmonic stenosis
   **c.** cleft mitral valve
   **d.** anomalous pulmonary venous drainage
   **e.** persistent left superior vena cava

56. Ostium primum ASD
57. Noonan's syndrome
58. Coronary sinus ASD
59. Williams syndrome
60. Sinus venosus ASD

## Questions 61–65

Match the characteristic chest radiography findings with the corresponding congenital disorder.

   **a.** Eisenmenger's syndrome
   **b.** coarctation of the aorta
   **c.** PDA
   **d.** Ebstein's anomaly
   **e.** tetralogy of Fallot

61. Prominent central PAs (possible calcifications) and peripheral PA pruning
62. Right aortic arch, RV enlargement, and a "boot-shaped" heart

**63.** Marked cardiomegaly, severe right atrial enlargement, and normal lung fields

**64.** Posterior rib notching and a "reverse E" or "3" sign

**65.** Pulmonary plethora, prominent ascending aorta, proximal PA dilatation, and opacity at the confluence of the aortic knob and descending aorta

## Questions 66–70

Match the following congenital cardiac disorder with the characteristic TTE finding (Figs. 9A–7 through 9A–11).

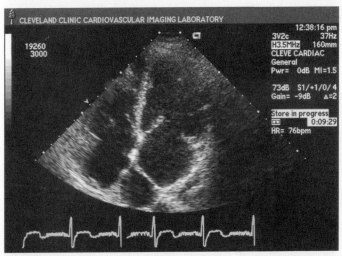

**FIGURE 9A–7**

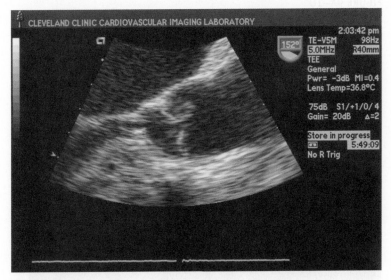

**FIGURE 9A–8**

NOTES

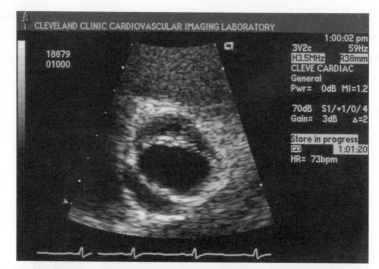

**FIGURE 9A–9**

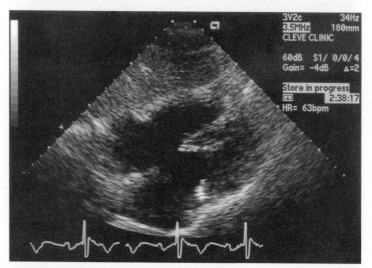

**FIGURE 9A–10**

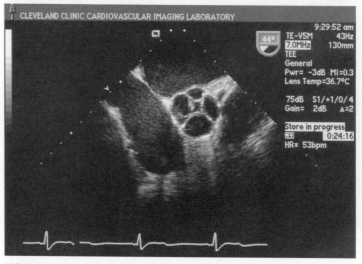

**FIGURE 9A–11**

    **a. FIGURE 9A–7**
    **b. FIGURE 9A–8**
    **c. FIGURE 9A–9**
    **d. FIGURE 9A–10**
    **e. FIGURE 9A–11**

**66.** Bicuspid aortic valve

**67.** Cor triatriatum

**68.** Ostium primum ASD

**69.** Quadricuspid aortic valve

**70.** Subaortic valve stenosis

# ANSWERS

1. **b.** Bicuspid aortic valve. Aortic coarctation is a common congenital defect that consists of a constriction just distal to the left subclavian artery at the site of residual ligamentum arteriosus. Bicuspid aortic valve is the most common coexisting anomaly. However, the presence of VSD, PDA, and malformations of the mitral valve apparatus is well documented. There is no association between aortic coarctation and Ebstein's anomaly.

2. **c.** Right-axis deviation is not a characteristic finding. Ostium primum ASD is usually associated with left-axis deviation. The other findings are characteristic physical and radiologic findings of ASD.

3. **e.** Unrecognized and untreated aortic coarctation causes premature death, with mean survival of 35 years and 75% mortality by age 50. Ninety percent of patients with this condition die before they reach the age of 60 years. Complications of aortic coarctation include systemic hypertension with LV hypertrophy, aortic dissection, premature CAD with MI, cerebral vascular complications, infective endocarditis, and CHF. SVT is most commonly associated with other congenital diseases, such as Ebstein's anomaly, ASD, or tetralogy of Fallot.

4. **c.** Asymptomatic adult patients have normal life expectancy. Bicuspid aortic valve has a male preponderance. In approximately 20% of cases, this condition is associated with congenital conditions, such as coarctation of the aorta and PDA. It is frequently associated with dilatation of the aortic root because of a congenital abnormality in the medial layer of the aorta. Percutaneous balloon valvotomy for congenital aortic stenosis has demonstrated good short-term results in children but not in adults.

5. **b.** Approximately 90% of cases are valvular in nature. Balloon valvuloplasty is the procedure of choice and has excellent long-term results. In approximately 10% to 15% of cases, the valve leaflets are dysplastic and may be thickened, immobile, or myxomatous. Valve replacement is reserved for dysplastic leaflets or if significant regurgitation is present. Adults are usually asymptomatic, and the condition is discovered through routine auscultation.

6. **b.** Apical displacement of tricuspid leaflets will not be seen in this condition. The most common cyanotic congenital heart defect is tetralogy of Fallot. The characteristic signs that are confirmed by two-dimensional TTE are obstruction of RV outflow tract (pulmonary stenosis), RV hypertrophy, an aorta that overrides the LV and RV, and a large VSD. Apical displacement of tricuspid leaflets is the hallmark of Ebstein's anomaly.

7. **d.** Surgical repair is recommended to patients with tetralogy of Fallot to relieve symptoms and improve survival. In one series, performed by Murphy et al., the rate of survival 32 years after surgery was 86% among patients with repaired tetralogy and 96% in an age-matched control population. Both supraventricular and ventricular arrhythmias are commonly seen in patients post-repair and are a significant cause of morbidity and mortality. Complete surgical correction with closure of VSD and relief of RV outflow obstruction is the preferred surgical strategy in the appropriate setting. Palliative shunting is performed in severely ill infants or in those patients who have underdeveloped PAs. Palliative surgery does not correct the underlying anatomic defects and is associated with long-term risk.

8. **a.** A PDA, unlike VSD, rarely closes spontaneously after infancy. It is associated with maternal rubella, perinatal hypoxemia, premature births, or births at high altitude. It causes left atrial and LV hypertrophy. With development of pulmonary hypertension, RV hypertrophy may develop, and the duration and intensity of the machinery murmur may diminish. Uncorrected, one third of patients die of heart failure, pulmonary hypertension, or endocarditis by the age of 40 years, and two thirds die by the age of 60 years.

9.  **e.** Fibromuscular diaphragm inferior to the left atrial appendage is not found in cor triatriatum. Cor triatriatum is a congenital disease that is characterized by the presence of a fibromuscular diaphragm in the left atrium that divides the left atrium into two chambers. It arises from the failure of resorption of the common pulmonary vein. There may be significant obstruction between the posterosuperior chamber that receives the pulmonary veins and the anteroinferior chamber that encompasses the left atrial appendage and the mitral valve. Pulmonary hypertension may result. The increased velocity across the diaphragm may cause diastolic fluttering of the mitral valve and increased flow through the distal atrial chamber and at the mitral orifice. The diaphragm arises superior to the left atrial appendage, unlike the supravalvular mitral ring.

10. **c.** BP control that includes a beta-blocker agent. This young man's aortic coarctation is mild to moderate and does not warrant surgical repair at this time. Surgical repair is indicated when the transcoarctation pressure gradient exceeds 30 mm Hg. Percutaneous balloon angioplasty is associated with a higher rate of recurrent coarctation and increased risk of subsequent aortic aneurysm and, therefore, is not the first therapeutic choice. Because this patient has hypertension and is at risk for aortic dissection, tight BP control with beta-blockers is advised. There is no role for EP study, and repeat cardiac catheterization is not indicated because of its invasive nature. A follow-up TTE every 6 months is recommended.

11. **a.** Congenital MR is associated with multiple congenital heart diseases, including ostium primum septal defect, coarctation of the aorta, congenitally corrected transposition of the great arteries, subaortic stenosis, hypertrophic obstructive cardiomyopathy, endocardial fibroelastosis, and anomalous pulmonary origin of the coronary artery. Cor triatriatum produces symptoms and findings similar to mitral stenosis but is not associated with congenital MR.

12. **c.** Left circumflex artery arising from the right coronary artery.

13. **e.** Valvular calcification. Both valvular and subvalvular aortic stenoses have male preponderance and may be associated with dilatation of the ascending aorta. The indications and risk of operation are similar. Although aortic regurgitation is more common in subvalvular aortic stenosis, it may also occur in valvular aortic stenosis. Valvular calcification is usually not observed in subvalvular aortic valve stenosis.

14. **a.** VSD. Two thirds of patients with PA stenosis, also known as supravalvar pulmonic stenosis, have associated cardiac anomalies. The most common are valvular pulmonic stenosis and VSD. PDA and ASD are common, especially in mothers with rubella. Tetralogy of Fallot is also seen.

15. **c.** Ebstein's anomaly is not associated with congenital rubella. The most common malformations associated with congenital rubella are PA stenosis and PDA. Other malformations include pulmonary valve stenosis, systemic arterial stenosis, hypoplasia of the abdominal aorta, VSD, ASD, tetralogy of Fallot, coarctation of the aorta, aortic valvular or supravalvar stenosis, transposition of the great arteries, tricuspid atresia, and multiple valvular scleroses.

16. **d.** Spontaneous closure rarely occurs. The most common origin of coronary arteriovenous fistula is the right coronary artery, with a fistulous communication into the RV, right atrium, or coronary sinus. Less commonly, it empties into the LV, left atrium, or PA. Complications may include CHF from left-to-right shunt, bacterial endocarditis, coronary ischemia, and rupture or thrombosis of the fistula. Surgical closure is associated with a good outcome. A fistula rarely closes spontaneously.

17. **a.** Elective surgical resection should be considered. Subaortic valve stenosis involves the presence of a membranous diaphragm in the LVOT that creates a turbulent flow across the LVOT. This frequently causes damage to the aortic valve and may cause aortic valve insufficiency, aside from creating LVOT obstruction. Because of the potential damage to the aortic valve, elective surgical resection is

advised even with mild stenosis, especially if damage to the aortic valve is already established. Although recurrences occur, surgical resection is frequently curative. Transluminal balloon dilatation may be appropriate in carefully selected patients, but the relief of obstruction is frequently not as durable or complete as surgical resection. Trauma to the aortic valve predisposes to bacterial endocarditis, and endocarditis prophylaxis should be advised.

18. **b.** Weber-Osler-Rendu syndrome. Pulmonary arteriovenous fistula involves direct communication between PAs and veins. Most patients have associated Weber-Osler-Rendu syndrome, a condition associated with the presence of multiple telangiectasias. Williams syndrome is associated with mental retardation, elfin facies, and supravalvular aortic and pulmonic stenosis. Bland-Garland-White syndrome involves the anomalous origin of the left coronary artery from the PA. Kartagener's syndrome is associated with situs inversus, sinusitis, and bronchiectasis. Crouzon's syndrome is associated with PDA and aortic coarctation.

19. **c.** Asymptomatic subaortic stenosis with severe aortic valve insufficiency. In subaortic stenosis, a high-velocity jet damages the aortic valve. Thus, even in the absence of symptoms, surgery is recommended because of progressive valve destruction. In VSD, surgical correction does not entirely eliminate the risk of endocarditis. In ASD, closure is not recommended solely for the purpose of preventing paradoxical embolization. In PDA, high pulmonary vascular resistance connotes poor survival, and surgical correction is not recommended. In coarctation of the aorta with a small transcoarctation gradient of 20 mm Hg or less, surgical treatment has not been proven to be superior to medical treatment.

20. **a.** It is not frequently associated with secundum-type ASD. Anomalous pulmonary venous drainage is frequently associated with sinus venosus–type ASD. In addition, in approximately 20% of cases, there is an associated cardiac anomaly, such as VSD or tetralogy of Fallot. The physiologic consequence increases with the number of pulmonary veins involved. TTE may miss this finding, and TEE may be needed for identification of the defect. Because of the contribution of oxygenated blood from the renal arteries, oximetry may be limited if the pulmonary vein drains into the inferior vena cava.

21. **a.** 50-mm Hg transcoarctation pressure gradient. A greater than 30-mm Hg transcoarctation gradient is a definite indication for surgical repair. Symptoms such as headaches, chest pain, and presyncope are nonspecific and by themselves do not warrant surgical repair. The site of discrete narrowing is commonly distal to the left subclavian artery; it should not cause right upper extremity claudication.

22. **d.** Ebstein's anomaly involves the tricuspid valve, with displacement of tricuspid leaflets (mainly posterior) into the RV, resulting in an "atrialized" small RV. Approximately 80% of patients with this form of congenital anomaly have an interatrial communication, with potential for right-to-left shunting of blood. On physical examination, there are widely split $S_1$ and $S_2$. $S_3$ and $S_4$ gallop sounds are often heard. Because of the incompetency of the tricuspid leaflets (deformed and abnormal attachments), a loud tricuspid regurgitation murmur can be heard, a holosystolic murmur at the left lower sternal border that accentuates in intensity with respirations. Approximately 20% of patients with Ebstein's anomaly develop Wolff-Parkinson-White syndrome with pre-excitation and supraventricular tachyarrhythmias. When surgical repair is indicated, replacement of the deformed tricuspid leaflets with a bioprosthetic valve has been shown to compare favorably with bioprosthesis durability in other cardiac valve positions.

23. **b.** Platypnea-orthodeoxia. In congenitally corrected transposition, there is AV discordance as well as ventriculoarterial discordance. Systemic and pulmonary circulations are in series, just like normal cardiopulmonary circulation, and in the absence of a shunt, the patient is acyanotic. Morphologic RV and tricuspid valves are aligned with the aorta and perform lifelong systemic work. Other accompanying defects include perimembranous VSD, pulmonary stenosis, and

Ebstein's anomaly. Clinical features that manifest themselves in adulthood include CHB, significant AV valve regurgitation with heart failure, and supraventricular arrhythmias. Platypnea (dyspnea induced by assumption of the upright position and relieved by assumption of a recumbent position) and orthodeoxia ($O_2$ desaturation and hypoxemia in the upright position) can be seen with aortic elongation and patent foramen ovale and is not a common presentation of congenitally corrected transposition.

24. **e.** Patients with Eisenmenger's syndrome develop irreversible pulmonary vascular disease, pulmonary hypertension, and right-to-left shunting with cyanosis. Erythrocytosis and hyperviscosity syndrome is a significant source of morbidity and increases risk of mortality. Dehydration, high altitude with lower partial $O_2$ pressure, heavy exertion, and vasodilators tend to worsen this condition and result in greater right-to-left shunting and hypoxemia. On the contrary, phlebotomy is therapeutic when patients present with hematocrit >60 and symptoms of hyperviscosity.

25. **c.** Ebstein's anomaly. The ECG demonstrates a short PR interval, presence of delta waves, and wide QRS interval that are all consistent with pre-excitation and Wolff-Parkinson-White syndrome. Wolff-Parkinson-White syndrome is most commonly associated with Ebstein's anomaly.

26. **a.** Ligation or closure of the PDA. There is no evidence by clinical or TTE examination of elevated pulmonary vascular resistance. The mortality rate for ligation and division of the PDA is exceedingly low, but the risk of endarteritis with unrepaired ductus is significant enough (0.45% per year after the second decade of life) that authorities recommend closure or ligation even with small PDA. Endocarditis prophylaxis is recommended but does not definitely address the problem. Direct visualization with TTE may be difficult, but if good visualization is achieved, a TEE is rarely needed.

27. **c.** LV dysfunction is unusual in the young, but the incidence is as high as 15% in patients older than age 50. The annual mortality rate increases to 10% in the sixth decade. Most patients are minimally symptomatic in the first three decades of life, but by the fifth decade, more than 70% are symptomatic. Pulmonary hypertension is unusual in patients younger than 20 years, but approximately 50% of patients older than 40 years of age develop it.

28. **a.** Coronary artery ectasia is not associated with hyperviscosity syndrome. Chronic hypoxemia and cyanosis lead to compensatory erythrocytosis and significant rise in hematocrit. Symptoms and signs of hyperviscosity syndrome include visual disturbances, headache, dizziness, fatigue, hemoptysis, thrombosis and bleeding, and paresthesias. Cerebral catastrophes may occur as a result of venous thrombosis of cerebral vessels, intracranial hemorrhage, or paradoxical embolization.

29. **c.** Secundum ASD is a very low-risk lesion and, therefore, does not require endocarditis prophylaxis. Current guidelines for prevention of bacterial endocarditis apply to most congenital heart lesions, with the exception of isolated secundum ASD and surgically repaired atrial and ventricular or ductal shunt without residual shunt beyond 6 months after repair.

30. **e.** All of the above. The conditions that result in greatest risk to the mother or the fetus, or both, include Eisenmenger's syndrome, severe pulmonary hypertension, severe LV outflow obstruction, Marfan's syndrome with an enlarged aortic root, and New York Heart Association class III or IV heart failure.

31. **c.** Pulmonary vascular resistance greater than 15 Wood units that does not diminish with vasodilators is not an indication for surgical closure. Surgery is not recommended in patients with ASD with elevated pulmonary vascular resistance, which is irreversible.

32. **a.** Dilatation at the aortic end is found in 65% of patients. Constriction of the PDA starts at the pulmonary end, where endocarditis frequently originates. Patients with clinically silent PDA detected by TTE do not appear to be at risk

**NOTES**

for endocarditis. PDA is most commonly located distal to the origin of the left subclavian artery. The fetal ductus is derived from the sixth aortic arch, the same origin as that of the left and right PAs.

33. **c.** Lateral and inferior displacement of the apex beat are not associated with ostium secundum ASD. Lateral and inferior displacement of the apex beat occur with LV enlargement. In secundum ASD, the major hemodynamic consequences occur to the RV and not to the LV. An RV impulse or precordial heave as well as pulmonary arterial impulse may be palpable. There is fixed splitting of the S$_2$ because the phasic changes in the systemic venous return that occurs with respiration and that is responsible for physiologic splitting are minimized by the accompanying reciprocal changes in shunted blood from the left atrium to the right atrium.

34. **d.** Eisenmenger's syndrome. Eisenmenger's syndrome is one of few conditions that pose an absolute contraindication to pregnancy. Pregnancy in patients with Eisenmenger's syndrome is associated with mortality rates of up to 50%.

35. **e.** Regular follow-up with repeat TTE in 6 months. The patient has moderately severe tricuspid regurgitation and mild pulmonary hypertension, with preserved RV systolic function. He has no symptoms and no evidence of CHF. There is no need to intervene at this time, and regular follow-up with TTE should suffice.

36. **b, e.** Blalock-Taussig and Fontan.

37. **c, d, f.** Senning or Mustard, arterial switch, and Rashkind.

38. **e, f.** Fontan and Rashkind.

39. **g.** None of the above.

40. **a.** Ross. Please refer to Table 9A–1, which provides a complete overview of common surgical procedures for congenital heart disease.

**TABLE 9A–1    Common Surgical Procedures for Congenital Heart Disease**

| Procedure | Description | Intent | Result |
|---|---|---|---|
| Blalock-Taussig | Subclavian artery to PA anastomosis | PAL | Increases pulmonary blood flow |
| Central shunt | Conduit or anastomosis between aorta and PA | PAL | Increases pulmonary blood flow |
| Damus-Kaye-Stansel | PA end-to-side anastomosis to aorta, valved conduit between RV and main PA | COR | Increases blood flow to aorta and PA when there is aortic stenosis and two ventricles; re-establishes RV to PA continuity |
| Fontan | Anastomosis or conduit between right atrium and PA | PAL | Increases pulmonary blood flow in cases of univentricular heart or tricuspid atresia |
| Glenn (bidirectional Glenn) | SVC to PA anastomosis | PAL | Increases pulmonary blood flow |
| Arterial switch or Jatene | Transection of aorta and PA with reimplantation onto the proper ventricles, coronary arteries reimplanted | COR | Creates normal relationship between the ventricles and great arteries in transposition |
| Hemi-Fontan | SVC to PA anastomosis with baffle placed in right atrium so that inferior vena cava blood flow goes across ASD to left heart | PAL | Increases pulmonary blood flow and sets the stage for eventual complete Fontan |
| Konno | Replacement of aortic valve with aortic valve annular enlargement | COR | Alleviates subaortic obstruction and replaces abnormal aortic valve |
| Mustard | Atrial switch with intra-atrial baffle made of pericardium | COR | Re-establishes proper flow sequence to PA and aorta in D-transposition of the great arteries |
| Norwood (first stage) | PA anastomosis to aorta, conduit from aorta to main PA | PAL | Increases flow to aorta for subaortic obstruction with single ventricle |

*(Continued)*

**TABLE 9A–1    Common Surgical Procedures for Congenital Heart Disease** *(Continued)*

| Procedure | Description | Intent | Result |
|---|---|---|---|
| Potts | Descending aorta-to-PA shunt | PAL | Increases pulmonary flow (rarely done anymore) |
| PA band | Constrictive band around main PA | PAL | Decreases pulmonary flow |
| Rashkind | Atrial septostomy with catheter balloon | PAL | Increases mixing of blood for transposition of the great arteries or tricuspid atresia |
| Rastelli | Valved conduit from RV to PA, closure of VSD | COR | Increases pulmonary flow, may re-establish proper sequence of flow to aorta and PA |
| Ross | Pulmonary autograft to aorta, pulmonary homograft | COR | Correction for aortic stenosis; avoids mechanical and bioprosthetic valve |
| Senning | Atrial switch with intra-atrial baffle made of atrial wall flaps | COR | Re-establishes proper flow sequence to PA and aorta in transposition of the great arteries |
| Waterston | Ascending aorta to right pulmonary anastomosis | PAL | Increases pulmonary blood flow (rarely done anymore) |

ASD, atrial septal defect; COR, total correction; PAL, palliation; SVC, superior vena cava. (From *ACC Current Journal Review*. March/April 1996:46, with permission.)

**41. c.** Equal preponderance.

**42. b.** Predominantly female.

**43. a.** Predominantly male.

**44. a.** Predominantly male.

**45. c.** Equal preponderance.

**46. d.** Pulmonic stenosis. A left lateral right ventriculogram demonstrates pulmonic stenosis with dilatation of the proximal main PA.

**47. a.** Coarctation of the aorta. Left lateral view of the LV and aorta. The catheter was advanced from the femoral vein and crossed a large patent foramen ovale to reach the left side of the heart. A discrete area of narrowing (coarctation) is seen in the upper descending aorta.

**48. e.** VSD. A left ventriculogram obtained in the left anterior oblique view allows optimal visualization of the interventricular septum and demonstrates a large VSD and a large left-to-right shunt.

**49. b.** PDA. An aortogram in straight lateral view. There is a large abnormal communication between the upper descending aorta and the main PA, confirming the diagnosis of PDA.

**50. c.** Hypertrophic cardiomyopathy. A left ventriculogram in right anterior oblique projection demonstrates a small ventricle with marked ventricular hypertrophy and narrow LVOT.

**51. e.** Tetralogy of Fallot. On cardiac palpation and auscultation, patients with tetralogy of Fallot demonstrate RV lift (RV hypertrophy) and a systolic ejection murmur over the pulmonic region caused by RV outflow tract obstruction. A soft, short systolic ejection murmur suggests severe obstruction. The intensity and severity of the ejection murmur are inversely related to the severity of RV obstruction. $P_2$ is absent, and only the aortic component of $S_2$ is audible.

**52. d.** Ebstein's anomaly. Patients with Ebstein's anomaly have widely split $S_1$ and $S_2$, with loud $T_1$ and extra heart sounds and ejection clicks. A tricuspid regurgitation murmur is usually present. Hepatomegaly caused by passive congestion and elevation right atrial pressure may be present.

**NOTES**

53. **b.** Coarctation of the aorta. Patients with coarctation of the aorta have systolic hypertension and higher BP in their arms than in their legs, resulting in delayed femoral arterial pulses. Because many patients also have bicuspid aortic valve, a systolic ejection click is frequently present, and the aortic component of $S_2$ is accentuated. A harsh systolic ejection murmur is audible along the left sternal border and radiates to the back, especially over the point of discrete coarctation.

54. **a.** Eisenmenger's syndrome. Patients with Eisenmenger's syndrome demonstrate cyanosis and digital clubbing, the severity of which depends on the magnitude of right-to-left shunting. An RV lift and loud $P_2$ caused by pulmonary hypertension are usually present. The murmur caused by ASD, VSD, or PDA is no longer present when Eisenmenger's syndrome develops. Many patients can have a tricuspid or pulmonary regurgitation murmur, or both.

55. **c.** PDA. Patients with PDA exhibit hyperdynamic LV impulse with wide pulse pressure. A continuous machinery murmur, heard best in the pulmonic region, is a characteristic finding.

56. **c.** Cleft mitral valve.

57. **b.** Supravalvular pulmonic stenosis.

58. **e.** Persistent left superior vena cava.

59. **a.** Supravalvular aortic stenosis.

60. **d.** Anomalous pulmonary venous drainage.

61. **a.** Eisenmenger's syndrome.

62. **e.** Tetralogy of Fallot.

63. **d.** Ebstein's anomaly.

64. **b.** Coarctation of the aorta.

65. **c.** PDA.

66. **c.** Figure 9A–9. This is a parasternal short-axis view at the aortic valve level using TTE. Two leaflets showing a "fish-mouth" opening during systole are seen instead of three leaflets.

67. **a.** Figure 9A–7. This is an apical four-chamber view using TTE. There is a membrane separating the left atrium into a posterior chamber, usually where the pulmonary veins empty, and an anterior chamber that contains the mitral valve.

68. **d.** Figure 9A–10. Subcostal TTE view showing the ASD in the lower atrial septum, with downward displacement of the AV valve.

69. **e.** Figure 9A–11. This is a parasternal short-axis view at the aortic valve level, using TTE. There are four visible leaflets.

70. **b.** Figure 9A–8. A magnified TEE long-axis view of the LVOT, aortic valve, and ascending aorta. There is a membrane visible in the LVOT, consistent with a subaortic membrane.

## Suggested Reading

Brickner ME, Hillis LD, Lange RA. Congenital heart disease in adults. *N Engl J Med.* 2000;342:256–263, 334–342.

Gregoratos G, ed. *Cardiovascular Medicine Medical Knowledge Self-Assessment Program.* Philadelphia: American College of Physicians; 1998.

Marelli AJ, Moodie DS. Adult congenital heart disease. In: Topel E, ed. *Textbook of Cardiovascular Medicine*, 2nd ed. Philadelphia: Lippincott Williams & Wilkins; 2002.

Moss AJ, Adams FH, Emmanouilides GC, eds. *Heart Disease in Infants, Children and Adolescents*, 2nd ed. Baltimore: Williams & Wilkins; 1977.

Murphy JG, Gersh BJ, Mair DD, et al. Long-term outcome in patients undergoing surgical repair of tetralogy of Fallot. *N Engl J Med.* 1993;329:593–599.

# Adult Congenital Heart Disease

## Part B

RICHARD A. KRASUSKI

## QUESTIONS

1. You are seeing a 27-year-old female postal employee in outpatient clinic. She has a history of asthma treated with inhalers, though her pulmonary function tests and methacholine challenge were recently normal. She has noted progressive fatigue over the past 6 months and finds that getting up large hills on her mail route gets her out of breath. On examination she has a fixed split second heart sound and soft systolic ejection murmur over the left upper sternal border. Her lungs are clear and all her extremity pulses are equal and of normal intensity. All the following would be expected to be present on her diagnostic studies *except*

   a. unexplained right heart enlargement on echocardiography
   b. an rSR′ (incomplete bundle branch block) pattern on an electrocardiogram
   c. unexplained mild pulmonary hypertension on echocardiography
   d. right to left shunt by bubble study on echocardiography
   e. decreased pulmonary vascularity on chest x-ray

2. You are evaluating a 35-year-old female librarian with a history of complex congenital heart disease. She tells you that she has a "hole in the heart" but was told about 10 years ago that it was "too late to operate." Her health has recently been stable and she denies worsening dyspnea, headaches, chest pain, or other symptoms. She is currently able to walk from her home to her mail box (approximately 300 ft) before she has to stop and rest. On exam she appears cyanotic but is breathing comfortably. She has a loud pulmonic closure sound and a II/VI holosystolic murmur at the right lower sternal border. There are no surgical scars over her back or chest and her pulses are equal in all four extremities. Her bloodwork demonstrates

   White blood cell count = 8,000
   Hemoglobin = 22.4
   Platelets = 295,000
   Urea nitrogen = 1
   Creatinine = 0.9

   Reasonable therapeutic considerations in this patient include all of the following *except*

   a. endocarditis prophylaxis with dental procedures
   b. supplemental oxygen to wear at night or with exertion
   c. phlebotomy of 2 units with equal volume repletion
   d. invasive assessment of cardiac hemodynamics followed by initiation of bosentan
   e. avoiding studies that require the administration of intravenous contrast dye

NOTES

3. Which of the following statements about atrial septal aneurysm (ASA) is true?

   a. The term ASA is used to describe a very floppy interatrial septum.
   b. An ASA occurs when there is overabundant tissue in the septum primum.
   c. The most widely accepted definition of an ASA is >15 mm excursion from left to right atrium on echocardiography.
   d. The presence of an ASA in patients with patent foramen ovale and presumed embolic stroke appears to increase the risk of subsequent stroke.
   e. All the above are true.

4. Which of the following statements about patent foramen ovale (PFO) is the most accurate?

   a. PFO is uncommon in the general population, less common in patients with cryptogenic stroke, and its optimal management is well defined and evidence based.
   b. PFO is common in the general population, more common in patients with cryptogenic stroke, and its optimal management in most cases remains to be defined.
   c. PFO is uncommon in the general population, more common in patients with cryptogenic stroke, and its optimal management in most cases remains to be defined.
   d. PFO is common in the general population, less common in patients with cryptogenic stroke, and its optimal management in most cases remains to be defined.
   e. PFO is common in the general population, more common in patients with cryptogenic stroke, and its optimal management is well defined and evidence based.

5. All of the following statements about anomalous pulmonary venous return are correct *except*

   a. Anomalous pulmonary venous return can lead to right heart enlargement and elevations in pulmonary arterial pressures.
   b. Sinus venosus atrial septal defects are often associated with anomalous pulmonary veins.
   c. Cardiac computed tomography, magnetic resonance imaging, and transesophageal echocardiography are all reasonable modalities to assess for anomalous pulmonary veins.
   d. A bubble study during transthoracic echocardiography can help detect an anomalous pulmonary vein.

6. You are seeing a 35-year-old flight attendant with a history of coarctation of the aorta. At age 10 the patient underwent a coarctation resection and end-to-end anastomosis. She has noted no limitations since that time but notes that in general she has had slightly "less stamina" than her friends and colleagues over the past several years. On exam she has equal blood pressures in all four extremities and a soft systolic ejection murmur. All of the following statements are true concerning this patient *except*

   a. It is likely that the patient has a bicuspid aortic valve.
   b. There is a 10% chance that the patient has a berry aneurysm in the brain.
   c. The type of surgery that the patient underwent makes the possibility of aneurismal dilatation at the surgical site very likely.
   d. The patient is at a higher risk of developing hypertension than the general population.
   e. All of the above are true.

7. The lesions that constitute tetralogy of Fallot include all of the following *except*

   a. a ventricular septal defect
   b. an overriding aorta

c. an atrial septal defect

d. right ventricular outflow obstruction

e. right ventricular hypertrophy

8. A 21-year-old college student presents for a routine medical checkup. He has never seen an adult cardiologist and last saw a pediatric cardiologist while in high school. He has been told he has congenitally corrected transposition with an intact ventricular septum and no known valvular dysfunction. All of the following concerns about this young man are valid *except*

   a. His systemic right ventricle is at risk for dilatation and failure.

   b. He has a 10% lifetime risk of developing Eisenmenger syndrome.

   c. His systemic tricuspid valve is at risk for developing significant regurgitation.

   d. He has a 32% lifetime probability of developing complete heart block.

   e. All of the above are correct.

9. All of the following syndromes and cardiac anomalies are closely associated *except*

   a. trisomy 21 and atrioventricular canal defects

   b. Noonan syndrome and pulmonic stenosis

   c. Holt-Oram syndrome and atrial septal defects

   d. Marfan syndrome and mitral valve prolapse

   e. Williams syndrome and ventricular septal defects

10. Which of the following statements regarding Ebstein anomaly is not correct?

    a. An atrial septal defect or patent foramen ovale is present in up to 80% of patients.

    b. The cardinal feature is an apically displaced tricuspid valve resulting in atrialization of ventricular tissue.

    c. Wolf-Parkinson-White syndrome is common in these patients and multiple tracts can exist.

    d. A bicuspid aortic valve is commonly present.

    e. A "sail sound" is a common finding on physical examination.

11. You are seeing a 34-year-old gentleman in clinic. He has a history of tetralogy of Fallot and underwent a palliative Blalock-Taussig at 10 months followed by a complete repair at age 3. He has been reasonably active for several years but recently has been "slowing down" a little bit. His physical examination demonstrates scars over his left scapulae and midsternum. He has a III out of VI systolic ejection murmur and a II out of IV diastolic murmur over the left upper sternum. He has clear lungs and equal pulses in all four extremities and no peripheral edema. An echocardiogram is somewhat limited in quality because of the fact he is a rather large individual, but you are able to see evidence that the right heart appears enlarged and there is some pulmonic regurgitation present. The electrocardiogram shows some widening of the QRS complex with right bundle branch block morphology. The most reasonable next step in the diagnostic evaluation of this patient would be

    a. a repeat echocardiogram with a saline microcavitation (bubble) study

    b. an electrophysiological study to look for ventricular arrhythmias

    c. a cardiac catheterization to formally examine the hemodynamics

    d. a cardiac magnetic resonance imaging study

    e. the initiation of diuretics and digitalis

12. You have been asked to see a 45-year-old woman with a ventricular septal defect. She has been in excellent health for many years and voices no particular complaints. She had been taking antibiotic prophylaxis with dental procedures but discontinued this as a result of the recent guideline changes. On examination she has a III/VI pansystolic murmur and normal intensity first and second heart sounds. Her lungs are clear and she has no jugular venous distention. All

of the following characteristics would argue for a benign clinical course in this patient *except*

**a.** a loud murmur
**b.** normal intensity heart sounds
**c.** a supracrystal (or subaortic) morphology
**d.** the absence of right or left heart enlargement
**e.** all are benign characteristics

**13.** A 28-year-old woman is referred to you for evaluation of a heart murmur. She states she is a long-distance runner and has not noted any significant symptoms. On examination you note very brisk pulses and her blood pressure is 100/40 mm Hg. Her murmur extends from systole into diastole and there is a near "machinery"-type quality to it. The remainder of her physical examination is essentially unremarkable, as is her bloodwork. The most likely cardiac anomaly in this case is

**a.** an atrial septal defect
**b.** coarctation of the aorta
**c.** a patent ductus arteriosus
**d.** congenitally corrected transposition with a VSD and pulmonic valve stenosis
**e.** ventricular septal defect

**14.** A 40-year-old man is referred to you for evaluation of a heart murmur. He had been active until about 3 years ago when he experienced severe pain in his right knee, which was eventually diagnosed as a ligamental tear. He underwent open knee surgery and has been limited by pain since that time. As a result he has gained approximately 30 lb and states he now gets out of breath with anything more than moderate activity. On examination he has a systolic ejection murmur heard beat over the left upper sternal border. There is no radiation to the carotid arteries. An echocardiogram is performed and demonstrates a doming pulmonic valve with trace regurgitation. The following Doppler tracing (Fig. 9B–1) is obtained across the pulmonic valve:

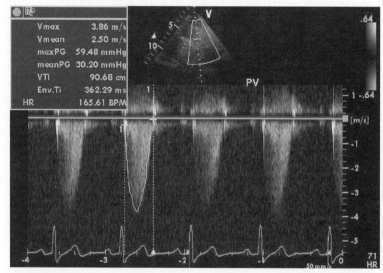

**FIGURE 9B–1**

The most appropriate next step would be

**a.** continued observation with yearly visits and echocardiography
**b.** referral for catheterization and likely pulmonic valvuloplasty
**c.** referral for surgery after diagnostic angiography
**d.** stress echocardiography
**e.** magnetic resonance imaging

15. A 19-year-old basketball player is brought to the emergency department after he collapsed on the court. He received bystander cardiopulmonary resuscitation and was apparently defibrillated using a AED. All of the following abnormalities should be part of the differential diagnosis for the cause of sudden death in this young man *except*

    a. anomalous origin of the left main coronary artery from the right coronary cusp
    b. hypertrophic cardiomyopathy
    c. congenitally prolonged QT syndrome
    d. atrial septal defect
    e. arrhythmogenic right ventricular dysplasia

# Answers

1. **e.** The chest x-ray in this case would be expected to demonstrate *increased* lung vascularity. The patient described in this case has an atrial septal defect. The telltale physical examination findings in atrial septal defect are a pulmonic outflow murmur resulting from increased pulmonary blood flow caused by left-to-right shunting and a fixed split second heart sound. Atrial septal defects, if sufficiently large, lead to right heart enlargement and an incomplete right bundle branch block pattern on electrocardiography. Pulmonary hypertension can result from increased blood flow and up to 10% may develop Eisenmenger physiology if uncorrected. As with any atrial flow communication a bubble study on echocardiography would be expected to be positive, providing the right atrial pressure can be made to exceed the left atrial pressure (such as following a Valsalva maneuver).

2. **c.** Phlebotomy should not be performed in patients with Eisenmenger physiology unless they have symptoms suggesting active sludging caused by polycythemia. Suggestive symptoms include headaches, visual changes, and mental status changes. Unnecessary phlebotomy can provoke iron deficiency, which can further increase the risk of sludging and its consequences. If phlebotomy is necessary, equal volume replacement with saline is essential. As with all cyanotic heart disease, endocarditis prophylaxis for dental procedures is recommended. The use of oxygen has not been well studied in this population but is reasonable if it affords the patient symptomatic benefit. An oral endothelin blockade, bosentan, has recently been demonstrated to improve functional capacity compared to placebo for patients with World Health Organization class III symptoms. Since the patient in this case seems fairly limited, bosentan may be a very reasonable therapeutic option for her. Any procedures requiring the use of anesthesia or contrast dye should be approached very carefully in patients with Eisenmenger syndrome because of the risk for adverse consequences.

3. **e.** An atrial septal aneurysm is a floppy interatrial septum resulting from overabundant tissue in the septum primum. A total septal excursion of >15 mm has been most widely accepted as the definition for this entity. If the septal excursion is less, it is generally referred to as a "redundant atrial septum." In patients with cryptogenic stroke and a patent foramen ovale, a concurrent atrial septal aneurysm appears to significantly increase the risk of future stroke.

4. **b.** The foramen ovale is the interface between the septum primum and septum secundum and in utero provides an important route that blood can take to bypass the fetal lungs (which are collapsed until birth). In about 25% of humans the flap of tissue making up the foramen ovale does not fuse after birth and results in a patent foramen ovale (PFO). Several studies have demonstrated an increased incidence of PFO in patients with cryptogenic (otherwise unexplained) stroke. Though several management strategies exist for patients with cryptogenic stroke and PFO, including anticoagulation, antiplatelet therapy, and percutaneous and surgical closure, no clear consensus regarding therapy exists, and studies are currently ongoing to try to shed light on this controversial subject.

5. **d.** A bubble study would not be expected to be abnormal in the presence of an anomalous pulmonary vein unless a concurrent atrial septal defect were present. Normally all four pulmonary veins drain back to the left atrium. Rarely one or multiple pulmonary veins can drain back to the right atrium and result in a left-to-right shunt. This can lead to right heart enlargement and even pulmonary hypertension. Anomalous pulmonary veins are present in most sinus venosus atrial septal defects and in up to 10% of secundum atrial septal defects. Though transthoracic echocardiography is generally unable to image an anomalous pulmonary vein, CT, MRI, and transesophageal echocardiography are all helpful in its detection.

**6.** **c.** End-to-end resection of an aortic coarctation is most likely to be complicated by eventual recoarctation, which can often be approached percutaneously. Another procedure that was previously popularized for coarctation repair, the so-called "patch aortoplasty," can lead to aneurismal dilatation, and these patients require very close monitoring. Coarctation of the aorta is believed to result from the migration of ductus arteriosus tissue into the aorta proper. As a result, constriction of the aorta occurs and leads to upper extremity hypertension and lower extremity hypoperfusion through activation of the renin-angiotensin-aldosterone system. In adults coarctation is most commonly identified during evaluation for secondary causes of hypertension. A bicuspid aortic valve is present in 50% to 85% of patients and ascending aortic enlargement can also be seen. There is also a 10% chance of having a concurrent berry aneurysm. Despite surgical or percutaneous repair, patients are at increased risk of developing hypertension later in life, even in the absence of an appreciable residual gradient (Figs. 9B–2 and 9B–3).

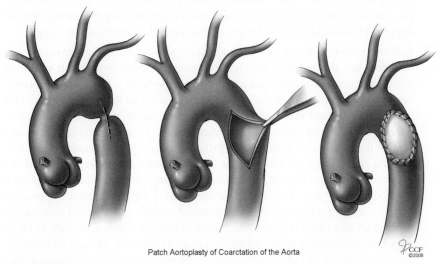

Resection and End-to-end Anastamosis of Coarctation of the Aorta

**FIGURE 9B–2**

Patch Aortoplasty of Coarctation of the Aorta

**FIGURE 9B–3**

7. **c.** The lesions of tetralogy of Fallot include a ventricular septal defect, an over-riding aorta, the presence of right ventricular outflow obstruction (valvular or subvalvular), and right ventricular hypertrophy. Concurrent presence of an atrial septal defect has been referred to as "pentalogy of Fallot," but is not generally accepted as part of the primary lesion complex.

8. **b.** In the absence of any significant shunt lesions, there is no risk to this patient of developing Eisenmenger syndrome. Congenitally corrected transposition of the great vessels implies that the patient has both atrioventricular and ventriculoarterial discordance. In other words, this patient's systemic venous drainage enters the right atrium, which is connected to a left ventricle and then is taken to the lungs via the pulmonary artery. Pulmonary venous return then enters the left atrium, which flows into the right ventricle and is subsequently pumped to the body through the aorta. Although this anatomy reproduces a near-normal circulation, the right ventricle has not been adequately designed to withstand the workload of being a systemic ventricle. As a result it eventually begins to dilate and fail. Also the tricuspid valve (the systemic AV valve—valves always follow their respective ventricles) begins to leak. Patients with congenitally corrected transposition also have conduction issues and are prone to developing heart block.

9. **e.** The characteristic cardiovascular lesion of Williams syndrome is supravalvular aortic stenosis, though coarctation of the aorta and peripheral pulmonary artery stenosis have also been described. The characteristic lesion of trisomy 21 (Down syndrome) is an atrioventricular canal defect (also known as a primum ASD/VSD), though ASD, VSD, and patent ductus arteriosus are also common. Noonan syndrome has most classically been associated with dysplastic or stenotic pulmonic valves. Holt-Oram syndrome is an autosomal-dominant disorder in which atrial septal defects and ventricular septal defects are most common. Marfan syndrome's most worrisome cardiovascular involvement is of the aorta, which can lead to dissection and even death. Many of these patients have concurrent mitral valve prolapse, though it is a less likely cause of morbidity or mortality.

10. **d.** A biscuspid aortic valve does not appear to be a common finding in most patients with Ebstein anomaly. Ebstein anomaly is characterized by apical displacement of the septal and posterior tricuspid valve leaflets, leading to atrialization of the right ventricle. An atrial flow communication (ASD or PFO) exists in up to 80% of patients. The electrocardiogram often demonstrates very large or "Himalayan" P waves. Wolf-Parkinson-White syndrome is present in up to 30% of patients, with half of these possessing multiple accessory tracts. The loud snapping sound of the ballooning tricuspid leaflets has been compared to that of a sail flapping in the wind, and can be a very characteristic examination finding.

11. **d.** Primary repair of tetralogy of Fallot entails not only closing the ventricular septal defect, but also resecting the right ventricular outflow obstruction and often placing a patch over the resected tissue. Because the valve is frequently dysplastic, significant regurgitation of the pulmonic valve remains following surgery. This patient demonstrates the typical examination of a patient with prior repair complicated by significant pulmonic valve regurgitation. These patients do remarkably well for many years, but then develop progressive right heart dilatation, heart failure, and arrhythmias. Widening of the QRS complex has been well described as a precursor to adverse clinical outcomes. The timing of reoperation to implant a pulmonic valve is very challenging, and the status of the right ventricle appears to be the most important determining factor. A bubble study would only clarify whether an atrial level or pulmonary shunt is present, which is unlikely to be an important contributor to the pathophysiology in this case. Though arrhythmias are a complication of right heart dilatation, the role of electrophysiological testing in this population of patients is far from clear, and in this patient, who is without a history of presyncope or palpitations, formal testing would not be indicated. It

is also unlikely that invasive hemodynamics would provide crucial diagnostic information. Finally, without evidence for significant volume overload, the initiation of diuretics and digoxin would not be recommended at this time.

12. **c.** Of the various types of ventricular septal defects, supracrystal (subaortic) defects should be monitored closely because of their predilection for spontaneous closure by aortic leaflet tissue, which can result in significant aortic regurgitation. The patient in this case has a small, restrictive, and asymptomatic ventricular septal defect. Flow in such cases is determined by the size of the shunt and the compliance of the ventricles. In general, smaller lesions will have increased turbulence and thus louder murmurs. Thus, a louder murmur isolated to systole is reassuring of a more benign clinical course, as is the presence of normal intensity heart sounds. In the presence of pulmonary hypertension the pulmonic component of the second heart sound is often accentuated. Cardiac chamber enlargement results from volume overload and its absence in this case again suggests a more benign lesion.

13. **c.** Patent ductus arteriosus is the persistence after birth of an in-utero communication between the aorta and the left pulmonary artery, which, along with the foramen ovale, is designed to bypass blood away from the collapsed lungs. It is the third most common congenital heart defect in adults and is generally found in isolation in the adult. Most adult patients with patent ductus are asymptomatic, though this depends on the pulmonary vascular resistance and the size of the ductus. Frequently, this lesion is discovered by the unusual quality of a continuous murmur at the left upper sternal border that can be mistaken for an innocent venous hum. Because a patent ductus is an aortopulmonary communication, however, the pulse pressure frequently is widened, and the pulses are brisk to bounding. Because of the risk of endocarditis, some advocate repair, even if the shunt is not significant, though this remains controversial. Fortunately, most ductus lesions can be now be closed in the catheterization laboratory without the need for surgery.

14. **b.** This patient has pulmonic stenosis with peak gradient in excess of 50 mm Hg. This by itself is an indication for an intervention in this gentleman, who appears to have some limitation, though his deconditioning does provide a confounding factor. Stress echocardiography would be of little utility as the rest gradient is already sufficient to recommend an intervention. In patients with less gradient and suggestive symptoms, a stress test can demonstrate a provokable gradient with associated symptoms, which would imply a benefit from intervention. Magnetic resonance is useful to establish the location of narrowing (valvular, subvalvular, or supravalvular) in difficult-to-image cases, but in this patient the echo images have already established that the narrowing is valvular. Though surgery can be performed in these patients, percutaneous balloon valvotomy is now the preferred therapy in the majority of patients with isolated valvular pulmonic stenosis.

15. **d.** Though an atrial septal defect does increase the risk of developing atrial fibrillation later in life and, unrepaired, may contribute to shortened lifespan, there has been no established link between ASD and sudden death. The most common lesions to exclude in a young person who suffers a sudden death include hypertrophic cardiomyopathy, an autosomal-dominant disorder that results in abnormal myocardial architecture and increases arrhythmogenic risk. Abnormal coronary artery origins appear to be a risk for sudden death as well, particularly a left main coronary artery arising from the right coronary artery cusp and passing between the great vessels, though the mechanism remains poorly understood and controversial. It may be caused by compression of the coronary artery between the great vessels, the result of an abnormal, slit-like orifice at the take-off of the vessel from the aortic cusp. Congenital QT-prolongation can result in sudden death and may occasionally be diagnosed from an electrocardiogram. Arrhythmogenic RV dysplasia and Brugada syndrome are other abnormalities that disturb the normal electrophysiological milieu and increase the risk for sudden death.

NOTES

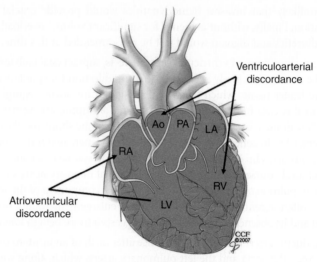

Ao = aorta; LA = left atrium; LV = left ventricle; PA = pulmonary artery;
RA = right atrium; RV = right ventricle

**FIGURE 9B–4**

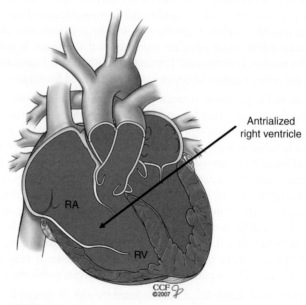

**FIGURE 9B–5**

# chapter 10

# Physiology/Biochemistry

MARC S. PENN

1. At the completion of a cycle of excitation-contraction coupling, cytosolic $Ca^{2+}$ is sequestered in the sarcoplasmic reticulum by what adenosine triphosphatase?

   a. glyceraldehyde phosphate dehydrogenase
   b. sarcoplasmic-endoplasmic reticulum calcium ATPase type 2 (SERCA2)
   c. adenylyl cyclase
   d. V-adenosine triphosphatase
   e. L-type calcium channels

2. In myocardium from patients with CHF, the SERCA2-to-phospholamban ratio has been shown to be

   a. increased
   b. unchanged
   c. decreased

3. Downregulation of signaling along the adrenergic pathway in failing myocardium is caused by all of the below *except*

   a. overexpression of beta-adrenoreceptor (β-AR) kinase
   b. downregulation of the $β_2$-receptor
   c. phosphodiesterase inhibitors
   d. beta-blocker therapy
   e. ACE inhibitors

4. The most efficient methodology for the delivery of cDNA for gene therapy presently being used in clinical trials is

   a. adeno-associated virus
   b. bacteriophage
   c. adenovirus
   d. plasmid DNA
   e. liposomes

5. All of the delivery vectors listed below allow for the possibility of stable integration of genetic material into chromosomal DNA *except*

   a. adeno-associated virus
   b. adenovirus
   c. plasmid DNA
   d. liposomes

6. Arterial thrombosis after plaque rupture is initiated by

   a. tissue plasminogen activator
   b. factor XIII

**c.** protein C
**d.** activated protein C
**e.** tissue factor

7. Blood-borne markers of inflammation that have been shown to predict the presence of CAD or acute coronary syndrome include all the following *except*

   **a.** high-sensitivity C-reactive protein
   **b.** interleukin-6
   **c.** myeloperoxidase
   **d.** interferon alpha
   **e.** serum amyloid A

8. Potential mediators of lipid oxidation in vivo include all of the following *except*

   **a.** myeloperoxidase
   **b.** lipoxygenase
   **c.** ceruloplasmin
   **d.** catalase
   **e.** ischemia

9. Low levels of gene expression can be detected by

   **a.** Northern blot
   **b.** Western blot
   **c.** reverse transcriptase-polymerase chain reaction (RT-PCR)
   **d.** Southern blot
   **e.** gene transfer

10. DNA can be cut at sites of specific sequences using

    **a.** hybridization
    **b.** restriction enzymes
    **c.** RT-PCR
    **d.** pepsin
    **e.** desalting column

11. Oxidized LDL can be characterized by the following *except*

    **a.** positive charge
    **b.** cytotoxicity
    **c.** high malondialdehyde levels
    **d.** recognition by the scavenger receptor
    **e.** low vitamin E

12. The final common pathway of platelet aggregation is mediated through

    **a.** adenosine diphosphate binding
    **b.** collagen
    **c.** thrombin
    **d.** $\alpha_v\beta_3$ receptor
    **e.** glycoprotein (GP) IIb/IIIa receptor

13. Inducers of smooth muscle cell proliferation include

    **a.** platelet-derived growth factor $\beta$
    **b.** basic fibroblast growth factor (bFGF)
    **c.** transforming growth factor $\beta$
    **d.** thrombin
    **e.** oxidized LDL

14. Apoptosis of a cell is indicated by all of the following *except*

    **a.** phosphatidylserine in the outer leaflet
    **b.** high caspase 3 activity
    **c.** low annexin-V binding
    **d.** DNA laddering
    **e.** low cytoplasmic cytochrome C levels

**15.** Inhibitors of cardiac myocyte apoptosis include
   **a.** insulin-like growth factor-1β
   **b.** dobutamine
   **c.** ischemia
   **d.** caspase 3
   **e.** Bid cleavage

# ANSWERS

1. **b.** SERCA2.

2. **c.** Decreased.

3. **d.** Intracellular calcium ($Ca^{2+}$) plays an integral role in contraction and relaxation in cardiac myocytes, a process tightly controlled by mechanisms that regulate its rise and fall. During depolarization, $Ca^{2+}$ entry through the L-type $Ca^{2+}$ channels triggers an exponential release of $Ca^{2+}$ from the sarcoplasmic reticulum (SR) through ryanodine receptors, resulting in activation of contractile proteins. At the completion of a cycle of excitation-contraction coupling, cytosolic $Ca^{2+}$ is sequestered in the SR by the SR-$Ca^{2+}$ adenosine triphosphatase (SERCA2a) pump (~75%) or exported extracellularly via the Na/Ca exchanger (~25%) located on the sarcolemmal membrane. Cardiomyocytes isolated from humans with CHF are characterized by contractile dysfunction as evidenced by decreased systolic force generation, prolonged relaxation, and elevated diastolic force. Abnormalities in $Ca^{2+}$ homeostasis, including reduced SR $Ca^{2+}$ release, elevated diastolic $Ca^{2+}$ levels, and a reduced rate of $Ca^{2+}$ removal, parallel the contractile dysfunction seen in the failing myocardium. Furthermore, a reduction in frequency-dependent systolic force and $Ca^{2+}$ can be witnessed in failing human myocytes. Key components in the development of the derangements in contraction and relaxation observed in CHF have been shown to be SERCA2a and its regulatory protein, phospholamban. SERCA2a controls function of $Ca^{2+}$ reuptake after myocyte contraction and serves to regulate $Ca^{2+}$ transients initiating diastolic relaxation. Phospholamban exerts an inhibitory effect on SERCA2a functioning, reducing its ability to assist in removal of cytosolic $Ca^{2+}$ after contraction, a mechanism believed to result in the diastolic dysfunction seen in CHF patients. The ratio of SERCA2a/phospholamban has been demonstrated to be decreased in patients with CHF, resulting in the derangements described previously. With this improved understanding of calcium homeostasis in failing hearts, interests have pointed toward methods of ameliorating these dysfunctional mechanisms. Heart failure results in dramatic changes in certain neurotransmitter and hormone receptors. The majority of the changes occur in the heart and generally can be classified as regulatory phenomena that withdraw the failing heart from adrenergic stimulation. However, these changes can also result in alterations of excitation-contraction coupling and, ultimately, contribute to CHF. Derangements in β-adrenergic signaling, including β-AR receptor downregulation, β-AR uncoupling from second messenger systems, and upregulation of β-AR kinase, have been demonstrated as significant components of heart failure. Phosphodiesterase inhibitors, such as milrinone, are used to increase β-adrenergic signaling by bypassing the β-AR. ACEIs have no effect on β-adrenergic signaling. Beta-blockers increase β-adrenergic signaling by increasing the density of β-AR on the cardiomyocyte cell surface.

4. **c.** Adenovirus.

5. **b.** Adenovirus does not allow for the possibility of stable integration. Replication-defective adenoviral vectors have emerged as the primary modality for gene transfer in a variety of preclinical and clinical studies of gene therapy. A number of properties have resulted in the popularity of these vectors for cardiovascular gene therapy. Adenoviral vectors are rendered replication incompetent by deleting the early (E1A and E1B) genes responsible for viral gene expression from the genome and are stably integrated into the host cells in an extrachromosomal form. This decreases the risk of integration into the host cell genome and mutagenesis. Adenoviral vectors have been shown to result in transient expression of therapeutic genes in vivo, peaking at 7 days and lasting approximately 4 weeks. Unlike replication-defective adenoviral vectors, adeno-associated virus vectors do not express any viral

gene products, rendering them significantly less immunogenic. This vector demonstrated efficient and stable integration of its transgene with a minimal inflammatory response. Multiple studies have demonstrated the feasibility of in vivo gene transfer into myocardial cells by direct injection of plasmid DNA. These vectors have the enticing qualities of being relatively nonimmunogenic and nonpathogenic, with the potential to stably integrate in the cellular genome, resulting in long-term gene expression in postmitotic cells in vivo. Furthermore, plasmid DNA is rapidly degraded in the bloodstream; therefore, the chance of transgene expression in distant organ systems is negligible. The use of bacteriophage for gene transfer is presently theoretical and not under consideration for clinical use at this time.

6. **e.** Tissue factor. Tissue factor binding to factor VII is the initiating event for the extrinsic blood coagulation cascade. The complex can also cleave factor IX and contribute to activation of the intrinsic cascade as well. Tissue factor is normally not expressed in the vasculature, but, in atherosclerotic vessels, tissue factor is expressed by macrophages and smooth muscle cells. Tissue factor expression is increased in the lesions of patients who present with unstable angina. On plaque rupture, the exposure of tissue factor to blood-borne coagulation factors leads to thrombus formation.

7. **d.** Interferon alpha has not been shown to predict the presence of CAD or acute coronary syndrome. Increased levels of each of these circulating markers have been found in patients with CAD compared to the levels found in control populations.

8. **d.** Lipoxygenase, myeloperoxidase, and ceruloplasmin are all expressed by activated macrophages and lead to lipid oxidation. Ischemia, in particular ischemia-reperfusion, leads to generation of free radicals and lipid peroxidation. Catalase is an antioxidant by reacting with hydrogen peroxide and releasing water.

9. **c.** RT-PCR. RT-PCR is capable of finding a single copy of RNA. Northern blot analysis requires at least 5 to 10 µg of total RNA. Western blot analysis is for determining protein levels. Southern blot analysis is for genotyping and requires multiple copies of DNA. Gene transfer is not a detection method.

10. **b.** Restriction enzymes. Restriction enzymes cleave DNA at sites of specific DNA sequences. Pepsin cleaves protein at specific sites. RT-PCR is discussed in the answer to question 9, and hybridization refers to the process of annealing DNA to RNA or DNA.

11. **a.** Oxidized LDL has a higher electrophoretic mobility compared to native LDL because of its negative charge. LDL does not oxidize until its vitamin E content is reduced. It is highly cytotoxic to cells in culture. Oxidized LDL is not recognized by the LDL receptor; rather, it is recognized by the scavenger receptor. The level of LDL oxidation is quantified by its ability to generate high malondialdehyde levels.

12. **e.** GP IIb/IIIa receptor. Adenosine diphosphate, collagen, and thrombin bind independently, leading to platelet activation and, ultimately, to expression of the GP IIb/IIIa receptor. GP IIb/IIIa receptor expression leads to platelet clumping by binding to surrounding activated platelets. The $\alpha_v\beta_3$ receptor does not lead to platelet aggregation.

13. **c.** Transforming growth factor β. Platelet-derived growth factor β, bFGF, and thrombin are all smooth muscle mitogens. Oxidized LDL causes smooth muscle cell proliferation through the autocrine release of bFGF. Transforming growth factor β alters the smooth muscle cell phenotype from a proliferative to a synthetic state and, thus, is antiproliferative.

14. **c.** Low annexin-V binding does not indicate apoptosis of a cell. Cellular apoptosis is characterized by increased phosphatidylserine expression in the outer leaflet of the plasma membrane that leads to increased annexin-V binding. Intracellular markers of apoptosis include increased caspase 3, decreased cytochrome C levels, and evidence of DNA laddering.

**NOTES**

**15. a.** Insulin-like growth factor-1β. Insulin-like growth factor-1β overexpression has been shown to be cardioprotective because of decreased apoptosis in the setting of myocardial ischemia. Dobutamine has been shown to induce cardiomyocyte apoptosis. Caspase 3 and Bid cleavage are cytoplasmic markers of apoptosis.

## Suggested Reading

Akhter SA, Skaer CA, Kypson AP, et al. Restoration of beta-adrenergic signaling in failing cardiac ventricular myocytes via adenoviral-mediated gene transfer. *Proc Natl Acad Sci USA.* 1997;94(22):12100–12105.

Annex BH. Differential expression of TF protein in directional atherectomy specimens from patients with stable and unstable coronary syndromes. *Circulation.* 1995;91:619–622.

Askari AT, Penn MS. Targeted gene therapy for the treatment of cardiac dysfunction. *Semin Thorac Cardiovasc Surg.* 2002;14:167–177.

Bristow MR, Ginsburg R, Minobe W, et al. Decreased catecholamine sensitivity and beta-adrenergic-receptor density in failing human hearts. *N Engl J Med.* 1982;307(4):205–211.

Chai YC, Howe PH, DiCorleto PE, et al. Oxidized low density lipoprotein and lysophosphatidylcholine stimulate cell cycle entry in vascular smooth muscle cells. Evidence for release of fibroblast growth factor-2. *J Biol Chem.* 1996;27:17791–17797.

Chisolm GM 3rd, Hazen SL, Fox PL, et al. The oxidation of lipoproteins by monocytes-macrophages. Biochemical and biological mechanisms. *J Biol Chem.* 1999;274:25959–25962.

del Monte F, Williams E, Lebeche D, et al. Improvement in survival and cardiac metabolism after gene transfer of sarcoplasmic reticulum Ca(2+)-ATPase in a rat model of heart failure. *Circulation.* 2001;104(12):1424–1429.

French B, Mazur W, Geske RS, et al. Direct in vivo gene transfer into porcine myocardium using replication-deficient adenoviral vectors. *Circulation.* 1994;90(5):2414–2424.

Guzman RJ, Lemarchand P, Crystal RG, et al. Efficient gene transfer into myocardium by direct injection of adenovirus vectors. *Circ Res.* 1993;73(6):1202–1207.

Gwathmey JK, Copelas L, MacKinnon R, et al. Abnormal intracellular calcium handling in myocardium from patient with end-stage heart failure. *Circ Res.* 1987;61(1):70–76.

Gwathmey JK, Slawsky MT, Hajjar RJ, et al. Role of intracellular calcium handling in force-interval relationships of human ventricular myocardium. *J Clin Invest.* 1990;85(5):1599–1613.

Hajjar RJ, Schmidt U, Kang JX, et al. Adenoviral gene transfer of phospholamban in isolated rat cardiomyocytes. Rescue effects by concomitant gene transfer of sarcoplasmic reticulum Ca(2+)-ATPase. *Circ Res.* 1997;81(2):145–153.

Hessler JR, Morel DW, Lewis LJ, et al. Lipoprotein oxidation and lipoprotein-induced cytotoxicity. *Arteriosclerosis.* 1983;3(3):215–222.

Kadambi VJ, Ponniah S, Harrer JM, et al. Cardiac-specific overexpression of phospholamban alters calcium kinetics and resultant cardiomyocyte mechanics in transgenic mice. *J Clin Invest.* 1996;97(2):533–539.

Kessler PD, Podsakoff GM, Chen X, et al. Gene delivery to skeletal muscle results in sustained expression and systemic delivery of a therapeutic protein. *Proc Natl Acad Sci USA.* 1996;93:14082–14087.

Kitsis RN, Buttrick PM, McNally EM, et al. Hormonal modulation of a gene injected into rat heart in vivo. *Proc Natl Acad Sci USA.* 1991;88(10):4138–4142.

Kohler C. Evaluation of caspase activity in apoptotic cells. *J Immunol Methods.* 2002;265:97–110.

Li Q, Li B, Wang X, et al. Overexpression of insulin-like growth factor-1 in mice protects from myocyte death after infarction, attenuating ventricular dilation, wall stress, and cardiac hypertrophy. *J Clin Invest.* 1997;100:1991–1999.

Lin H, Parmacek MS, Morle G, et al. Expression of recombinant genes in myocardium in vivo after direct injection of DNA. *Circulation.* 1990;82(6):2217–2221.

Losordo DW, Vale PR, Symes JF, et al. Gene therapy for myocardial angiogenesis: initial clinical results with direct myocardial injection of phVEGF$_{165}$ as sole therapy for myocardial ischemia. *Circulation.* 1998;98:2800–2804.

Lowes BD, Gilbert EM, Abraham WT, et al. Myocardial gene expression in dilated cardiomyopathy treated with beta-blocking agents. *N Engl J Med.* 2002;346(18):1357–1365.

Mercadier JJ, Lompre AM, Duc P, et al. Altered sarcoplasmic reticulum Ca2(+)-ATPase gene expression in the human ventricle during end-stage heart failure. *J Clin Invest.* 1990;85(1):305–309.

Morel DW, Hessler JR, Chisolm GM. Low density lipoprotein cytotoxicity induced by free radical peroxidation of lipid. *J Lipid Res.* 1983;24:1070–1076.

Moreno PR, Bernardi VH, Lopez-Cuellar J, et al. Macrophages, smooth muscle cells, and tissue factor in unstable angina. Implications for cell-mediated thrombogenicity in acute coronary syndromes. *Circulation.* 1996;94:3090–3097.

Morgan JP. Abnormal intracellular modulation of calcium as a major cause of cardiac contractile dysfunction. *N Engl J Med.* 1991;325:625.

Nilsson J. Cytokines and smooth muscle cells in atherosclerosis. *Cardiovasc Res.* 1993;27:1184–1190.

Reidy MA, Fingerle J, Lindner V. Factors controlling the development of arterial lesions after injury. *Circulation.* 1992;86(6 Suppl):III43–III46.

Reutelingsperger CP. Visualization of cell death in vivo with the annexin V imaging protocol. *J Immunol Methods.* 2002;265:123–132.

Rifai N, Ridker PM. Inflammatory markers and coronary heart disease. *Curr Opin Lipidol.* 2002;13(4):383–389.

Robbins M, Topol EJ. Inflammation in acute coronary syndromes. *Cleve Clin J Med.* 2002;69(Suppl 2):SII130–SII142.

Rosenberg RD, Aird WC. Vascular-bed-specific hemostasis and hyper-coagulable states. *N Engl J Med.* 1999;340(20):1555–1564.

Schmidt U, Hajjar RJ, Helm PA, et al. Contribution of abnormal sarcoplasmic reticulum ATPase activity to systolic and diastolic dysfunction in human heart failure. *J Mol Cell Cardiol.* 1998;30(10):1929–1937.

Schwinger RH, Munch G, Bolck B, et al. Reduced Ca(2+)-sensitivity of SERCA 2a in failing human myocardium due to reduced serin-16 phospholamban phosphorylation. *J Mol Cell Cardiol.* 1999;31(3):479–491.

Svensson EC, Marshall DJ, Woodard K, et al. Efficient and stable transduction of cardiomyocytes after intramyocardial injection or intracoronary perfusion with recombinant adeno-associated virus vectors. *Circulation.* 1999;99(2):201–205.

Topol EJ, Byzova TV, Plow EF. Platelet GPIIb-IIIa blockers. *Lancet.* 1999;353:227–231.

Toschi V, Gallo R, Lettino M, et al. Tissue factor modulates the thrombogenicity of human atherosclerotic plaques. *Circulation.* 1997;95:594–599.

Vale PR, Losordo DW, Milliken CE, et al. Randomized, single-blind, placebo-controlled pilot study of catheter-based myocardial gene transfer for therapeutic angiogenesis using left ventricular electromechanical mapping in patients with chronic myocardial ischemia. *Circulation.* 2001(103):2138–2143.

Whitmer JT, Kumar P, Solaro RJ. Calcium transport properties of cardiac sarcoplasmic reticulum from cardiomyopathic Syrian hamsters (BIO 53.58 and 14.6): evidence for a quantitative defect in dilated myopathic hearts not evident in hypertrophic hearts. *Circ Res.* 1988;62(1):81–85.

Wolff JA, Malone RW, Williams P, et al. Direct gene transfer into mouse muscle in vivo. *Science.* 1990;247(4949 Pt 1):1465–1468.

Zhang R, Brennan ML, Fu X, et al. Association between myeloperoxidase levels and risk of coronary artery disease. *JAMA.* 2001;286(17):2136–2142.

**NOTES**

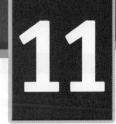

chapter **11**

# *Hypertension*

CHRISTOPHER INGELMO  •  ARMAN T. ASKARI

## QUESTIONS

1. A 30-year-old male with no past medical history presents to his primary care physician complaining of new onset morning headaches that have been ongoing for the past few weeks. His blood pressure is noted to be 220/100 mm Hg with a gradient between his brachial and popliteal arteries. On auscultation there is a II/VI systolic crescendo-decrescendo murmur heard across the precordium. His electrocardiogram is significant for left ventricular hypertrophy. A chest x-ray shows cardiomegaly with evidence of rib notching. The patient most likely has what valvular abnormality?

   a. bicuspid aortic valve
   b. mitral regurgitation
   c. tricuspid regurgitation
   d. pulmonary stenosis

2. A 55-year-old male with diabetes mellitus presents to his cardiologist with a blood pressure of 165/95 mm Hg. According to the JNC 7 guidelines, he would be classified as what stage of hypertension and what is his target blood pressure measurement?

   a. prehypertension, 140/90 mm Hg
   b. stage 2, 130/80 mm Hg
   c. stage 1, 140/90 mm Hg
   d. stage 2, 110/70 mm Hg

3. What is the mechanism of action of the antihypertensive medication Aliskiren?

   a. angiotensin-converting enzyme inhibitor
   b. nonselective beta-blockade
   c. angiotensin receptor blocker
   d. direct renin inhibitor

4. A 35-year-old female with no past medical history, not on oral contraceptives, and with a family history of hypertension presents with a gradual increase in blood pressure over the past few years. Today in clinic her blood pressure is 155/95. What is the most appropriate next step?

   a. Patient has essential hypertension; start thiazide diuretic.
   b. She is asymptomatic; therefore, observe patient and have her follow-up in 1 year.
   c. Have her follow-up in a few weeks for repeat blood pressure measurements.
   d. MRI of kidneys.

5. A 68-year-old male with coronary artery disease, hypertension, diabetes mellitus, and stage II hypertension presents for routine follow-up in the cardiology clinic. His blood pressure is 180/100 mm Hg. He is compliant with all his medications and

is currently on hydrochlorothiazide, lisinopril, metoprolol, amlodipine, and isosorbide mononitrate. He recently has had two episodes of noncardiogenic pulmonary edema in the setting of an ejection fraction of 55% with no evidence of nonsystolic heart failure. What is the most appropriate next step in the management of his hypertension?

**a.** addition of minoxidil
**b.** renal MRI
**c.** discussion of medical adherence
**d.** addition of hydralazine

6. A 42-year-old female with chronic obstructive pulmonary disease is found on multiple office visits to have elevated blood pressure measurements. Which of the following medications is contraindicated?

**a.** hydrochlorothiazide
**b.** metoprolol
**c.** lisinopril
**d.** none of the above

7. Which of the following pairs of medical conditions and antihypertensive medications would be incorrect to use in a patient with essential hypertension?

**a.** beta-blocker and history of myocardial infarction
**b.** alpha-blocker and prostatic hypertrophy
**c.** thiazide diuretic and gout
**d.** angiotensin-converting enzyme and diabetes mellitus

8. A 44-year-old female had a blood pressure of 115/75 mm Hg a few years ago. She now has a blood pressure of 155/75 mm Hg, which was confirmed on a repeat visit. How much has her risk for cardiovascular disease increased?

**a.** no change
**b.** twofold
**c.** fourfold
**d.** tenfold

9. The concomitant use of an angiotensin-converting enzyme (ACE) inhibitor and an NSAID will result in decreased effectiveness of the ACE inhibitor. True or false?

**a.** true
**b.** false

10. Which of the following antihypertensive agents is a known cause of autoimmune hemolytic anemia?

**a.** metoprolol
**b.** methyldopa
**c.** captopril
**d.** losartan

11. A 52-year-old male status post orthotopic heart transplantation develops hypertension. What of the following is the most appropriate antihypertensive agent?

**a.** hydrochlorothiazide
**b.** captopril
**c.** amlodipine
**d.** all of the above

12. Which of the following behavioral modifications have been shown to decrease blood pressure?

**a.** weight reduction
**b.** daily physical activity
**c.** diet rich in potassium and calcium
**d.** all of the above

**13.** A patient is initiated on an angiotensin-converting enzyme (ACE) inhibitor. What is the recommended cutoff for rise in creatinine before stopping the medication?

  **a.** 10% increase in creatinine
  **b.** 20% increase in creatinine
  **c.** 35% increase in creatinine
  **d.** 50% increase in creatinine

**14.** A 68-year-old male with hypertension and history of a stroke presents for further management of his hypertension. He is currently prescribed a thiazide diuretic; however, his blood pressure remains elevated. From the standpoint of decreasing his future risk of stroke, which of the following drug classes would be most beneficial?

  **a.** calcium channel blocker
  **b.** ACE inhibitor
  **c.** angiotensin receptor blocker
  **d.** beta-blocker

**15.** The antihypertensive agent fenoldopam is what class of agent?

  **a.** beta-blocker
  **b.** thiazide diuretic
  **c.** dopamine receptor subclass 1 receptor agonist
  **d.** angiotensin receptor blocker

**16.** A 50-year-old male with uncontrolled hypertension presents for initiation of blood pressure control. Achieving target blood pressure measurements would result in a decreased incidence of which of the following conditions?

  **a.** myocardial infarction
  **b.** stroke
  **c.** heart failure
  **d.** all of the above

**17.** A 50-year-old male with hypertension presents to the clinic office for his yearly physical examination. He informs you that he has been measuring ambulatory daytime blood pressure and it is typically 160/95 mm Hg, while in the clinic it is 140/80 mm Hg. Ambulatory blood pressure measurements are an independent predictor of cardiovascular events. True or false?

  **a.** true
  **b.** false

**18.** A 56-year-old female presents to your clinic for physical examination. She has no significant past medical history and is asymptomatic. Her vital signs are significant for a blood pressure of 145/95 mm Hg. What are the next steps in her evaluation for hypertension?

  **a.** She should return in 1 year for her yearly physical examination.
  **b.** She should have a repeat blood pressure measurement at a later time point during her visit and return in a few weeks to obtain repeat testing if that measurement is elevated.
  **c.** Start patient on thiazide diuretic at the initial clinic visit.
  **d.** Begin evaluation for secondary causes of hypertension.

**19.** A 45-year-old female with no significant past medical history is noted to have a blood pressure of 145/90 mm Hg in the outpatient clinic. This is confirmed on repeat visits. Which of the following tests would not be indicated at this time?

  **a.** electrocardiogram
  **b.** urinalysis
  **c.** creatinine
  **d.** urine metanephrines

**20.** A 26-year-old male with no significant history presents to his primary care physician with complaints of episodic palpitations, morning headaches, and diaphoresis.

He denies any illicit drug use. His physical examination is notable for a blood pressure of 230/120 mm Hg. His ophthalmologic examination is significant for AV nicking. What is the most appropriate next step?

**a.** toxicology screen
**b.** urine metanephrines
**c.** MRI thorax
**d.** start thiazide diuretic with follow-up in 1 month

21. A 65-year-old male with history of hypertension and dyslipidemia is admitted to the coronary care unit with a diagnosis of a myocardial infarction. He undergoes an emergent cardiac catheterization with insertion of a bare metal stent to his left anterior descending coronary artery. His vital signs show a blood pressure of 170/90 with a heart rate of 90 bpm and no evidence of heart failure on examination. Which of the following medications would be most appropriate to treat this patient's hypertension?

**a.** amlodipine
**b.** verapamil
**c.** metoprolol
**d.** nitroprusside

22. Which of the following antihypertensive drug classes is most effective at reducing carotid intimal thickness?

**a.** calcium channel blocker
**b.** beta-blocker
**c.** angiotensin-converting enzyme inhibitor
**d.** thiazide diuretic

23. The antihypertensive agent ramipril is effective at reducing the incidence of diabetes mellitus in patients with prediabetes. True or false?

**a.** true
**b.** false

24. What is the long-term antihypertensive mechanism of action for thiazide diuretics?

**a.** decreased plasma volume
**b.** natriuresis
**c.** decreased cardiac output
**d.** decreased peripheral resistance

25. A 76-year-old male with isolated systolic hypertension should not be treated for his hypertension. True or false?

**a.** true
**b.** false

26. A 46-year-old female, status post orthotopic heart transplantation, is currently taking mycophenolate, prednisone, and tacrolimus as an immunosuppressive regimen. On routine laboratory evaluation she is found to have leukopenia. Mycophenolate levels have not been elevated in the past few months. Which of the following antihypertensive agents is the most likely culprit?

**a.** hydrochlorothiazide
**b.** metoprolol
**c.** captopril
**d.** clonidine

27. A 34-year-old male with isolated essential hypertension presents to clinic and is found to have a blood pressure of 180/100 mm Hg after failure of behavioral modifications. What is the most appropriate next step?

**a.** start hydrochlorothiazide
**b.** start hydrochlorothiazide and lisinopril

**c.** repeat blood pressure in 4 weeks

**d.** start amlodipine

**28.** A 62-year-old male with isolated essential hypertension, currently taking hydrochlorothiazide 25 mg PO daily, comes to you for his first clinic visit. He notes that his blood pressure at home is always less than 140/80 mm Hg, but in clinic it is always at least 155/95 mm Hg. What is the next step?

    **a.** increase dose of thiazide

    **b.** addition of second antihypertensive medication

    **c.** do nothing as he has white coat hypertension

    **d.** evaluate for secondary causes of hypertension

**29.** A 48-year-old male with diabetes mellitus, hypertension, and hyperlipidemia presents to the emergency room with hypertensive emergency. His mean arterial pressure is 150 mm Hg. Which medications would be most appropriate therapy for this patient?

    **a.** nitroprusside

    **b.** enteral metoprolol

    **c.** fenoldopam

    **d.** intravenous nitroglycerin

**30.** A 60-year-old male with left ventricular hypertrophy secondary to hypertension is currently on the angiotensin receptor blocker (ARB) losartan. Which of the following statements is false?

    **a.** Losartan is as effective as atenolol.

    **b.** Angiotensin-converting enzyme (ACE) inhibitors and calcium channel blockers are equally effective.

    **c.** ARBs and ACE inhibitors are equally effective at reducing left ventricular hypertrophy.

    **d.** b and c are true.

**31.** A 48-year-old obese male with hypertension, dyslipidemia, and diabetes mellitus presents to the outpatient clinic for his yearly physical. He has refused medications in the past, but now is willing to consider treatment. His blood pressure is 145/95 with a heart rate of 80 bpm. His laboratory data a significant for a creatinine of 1.3 mg/dL with the presence of microalbuminuria. Which of the following mediations would be most appropriate?

    **a.** carvedilol

    **b.** lisinopril

    **c.** chlorthalidone

    **d.** terazosin

**32.** A 34-year-old female with essential hypertension is considering becoming pregnant. Which of the following medications would be absolutely contraindicated to control her blood pressure during pregnancy?

    **a.** methyldopa

    **b.** labetolol

    **c.** captopril

    **d.** nifedipine

**33.** A 48-year-old Caucasian male with impaired fasting glucose presents to his physician for a follow-up visit after he was noted to have a blood pressure of 150/95 mm Hg. On repeat evaluation his blood pressure is 155/95 mm Hg. Which of the following medications would be the least favored?

    **a.** hydrochlorothiazide 25 mg PO daily

    **b.** lisinopril 10 mg PO daily

    **c.** atenolol 25 mg PO daily

    **d.** chlorthalidone 25 mg PO daily

**34.** A 65-year-old African American male with isolated hypertension presents to clinic for his yearly physical examination. He is noted to have a blood pressure of 170/95 mm Hg. He is currently prescribed lisinopril and metoprolol. Which of the following medication changes would be most appropriate?

   **a.** continue current medications at increased doses
   **b.** conversion of patient to a calcium channel blocker and thiazide diuretic
   **c.** addition of clonidine
   **d.** stopping lisinopril because of concern for renal artery stenosis

**35.** A 42-year-old female with a new diagnosis of diabetes mellitus presents for management of hypertension. She was previously an avid athlete, but over the past few years has noted increased weight gain, a radial fracture after a minor fall, and increasing hirsutism. She is currently on hydrochlorothiazide, amlodipine, and lisinopril. What is the most appropriate next step in the management of this patient's hypertension?

   **a.** referral to nutrition specialist to assist her with weight loss
   **b.** addition of clonidine
   **c.** 24-hour urine cortisol test
   **d.** MRI brain

**36.** A 69-year-old female with diabetes mellitus and hyperlipidemia and no history of hypertension is noted at her yearly clinic visit to have new onset hypertension with a blood pressure of 180/110 mm Hg. She undergoes screening for secondary causes of hypertension and is found to have a pheochromocytoma. What of the following medications is contraindicated as monotherapy?

   **a.** metoprolol
   **b.** lisinopril
   **c.** phentolamine
   **d.** hydrochlorothiazide

**37.** A 42-year-old male comes in for a routine physical examination. He is noted to have a BMI of 30, impaired fasting glucose, and a blood pressure of 135/85 mm Hg. What is the best treatment plan for this individual?

   **a.** aggressive lifestyle modification
   **b.** institute thiazide diuretic regimen
   **c.** no treatment at this time
   **d.** initiate angiotensin-converting enzyme inhibitor

**38.** A 50-year-old male with chronic kidney disease and hypertension has a blood pressure of 165/110 mm Hg. What is this patient's target blood pressure according to the JNC 7 guidelines?

   **a.** 140/90 mm Hg
   **b.** 130/80 mm Hg
   **c.** 120/80 mm Hg
   **d.** 110/70 mm Hg

**39.** A 36-year-old patient, status post heart transplantation, is found to have hypertension. He is currently taking prednisone, mycophenolate, and cyclosporine. Which of the following antihypertensive medications would increase cyclosporine levels?

   **a.** lisinopril
   **b.** hydrocholothiazide
   **c.** diltiazam
   **d.** metoprolol

**40.** A 48-year-old male presents with hypertensive urgency. He receives fenoldopam with improved blood pressure control. A repeat electrocardiogram reveals new-onset T-wave flattening in the anterior and lateral leads. His cardiac biomarkers were unremarkable on admission. He is currently asymptomatic.

Your medical student indicates that this is a known complication of fenoldopam. True or false?

**a.** true
**b.** false

41. A 56-year-old male with resistant hypertension begins to take a new antihypertensive agent. Within the next few weeks he is diagnosed with pericarditis. Which of the following agents is most likely responsible?

**a.** carvedilol
**b.** minoxidil
**c.** amlodipine
**d.** captopril

42. A 27-year-old female presents to the cardiology clinic for evaluation of uncontrolled hypertension. She was diagnosed 2 years ago and is currently taking hydrochlorothiazide, lisinopril, and amlodipine. She denies nonadherence and has a blood pressure of 170/100 mm Hg that is equal in both arms. On routine laboratory examination she has a potassium level of 2.9 mEq/L with a sodium level of 148 mEq/L. What is the most appropriate diagnostic test?

**a.** renal MRI/MRA
**b.** morning renin and aldosterone concentrations
**c.** adrenal vein sampling
**d.** 24-hour urine cortisol concentration

43. A 58-year-old obese male with hypertension, diabetes mellitus, hyperlipidemia, and recent myocardial infarction presents for his yearly physical examination. He is currently prescribed atenolol, hydrochlorothiazide, amlodipine, and quinapril. His blood pressure is at target values. His HgA1c is at goal. However, he has noted increasing lower extremity edema over the past few months and had a near-fatal car accident after falling asleep while driving. His echocardiogram reveals an ejection fraction of 65% with no evidence of nonsystolic dysfunction. Which of the following management decisions would be most appropriate at this time?

**a.** discontinue calcium channel blocker
**b.** overnight sleep study
**c.** addition of loop diuretic
**d.** maintain current regimen with advisement that his symptoms are typical with aging

44. A 69-year-old male presents to the emergency room with complaints of chest pain. His electrocardiogram is significant for left ventricular hypertrophy, and serum troponin T measurements are mildly positive. His blood pressure is 240/140 mm Hg. He admits to recent cocaine use. Which of the following medications would be contraindicated?

**a.** metoprolol
**b.** nifedipine
**c.** nitroprusside
**d.** nitroglycerin

45. A 57-year-old female taking carvedilol for hypertension and congestive heart failure wants to know about the possible side effects. Which of the following are known side effects of carvedilol?

**a.** bradycardia
**b.** renal failure
**c.** increased liver function tests
**d.** all of the above

46. A 58-year-old male with diabetes mellitus and hypertension indicates that his insurance company would like him to change from his ACE inhibitor to an

angiotensin receptor blocker. His insurance company indicates that blood pressure outcomes are equivalent. True or false?

**a.** true
**b.** false

**47.** A 56-year-old male on hydralazine, hydrochlorothiazide, lisinopril, and metoprolol begins to develop a malar rash and arthralgias. Which of the above antihypertensive agents is known to cause drug-induced lupus?

**a.** hydralazine
**b.** hydrochlorothiazide
**c.** lisinopril
**d.** metoprolol

**48.** A 47-year-old male with coronary artery disease, diabetes mellitus, and hypertension is currently taking clonidine. He is found to have a blood pressure of 170/90 mm Hg after forgetting to take his medication for 48 hours. What is the best strategy to control his blood pressure?

**a.** restart clonidine
**b.** start nitroprusside
**c.** start esmolol
**d.** add thiazide diuretic

**49.** A 38-year-old male with hypertension and atrial fibrillation who is on digoxin began to experience blurred vision, nausea, and diarrhea after starting a new blood pressure medication. His electrocardiogram is significant for complete heart block with a junctional tachycardia. Which of the following antihypertensive agents is responsible for the above symptoms?

**a.** metoprolol
**b.** verapamil
**c.** candesartan
**d.** lisinopril

**50.** Which of the following statements regarding antihypertensive agents and atrial fibrillation is true?

**a.** Losartan has been shown to decrease new-onset atrial fibrillation more effectively than atenolol.
**b.** Valsartan has been shown to decrease new-onset atrial fibrillation more effectively than amlodipine.
**c.** Atenolol has been shown to decrease new-onset atrial fibrillation more effectively than captopril.
**d.** All of the above are false.

## ANSWERS

1. **a.** The young man in this vignette has a classic presentation of coarctation of the aorta. This secondary cause of hypertension is the result of stenosis of the aorta, usually at the embryonic site of the ligamentum arteriosum, and is typically distal to the origin of the left subclavian artery. The presentation in adulthood is varied and is twice as common in men. Symptoms of hypertension or congestive heart failure are common. The electrocardiogram is characterized by left ventricular hypertrophy. Right ventricular hypertrophy is common if a concomitant ventricular septal defect is present. The most common associated valvular abnormality is a bicuspid aortic valve seen in 22% to 42% of cases. Intracranial aneurysms are seen in up to 10% of cases. Patients will often have a characteristic systolic precordial murmur secondary to the development of collateral arteries. Long-term management involves surgical or transcatheter correction. Patients will often continue to have systemic hypertension after repair and should be treated accordingly.

2. **b.** The most recent JNC 7 guidelines reclassified the stages of hypertension. Normal blood pressure was defined as a systolic blood pressure less than 120 mm Hg or a diastolic blood pressure less than 80 mm Hg. The prehypertension stage is defined as a systolic blood pressure of 120 to 129 mm Hg or a diastolic blood pressure of 80 to 89 mm Hg. Stage 1 hypertension is classified as a systolic blood pressure of 130 to 159 mm Hg or a diastolic blood pressure of 90 to 99 mm Hg. Stage 2 hypertension is defined as a systolic blood pressure of 160 mm Hg or greater or a diastolic blood pressure of 100 mm Hg or greater. Target blood pressure recommendations are 140/90 mm Hg for those without comorbid conditions, such as diabetes mellitus or chronic kidney disease. In those conditions, the target blood pressure is 130/80 mm Hg. Our patient has stage 2 hypertension with a target blood pressure of 130/80 mm Hg.

3. **d.** Aliskiren is the first FDA-approved direct renin inhibitor. Aliskiren is a competitive inhibitor of the enzyme renin. The enzyme controls the rate-limiting step in the generation of angiotensin II. It reaches peak concentration in 2 to 4 hours with a half-life of 24 to 36 hours. It is 50% protein bound. Diarrhea is the most common side effect occurring in up to 9.5% of patients. A dose of 150 mg daily will decrease systolic blood pressure on average 12.5 mm Hg with a further 2.7 mm Hg decrease when the dose is increased to 300 mg PO daily as compared to placebo. Aliskiren has been shown to have similar blood-pressure–lowering effects when compared to thiazide diuretics as well as angiotensin-converting enzyme inhibitors. However, to date there are limited data on the effect of aliskiren on hypertension-induced end-organ damage and clinical outcomes.

4. **a.** The patient likely has essential hypertension. The age of onset is typically between the early 20s to the late 50s. The presence of a family history of hypertension, the mild elevation in blood pressure, and the gradual onset make the diagnosis of essential hypertension more likely. First-line therapy in this individual, assuming she is not trying to become pregnant, is the use of a thiazide diuretic. Re-evaluation in 1 year would not be appropriate given the long-term complications associated with uncontrolled hypertension. A repeat evaluation in a few weeks is not necessary given the documented hypertension over the past few years. The presence of unilateral renal artery stenosis from vascular hyperplasia is a possibility; however, the clinical history is most consistent with essential hypertension.

5. **b.** The distinction between essential hypertension and secondary causes is critical in the management of a patient with long-standing hypertension that is difficult to control. In this scenario, the inability to control the patient's blood pressure with multiple medications increases the pretest probability of a secondary etiology. In this individual, the presence of multiple cardiac risk factors, along with

repeat episodes of noncardiogenic pulmonary edema, suggests the diagnosis of bilateral renal artery stenosis. Addition of further antihypertensive medications would be indicated, but not prior to initiating a workup for renal artery stenosis. A renal MRI would be the most appropriate of the above answers.

6. **d.** None of the medications listed are contraindicated. A recent Cochrane review in patients with COPD defined as an $FEV_1$ <80% predicted found no changes in $FEV_1$ or symptoms with single or continuous dosing of beta-blockers. A subsequent meta-analysis confirmed this finding even in patients with severe COPD defined by an $FEV_1$ of <50% predicted. The presence of moderate to severe reactive airway disease would be a contraindication to beta-blockade, but the patient in the clinical vignette does not have an asthma component to her pulmonary disease.

7. **c.** According to the JNC 7 guidelines, the initial choice of antihypertensive medication is typically a thiazide diuretic unless altered by comorbid conditions. Beta-blockers would be an acceptable alternative in a patient with known coronary artery disease. Alpha-blockers would be beneficial to treat hypertension patients who have concomitant prostatic hypertrophy. Angiotensin-converting enzyme inhibitors are first-line therapy for treatment of hypertension in patients with diabetes mellitus. Thiazide diuretics should be used with caution in patients with history of gout as these medications can induce a state of hyperuricemia that would exacerbate the underling condition.

8. **b.** Increasing blood pressure beginning at 115/75 mm Hg is noted to be a risk factor for stroke, heart failure, and myocardial infarction. For every 20 mm Hg increase in systolic blood pressure and for every 10 mm Hg in diastolic blood pressure there is a twofold increase in the risk of cardiovascular disease. For the above patient, her risk of cardiovascular disease has increased by twofold.

9. **a.** True. The antihypertensive effect of an angiotensin-converting enzyme (ACE) inhibitor may be blunted by the use of NSAIDs. Of the available antihypertensive agents, calcium channel blockers are the least affected by NSAID use.

10. **b.** The central alpha agonist methyldopa is known to cause an autoimmune hemolytic anemia in up to 20% of patients taking the medication. Other common side effects include sedation, insulin resistance, and galactorrhea. Methyldopa is not a first-line agent for treatment of hypertension and is usually reserved for pregnant patients and those with resistant hypertension.

11. **d.** Hypertension is common status post heart transplantation. Anywhere from 50% to 95% of heart transplant patients have a diagnosis of hypertension. Many have pre-existing hypertension while others develop it post-transplant. This is often attributed to the immunosuppressive medications such as steroids, cyclosporine, and tacrolimus, all of which have been implicated as having a causal link with post-transplant hypertension. Currently there are no clinical trials that show superiority of one antihypertensive over another in heart transplant patients, but given the loss of the circadian rhythm of blood pressure, treatment is critical. Therefore, any of the above medications would be appropriate. Selection should be based on comorbidities and possible interactions with immunosuppressive medications.

12. **d.** Lifestyle modifications endorsed by JNC 7 include weight reduction, Dietary Approach to Stop Hypertension (DASH) diet, low sodium diet, physical activity, and moderate alcohol consumption. Each kilogram of weight loss is associated with a 5- to 20- mm Hg decrease in blood pressure. The DASH diet, rich in potassium and calcium, is associated with an 8- to 14- mm Hg decrease in blood pressure. Sodium restriction results in a 2- to 8- mm Hg decrease in blood pressure. Physical activity and moderate alcohol consumption decrease blood pressure by 4- to 9- mm Hg and 2- to 4- mm Hg, respectively. These behavioral modifications, when optimized, enhance the antihypertensive effectiveness of pharmacotherapy.

**13. c.** According to the JNC 7 guidelines, patients initiated on an ACE inhibitor should be continued on that medication unless the creatinine increases by more than 35% or another indication for discontinuation presents itself.

**14. a.** The Blood Pressure Lowering Treatment Trialist Collaboration Study found that calcium channel blockers provided a greater benefit in the reduction of stroke when compared to other antihypertensive agents. However, there was no difference in cardiovascular mortality or overall cardiovascular events.

**15. c.** Fenoldopam is a selective dopamine 1 receptor agonist. It causes peripheral vasodilation and diuresis. It does not penetrate the blood–brain barrier. It has 6% bioavailability and a half-life of 10 minutes. It reaches its peak effect in 1 to 4 hours, with tachyphylaxis at 24 hours. There is no evidence of rebound hypertension. Side effects include nausea, vomiting, tachycardia, and flushing. It has been shown to be as effective as nitroprusside in treating severe hypertension. It appears to improve renal function, but there is no evidence of long-term renal benefit.

**16. d.** Lowering blood pressure has multiple benefits, in particular with regard to decreased risk of stroke, myocardial infarction, and heart failure. Achieving target blood pressure is known to result in a 35% reduction in stroke, 25% in myocardial infarction, and 50% in heart failure, as noted in the JNC 7 guidelines.

**17. a.** True. Recent data suggest that patients who have a diagnosis of hypertension with normotensive measurements in the clinic setting, but with elevated ambulatory blood pressure (masked hypertension), are at greater risk of cardiovascular events independent of traditional risk factors. The JNC 7 guidelines recommend the use of ambulatory blood pressure measurements for any patient you suspect has white-coat hypertension, labile hypertension, postural hypotension, resistant hypertension, or hypotensive episodes.

**18. b.** The Joint National Committee 7 guidelines suggest that the diagnosis of hypertension requires at least two separate blood pressure measurements during a clinic visit. The patient should be resting in a chair for at least 5 minutes and should have her arm supported at heart level when the blood pressure is measured. Blood pressure measurements should be evaluated in the contralateral arm and while standing as well. Elevations in blood pressure should be confirmed in a timely manner on a repeat visit, the timing of which is dependent on the level of hypertension and the presence of comorbid conditions. The patient in this vignette has mild isolated hypertension and should return in a few weeks (6-8 wk). Those with more elevated blood pressure should return sooner. Antihypertensive medications should not be initiated on this initial visit as diurnal variations in blood pressure are common and she may not have hypertension. Ambulatory monitoring of blood pressure should be attempted. An evaluation for secondary cause is premature as the diagnosis of hypertension is not confirmed. Waiting to re-evaluate the patient in 1 year's time is unacceptable, as hypertension, if left untreated, increases the risk of stroke, myocardial infarction, heart failure, and renal insufficiency.

**19. d.** The initial assessment of any patient with a new diagnosis of hypertension requires evaluation for evidence of hypertension-induced end organ damage. All patients with a new diagnosis of hypertension should have the following testing: serum hematocrit, blood urea nitrogen, serum creatinine, serum potassium, serum calcium, blood glucose, an electrocardiogram, an ophthalmologic examination, a fasting lipid panel, and a urinalysis. Evaluation for secondary causes of hypertension should be limited to those with uncontrolled hypertension after treatment.

**20. b.** This patient's medical history is consistent with a diagnosis of pheochromocytoma. Pheochromocytomas arise from chromaffin cells. These tumors are most commonly found in the adrenal glands, but may be present anywhere there are sympathetic nerves. Classic symptoms are episodic palpitations, headaches, and diaphoresis. Rarely, patients may present with orthostatic hypotension.

Initial diagnostic testing would involve the evaluation of a urine specimen for urine metanephrines. A toxicology screen is not indicated given his clinical history. An MRI of the abdomen would be helpful to evaluate for intra-abdominal masses, but an MRI thorax would be of limited benefit. Starting a thiazide diuretic would be beneficial, but ultimately the patient requires surgical therapy for correction of his hypertension.

21. **c.** The initial choice of antihypertensive medication in this patient should be a beta-blocker. Multiple studies have shown the benefit of beta-blockers in the post–myocardial infarction period. The MIAMI-1 and ISIS-1 trials in the fibrinolytic era both showed trends toward a decrease in mortality with the use of intravenous beta-blockers. The COMMIT trial found decreases in the rate of reinfarction and ventricular fibrillation with intravenous metoprolol followed by oral metoprolol; however, there was a 30% increase in the risk of cardiogenic shock. A meta-analysis of the post–myocardial infarction use of beta-blockers has shown up to a 40% decrease in cardiovascular mortality. The American Heart Association 2007 STEMI guidelines classify perimyocardial infarction beta-blocker usage as a class I indication; however, intravenous beta-blockers are a class IIa indication given the concern for possible complications.

22. **a.** Calcium channel blockers are the most effective of the antihypertensive regimens at reducing carotid atherosclerosis. Studies comparing various calcium channel blockers to thiazide diuretics, angiotensin-converting enzyme inhibitors, and beta-blockers have shown that calcium channel blockers have greater ability to decrease carotid intimal thickness.

23. **b.** False. It has been hypothesized that blockage of the renin-angiotensin system may decrease the incidence of diabetes mellitus in those at increased risk of developing diabetes. The DREAM study evaluated the effectiveness of ramipril over a period of 3 years at decreasing the incidence of diabetes mellitus in those with impaired glucose intolerance and fasting glucose and found that during a period of 3 years there was no difference in the incidence of diabetes mellitus (18.1% in ramipril group vs. 19.1% in placebo group). There was an increase in return to normoglycemia in the ramipril group; however, this was not the primary outcome designated.

24. **d.** The initial mechanism of action for lowering blood pressure is a decrease in plasma volume secondary to natriuresis. This triggers an increase in the activity of the rennin-angiotensin system resulting in a return of plasma volume to normal. However, there is a long-term decrease in peripheral resistance that produces the chronic antihypertensive effects of thiazide diuretics.

25. **b.** False. According to the JNC 7 guidelines, those with isolated systolic hypertension with systolic blood pressure greater than 140 mm Hg should be treated with antihypertensive therapy. Isolated systolic hypertension is a known risk factor for cardiovascular disease. Treatment of elderly patients with the diuretic chlorthalidone for 4.5 years resulted in decreases in the incidence of stroke, heart failure, and coronary artery disease.

26. **c.** Aside from mycophenolate, the angiotensin-converting enzyme (ACE) inhibitor captopril is the most likely cause of this patient's leukopenia. When immunosuppressive therapy is combined with ACE inhibitors, there are reports of the development of anemia, neutropenia, leukopenia, and agranulocytosis. The best treatment strategy in this patient would be to use an alternative antihypertensive agent and monitor blood counts closely.

27. **b.** The most appropriate initial step in the management of the patient in this clinical vignette is the initiation of two antihypertensive medications as recommended in the JNC 7 guidelines. In general, if patients have a blood pressure of greater than 20/10 mm Hg above goal they should be initiated on two antihypertensive agents because monotherapy will typically be ineffective in achieving target blood pressure.

Most patients should be started on a thiazide diuretic when commencing treatment of hypertension, as confirmed by the results of the Antihypertensive and Lipid Lowering Treatment to Prevent Heart Attack Trial. Care should be taken in patients at risk for hypotension, specifically elderly patients, those with diabetes, and those with autonomic dysfunction.

28. **c.** The patient in the above clinical vignette has a diagnosis of white coat hypertension. It is defined as a clinic blood pressure of >140/80 mm Hg in at least three clinic settings, with blood pressure measurements of <140/80 mm Hg in at least two nonclinic settings, and with absence of end-organ damage. Multiple studies have been undertaken to evaluate if isolated elevations in blood pressure in the medical setting are associated with increased cardiovascular events. A 10-year follow-up study comparing cardiovascular events between patients with white coat hypertension and those with sustained hypertension found worse outcomes in those with sustained hypertension. The risk of myocardial infarction was two times greater and the risk of a cerebral vascular event was four times greater in the sustained hypertension group. Comparison of normotensive patients versus those with white coat hypertension has noted a greater prevalence of left ventricular hypertrophy in the white coat hypertension group. However, there are no clear data that white coat hypertension increases long-term cardiovascular events. Treatment of white coat hypertension is associated with decreases in clinic blood pressure with no significant decrease in ambulatory blood pressure. Patients with white coat hypertension should be monitored closely for development of sustained hypertension, but do not need to be initiated on antihypertensive therapy.

29. **a.** Treatment of hypertensive emergency requires the use of intravenous medications to decrease the mean arterial blood pressure by 25% in the first few hours. Lower target blood pressure goals increase the risk of inducing a cerebral vascular event from decreased cerebral perfusion. Nitroprusside, fenoldopam, and nitroglycerin are all possible options. However, given the rapid onset and offset of nitroprusside this would be the most appropriate medication for rapid and safe titration of blood pressure.

30. **a.** Multiple studies have evaluated the comparative ability of different antihypertensive agents at reducing left ventricular hypertrophy (LVH). Evidence from the Losartan Intervention for End Point Reduction in Hypertension (LIFE) trial has shown that losartan is more effective than atenolol at reducing LVH. Comparison of ARBs and ACE inhibitors have shown similar reductions in LVH. Trials of calcium channel blockers and ACE inhibitors have shown similar reductions in LVH.

31. **b.** The patient in the vignette has a target blood pressure of 130/80 mm Hg according to the most recent JNC 7 guidelines. The correct choice of initial blood pressure medication in this patient would be an angiotensin-converting enzyme inhibitor (ACEI). The ALLHAT study suggested that patients with diabetes mellitus have better long-term outcomes when using a thiazide diuretic compared to an ACEI. However, the patient in this vignette has evidence of protein in his urine. Current guidelines indicate that a thiazide diuretic should be first-line therapy, unless there is a specific indication. In this patient, the presence of proteinuria and diabetes mellitus makes the choice of an ACEI a better option than the thiazide. Alpha-blockers are not considered first-line therapy in hypertensive patients. In the ALLHAT study there was an increased incidence of heart failure when comparing the alpha-blocker group (doxazosin) versus the thiazide group.

32. **c.** ACE inhibitors and angiotensin receptor blockers are contraindicated during pregnancy, because of the increased risk of congenital malformations. Methyldopa is the medication most commonly used to control blood pressure in pregnancy. There is significant evidence that it does not produce any harmful outcomes to the fetus. Beta-blockers have been used in pregnancy with what appear to be safe results.

However, the data are contradictory. There is some evidence that beta-blockers, especially when used early in pregnancy, may increase the risk of fetal bradycardia, hypoglycemia, small placental weight, and a small-for-gestational-age fetus. Calcium channel blockers have been used in pregnancy without deleterious results, but the number of published cases is small. In general, methyldopa is the safest antihypertensive during pregnancy. Beta-blockers and calcium channel blockers may be used with caution. ACE inhibitors and angiotensin receptor blockers are contraindicated.

**33. c.** The least likely choice is atenolol. The ALLHAT study showed that the use of thiazide diuretics as first-line therapy for treatment of uncomplicated hypertension was as effective as, if not superior to, amlodipine and lisinopril in preventing fatal coronary artery disease and nonfatal myocardial infarction. The choice of an angiotensin-converting enzyme inhibitor would be reasonable given the presence of glucose intolerance. Beta-blockers would not be indicated as first-line therapy in this patient. Multiple meta-analysis comparing beta-blockers to placebo or other antihypertensive agents has shown no statistically significant decreases in mortality, myocardial infarction, and stroke. The ASCOT trial comparing atenolol with amlodipine found a 23% greater risk of stroke in the atenolol group versus the amlodipine-based regimen.

**34. b.** Analysis of the clinical trials in hypertension has noted that there are differences in the effectiveness of antihypertensive medications between different ethnic groups. African Americans are more responsive to calcium channel blockers and thiazide diuretics than other antihypertensive agents. This patient is on an angiotensin-converting enzyme inhibitor and a beta-blocker. Altering his regiment to include more effective antihypertensive agents would be indicated rather than increasing his medications, adding additional medications, or evaluating him for secondary causes of hypertension.

**35. c.** This patient's medical history is consistent with a secondary cause of hypertension, in particular, Cushing's syndrome. This syndrome is characterized by an excess of cortisol. It may be secondary to a pituitary tumor/hyperplasia (Cushing's disease), an adrenal tumor, or ectopic ACTH production. Clinical manifestations include diabetes mellitus, hypertension, obesity, hypokalemia, osteoporosis, and fungal infections. The initial step in diagnosis is a 24-hour urine free cortisol test. Treatment is surgical.

**36. a.** Pheochromocytoma is a rare cause of hypertension. Treatment ultimately requires surgical removal. The use of beta-blocker monotherapy is contraindicated as part of the medical management of pheochromcytomas. The catecholamines secreted by these tumors activate both peripheral alpha and beta receptors. Blockage of these peripheral beta receptors results in unopposed alpha activation. This can result in severe hypertension. Typical medical management of pheochromocytomas involves the use of antihypertensives with alpha-blocking capability. For example, prazosin or phenoxybenzamine may be used. Only once alpha-blockade is established should the use of a beta-blocker be entertained.

**37. a.** Patients with prehypertension are at increased risk of cardiovascular events compared to normotensive individuals; therefore, care of these patients should be focused on aggressive control of all cardiovascular risk factors. Analysis of the Women's Health Initiative compared cardiovascular outcomes in prehypertension patients versus normotensive patients and found that the prehypertension patients had hazard ratios indicating a 1.58 (95% confidence interval [CI], 1.12 to 2.21) greater risk for cardiovascular death; 1.76 (95% CI, 1.40 to 2.22) greater risk for myocardial infarction; 1.93 (95% CI, 1.49 to 2.50) greater risk for stroke; 1.36 (95% CI, 1.05 to 1.77) greater risk for hospitalized heart failure; and a 1.66 (95% CI, 1.44 to 1.92) greater risk for any cardiovascular event. Not only are these patients at increased risk of cardiovascular outcome, but they have a high incidence of developing hypertension. In the TROPHY trial, patients with prehypertension were randomized to candesartan or placebo. Over a period of 4 years,

67% of the untreated group developed hypertension as defined by the JNC 7 guidelines. These data suggest that patients with prehypertension are a high-risk population and should be treated aggressively. According to the JNC 7 guidelines, these individuals should increase their activity level, modify their diet, avoid excessive alcohol, and attempt weight loss. Initiation of antihypertensive medications should be reserved for those who progress to evident hypertension.

**38. b.** Current JNC 7 guidelines recommend that in patients with chronic kidney disease or diabetes mellitus, the target blood pressure should be <130/80 mm Hg.

**39. c.** Patients who have undergone a heart transplantation often have pre-existing hypertension or develop hypertension subsequent to the heart transplant. This is a unique patient population as many of the immunosuppressive medications used after transplantation have multiple drug interactions. With respect to antihypertensive agents, most if not all calcium channel blockers have been shown to increase cyclosporine levels. Diltiazem and verapamil, in particular, are potent inhibitors of protein P-glycoprotein and CYP 3A4. These enzymes are critical for the metabolism of diltiazem, and their inhibition can increase cyclosporine levels up to sixfold. It is recommended that patients who require diltiazem and are on cyclosporine have their cyclosporine dose decreased by 25% to 50%. Diltiazem can also increase tacrolimus levels.

**40. a.** True. Fenoldopam is a selective dopamine 1 receptor agonist that can be used effectively to treat hypertensive emergency. A known complication of this medication is the development of T-wave inversions or flattening in the anterior and lateral leads. They are of no clinical significance and are not thought to be related to ongoing ischemia. Patients with glaucoma should not receive fenoldopam as it can increase intraocular pressure.

**41. b.** Peridarditis is a known complication of the direct vasodilator minoxidil often accompanied by a pericardial effusion. Its other major side effect is hirsutism. Prompt withdrawal of the medication once the diagnosis of a pericardial effusion or pericarditis is made is recommended. Minoxidil is a potent peripheral vasodilator and is typically reserved for patients with severe or difficult-to-control hypertension.

**42. b.** The patient in this vignette has secondary hypertension from Conn's syndrome. This is primary hyperaldosteronism from uncontrolled secretion of aldosterone. Classic laboratory findings include hypokalemia and mild hypernatremia. The initial diagnostic test of choice is an aldosterone-renin ratio. A ratio of >20 is considered diagnostic. In this patient, the presence of lisinopril complicates the testing. Angiotensin-converting enzyme (ACE) inhibitors are known to decrease renin levels, and ideally the test should be done in the early morning after withdrawal of ACE inhibitor therapy. Adrenal vein sampling would be helpful in the diagnosis of primary hyperaldosteronism; however, it is not the initial test of choice. A 24-hour urine test would be more appropriate if Cushing's syndrome were suspected. The patient clinical description is not consistent with this diagnosis. The presence of fibromuscular dysplasia should be suspected in any young female with suspected secondary hypertension. However, the laboratory abnormalities are more suggestive of Conn's syndrome than renal artery stenosis.

**43. b.** The patient's clinical history is consistent with the presence of obstructive sleep apnea; therefore, an overnight sleep study would be the best option. Multiple studies have found evidence for increased risk of hypertension in patients with obstructive sleep apnea. There is no definitive evidence that treating patients with sleep apnea can lower blood pressure; however, there is an increasing hypertension risk as the number of overnight apneic episodes increases. Patients with >30 apnea or hypopnea episodes per hour have an odds ratio of 1.37 of developing hypertension versus those patients with <1.5 apnea or hypopnea episodes per hour.

**44. a.** Beta-blockers are contraindicated in the management of patients with hypertension secondary to cocaine use, especially when evidence of ongoing ischemia is present. Cocaine causes myocardial ischemia and hypertension partly through alpha-receptor–mediated vasoconstriction. The use of beta-blockers may exacerbate the vasoconstriction and make hypertension and coronary ischemia worse. In patients with ongoing cocaine use nitroglycerin and labetolol are recommended for antihypertensive management. Verapamil and benzodiazepines are also possible alternatives.

**45. d.** All of the above. Carvedilol is a combination alpha- and beta-blocker that is most commonly used for management of congestive heart failure. Patients on carvedilol should be monitored for bradycardia, nausea, vomiting, blurred vision, and worsening heart failure. Increases in liver function tests and worsening renal failure are also known complications.

**46. a.** True. There is no direct comparison of angiotensin receptor blockers (ARBs) and angiotensin-converting enzyme (ACE) inhibitors in hypertension patients. Data from heart failure and coronary artery disease trials suggest no difference in stroke, heart failure, and coronary artery disease outcomes between the two drug classes. In a recent meta-analysis, the two drug classes appear to exert similar blood-pressure–lowering reduction effects on heart failure, stroke, and coronary artery disease. However, ACE inhibitors produce a 9% relative risk reduction in coronary artery disease independent of blood pressure lowering. Overall, there appears to be no substantial difference when comparing ACE inhibitors and ARBs in blood pressure reduction.

**47. a.** Hydralazine is known to cause a lupus-like syndrome in 5% to 20% of patients taking the medication. This syndrome is characterized by arthralgias, myalgias, pericariditis, fever, and rash. Lisinopril, metoprolol, and hydrochlorothiazide are not known to induce lupus. Other side effects of hydralazine include nausea, vomiting, tachycardia, anorexia, flushing, and diarrhea. Treatment of hydralazine-induced lupus involves withdrawal of the medication.

**48. a.** Rebound hypertension is a known complication of clonidine. Immediate treatment of clonidine withdrawal involves reinstitution of therapy with a slow taper. The mechanism of action is thought to be an increase in sympathetic nervous system activity.

**49. b.** The patient in this scenario has a classic case of digoxin toxicity. Verapamil interferes with the P-glycoprotein transport and clearance of digoxin and increases drug levels, predisposing patients to digoxin toxicity. Metoprolol, candesartan, and lisinopril are not known to interfere with digoxin clearance unless they affect renal function. Any patient on digoxin who is initiated on verapamil should have digoxin levels checked to monitor for elevated levels that may be toxic.

**50. a.** In the LIFE trial, the angiotensin receptor blocker losartan was more effective than atenolol at decreasing the incidence of atrial fibrillation. Over a period of 4.8 years, the losartan group had a 6.8% risk of developing atrial fibrillation while the atenolol group had a 10.1% risk of developing atrial fibrillation.

## Suggested Reading

ALLHAT Officers and the Coordinators for the ALLHAT Collaborative Research Group. Major outcomes in high risk hypertensive patients randomized to angiotensin converting enzyme inhibitors or calcium channel blockers vs. diuretic. *JAMA.* 2002;288:2981–2997.

Blood Pressure Lowering Treatment Trialists' Collaboration. Blood pressure dependent and independent effects of agents that affect the renin angiotensin system. *J Hypertens.* 2007;25:951–958.

Blood Pressure Lowering Treatment Trialists' Collaboration. Effects of ACE inhibitors, calcium antagonists, and other blood-pressure-lowering drugs: results of prospectively designed overviews of randomized trials. *Lancet.* 2000;356:1955–1964.

Blood Pressure Lowering Treatment Trialists' Collaboration. Effects of different blood pressure regimens on cardiovascular events: results of prospectively designed overview of randomized trials. *Lancet.* 2003;362:1527–1535.

Chobanian AV. Isolated systolic hypertension in elderly. *N Engl J Med.* 2007;357:789–796.

Chobanian AV, Bakris GJ, Black HR, et al. The Seventh Report of the Joint National Committee on Prevention, Detection, Evaluation, and Treatment of High Blood Pressure: The JNC 7 Report. *JAMA.* 2003;289:2560–2572.

Clement DC, Buyzere MD, Bacquer DA, et al. Prognostic value of ambulatory blood pressure recordings in patients with treated hypertension. *N Engl J Med.* 2003;348:2407–2415.

Dahlof B, Sever PS, Poulter NR, et al. Prevention of cardiovascular events with an antihypertensive regimen of amlodipine adding perindopril as required versus atenolol adding benoflumethiazide as required, in the Anglo Scandinavian Cardiac Outcomes Trial-Blood Pressure Lowering Arm (ASCOT-BLA). *Lancet.* 2005;366:895–906.

Devereux RB, Dahlof B, Gerdts E, et al. Regression of hypertensive left ventricular hypertrophy by losartan compared to atenolol: the Losartan Intervention for End Point Reduction in Hypertesion (LIFE) Study. *Circulation.* 2004;110:1456–1462.

Devereux RB, Palmieri V, Sharpe N, et al. Effects of once daily angiotensin converting enzyme inhibition and calcium channel blockade based antihypertensive treatment regimens on left ventricular hypertrophy and diastolic filling in hypertension. *Circulation.* 2001;19:303–309.

DREAM Trial Investigators. Effectiveness of ramipril on the incidence of diabetes. *N Engl J Med.* 2006;355:1551–1562.

Gradman AH, Kad R. Renin inhibition in hypertension. *J Am Coll Cardiol.* 2008;51:519–528.

Hsia J, Margolis KL, Eaton CB, et al. Prehypertension and cardiovascular disease risk in the Women's Health Initiative. *Circulation.* 2007;115:855–860.

Julius S, Nesbitt S, Egan BM, et al. Feasibility of treating prehypertension with an angiotensin receptor blocker. *N Engl J Med.* 2006;354:1685–1697.

Khattar RS, Senior R, and Lahiri A. Cardiovascular outcome in white-coat versus sustained mild hypertension: a 10-year follow-up study. *Circulation.* 1998;98:1892–1897.

Lidenfield J, Page RL, Zolty R, et al. Drug therapy in the heart transplant recipient part III: common medical problems. *Circulation.* 2005;113:113–117.

Murphy MB, Murray C, Shorten GD. Fenoldopam—a selective peripheral dopamine receptor agonist for the treatment of severe hypertension. *N Engl J Med.* 2001;345:1548–1557.

Nieto FJ, Young TB, Lind BK, et al. Association of sleep disordered breathing, sleep apnea and hypertension in a large community based study. *JAMA.* 2000;283:1829–1836.

Page RL, Miller GG, Lidenfield J. Drug therapy in the heart transplant recipient part IV: drug-drug interactions. *Circulation.* 2005;111:230–239.

Prospective Studies Collaboration. Age-specific relevance of usual blood pressure to vascular mortality: a meta-analysis of individual data for one million adults in 61 prospective studies. *Lancet.* 2002;360:1903–1913.

Salpeter S, Ormiston T, Salpeter E. Cardioselective beta-blockers for chronic obstructive pulmonary disease. *The Cochrane Library.* 2006;3:1–25.

Salpeter S, Ormiston T, Salpeter E. Cardioselective beta-blockers in reactive airway disease. *The Cochrane Library.* 2006;3:1–45.

Sega R, Trocino S, Lanzarotti A, et al. Alterations in cardiac structure in patients with isolated office, ambulatory or home hypertension: data from the general population Pressione Arteriose Monitorate E Loro Associazioni [PAMELA] Study *Circulation.* 2001;104(12):1385–1392.

Simon A, Gariepy J, Moyse D, et al. Differential effects of nifedipine and co-amilozide on the progression of early carotid wall changes. *Circulation.* 2001;103:2949–2954.

Terpesta WF, May JF, Smit AJ, et al. Effect of amlodipine and lisinopril on intima media thickness in previously untreated elderly hypertensive patients (the ELVERA Trial). *J Hypertens.* 2004;22:1309–1316.

Wachtell K, Lehto N, Gerdts E, et al. Angiotensin II receptor blockade reduces new onset atrial fibrillation and subsequent stroke compared to atenolol: the Losartan Intervention for End Point Reduction in Hypertension (LIFE) Study. *J Am Coll Cardiol.* 2005;45:712–719.

**NOTES**

# chapter 12

# Pericardial Disease

MONVADI B. SRICHAI · WAEL A. JABER

## QUESTIONS

1. An 82-year-old man, who has a history of CAD with two surgical coronary revascularizations, is presenting with a few months' history of dyspnea on exertion, increased abdominal girth, and pedal edema. An evaluation performed in the office of his local cardiologist showed a slightly depressed LV EF of 45%. His cardiologist refers him to your center with the differential diagnosis of constrictive versus restrictive heart disease. All of the following echocardiographic markers support constrictive physiology *except*

   a. dissociation between intracardiac and intrathoracic pressures
   b. exaggerated ventricular interdependence in diastolic filling
   c. respiratory difference >20 cm/second in superior vena cava flow velocities
   d. increased atrial pressures and equalization of end-diastolic pressures

2. A 32-year-old white man presented initially with low-grade fever, cough, and pleuritic chest pain. He was found on ECG to have diffuse ST-segment elevation. A TTE revealed a large pericardial effusion, and serologies were positive for coxsackievirus B infection. He was diagnosed with acute viral pericarditis and treated with indomethacin. He returns 4 weeks later for follow-up and states that he no longer has any pain, but he notes some mild ankle swelling. His ECG is normal. A repeat TTE shows resolution of the effusion but new findings consistent with mild constriction. What is the next step in managing this patient?

   a. Obtain cardiac MRI to better assess the pericardium.
   b. Have a cardiothoracic surgical consultation for pericardectomy.
   c. Reassure the patient and observe him over the next 3 months for worsening of symptoms.
   d. Start a course of steroids.

3. All of the following statements concerning pericarditis post-MI are true *except*

   a. Thrombolytic therapy has reduced the incidence by 50%.
   b. It occurs most commonly after inferior infarctions.
   c. Typical diagnostic electrocardiographic changes of acute pericarditis are rare.
   d. Atrial tachyarrhythmias are common.

4. A 45-year-old woman with a history of treated carcinoma of the breast presents to the local emergency department with a few days of severe chest pain. In the emergency department, she appears ill and pale and in moderate discomfort. Her BP is 135/60 mm Hg; her respiratory rate is 24 breaths per minute; her heart rate is 82 bpm; and her temperature is 100.8°F. The resident on call reads her CXR as unremarkable. Her ECG is shown in Figure 12–1. What is the most reasonable next step?

**NOTES**

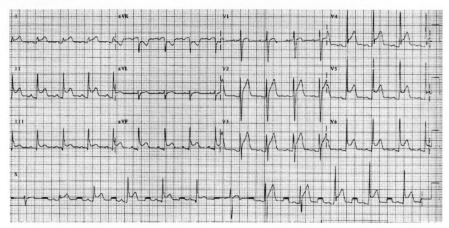

**FIGURE 12–1**  (From Wagner GS, ed. *Marriott's Practical Electrocardiography*, 9th ed. Baltimore: Williams & Wilkins; 1994, with permission.)

**a.** Give aspirin and nitroglycerin and prepare to administer thrombolytics.
**b.** Call the cardiac intervention team and rush the patient to the catheterization laboratory for emergency coronary intervention.
**c.** Give a nonsteroidal anti-inflammatory medication.
**d.** Discharge the patient and refer her for a gastroenterology follow-up as an outpatient.

5. You are called to see a 21-year-old female immigrant from Russia who presents to the emergency department with worsening left-sided chest pain of 6 months' duration. She also reports marked shortness of breath while walking to her daily job in a local supermarket. In addition, she has noticed "puffiness" in her lower extremities. However, she has attributed most of her symptoms to long hours of standing and dust in the warehouse. In addition to normal vital signs, her physical examination reveals quiet heart sounds. The rest of her examination is significant for distended neck veins, marked hepatosplenomegaly, and 3+ lower extremities edema. Her CXR is shown in Figure 12–2. All of the following are appropriate diagnostic tests *except*

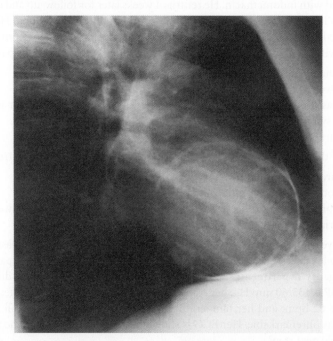

**FIGURE 12–2**  (From Pohost GM, O'Rourke GA, Berman DS, et al., eds. *Imaging in Cardiovascular Disease.* Philadelphia: Lippincott Williams & Wilkins; 2000, with permission.)

a. right and left cardiac catheterization
b. TEE
c. blood samples for liver function testing and hepatitis
d. cardiac CT
e. MRI

6. A 59-year-old man with a history of CAD and remote coronary bypass surgery presents with progressive dyspnea and vague chest pain. He had a stress echocardiogram for these symptoms that demonstrated normal LV function with no stress-induced wall motion abnormalities. However, he returned to the emergency department a few days later with recurrent symptoms. This time the house officer examining the patient notes 3+ pedal edema. The patient is admitted and started on diuretics. His blood tests are as follows:

White blood cell count = 11,000
Hemoglobin = 14.2
Platelets = 172,000
Albumin = 4.6
Urea = 11
Creatinine = 0.9

Owing to the recurrent symptoms, his cardiologist decides to refer him for a right and left heart catheterization. The coronary grafts are all patent. The tracings from the study are shown in Figure 12–3. What is the most logical explanation for this patient's symptoms?

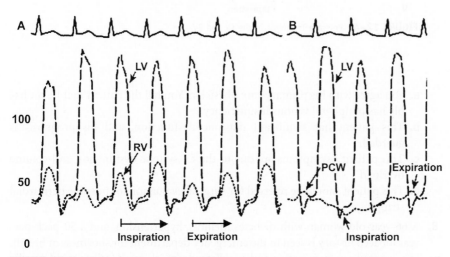

**FIGURE 12–3**   PCW, pulmonary capillary wedge.

a. constrictive pericardial disease
b. small vessel CAD
c. diastolic dysfunction related to his chronic CAD
d. cardiac amyloid
e. cardiac tamponade

7. A 73-year-old man with no cardiac history presents with chronic lower extremities edema. His primary care physician attributed his symptoms to old age. He was treated with hydrochlorothiazide. Initially, he reported a good response to the therapy, but, over the past few months, his edema recurred, and doubling the diuretic dose did not alleviate his symptoms. On his initial examination, you notice distended neck veins and a quiet precordium. He has mild hepatomegaly and 4+ pedal edema. A TTE is suboptimal because of the patient's inability to lie flat and obstructive lung disease. His blood work is as follows:

White blood cell count = 6,000
Hemoglobin = 12.7
Platelets = 225,000
Urea = 43
Creatinine = 2.4
Albumin = 3.6

A cardiac catheterization is performed. He has normal coronary arteries with mild impairment in LV systolic function. The tracings from the study are shown in Figure 12–4. What is your explanation of his symptoms?

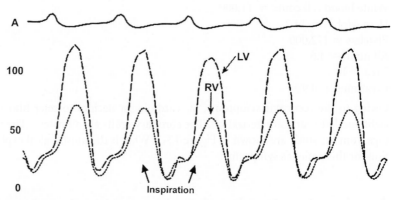

**FIGURE 12–4**   Pressure Tracinggs in the LV and RV.

**a.** You agree with his primary care physician. You tell the patient that he probably has peripheral venous insufficiency.
**b.** This patient has significant diastolic dysfunction, and his prognosis is guarded.
**c.** This patient's symptoms are due to the LV systolic dysfunction and volume overload.
**d.** This patient should be referred for surgical evaluation for possible pericardial stripping.

**8.** A 66-year-old woman with diabetes mellitus, hypertension, and a 50-pack-per-year tobacco history is seen in the emergency department for shortness of breath. She is noted on examination to have distended neck veins (16 cm), tachycardia with distant heart sounds, clear lungs, and pulsus paradoxus of 20 mm Hg. A CXR shows normal heart size. All of the following should be included on the differential *except*

**a.** hypertrophic obstructive cardiomyopathy
**b.** partial obstruction of the superior vena cava
**c.** cardiac tamponade
**d.** chronic obstructive pulmonary disease

**9.** A 56-year-old male smoker with a family history significant for CAD is presenting with dyspnea on exertion and nonexertional vague chest pain. His physical examination and his initial ECG are unremarkable. His CXR demonstrates an increased cardiac silhouette. There is also a small nodule seen in his right upper lobe. The radiologist is not certain about its significance. Given his risk factors and symptoms, he is referred for a perfusion stress test. The images from the stress test are shown in Figure 12–5. Which of the following does the patient clearly have?

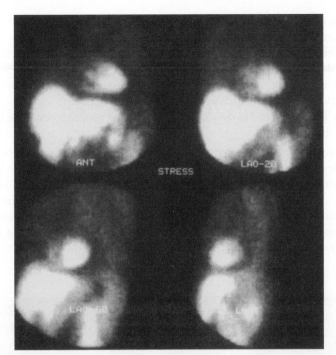

**FIGURE 12–5** (From Pohost GM, O'Rourke GA, Berman DS, et al., eds. *Imaging in Cardiovascular Disease*. Philadelphia: Lippincott Williams & Wilkins; 2000, with permission.)

**a.** He has coronary ischemia and should be referred for coronary angiography.
**b.** There is no evidence of pathology to justify his symptoms.
**c.** His symptoms are related to impairment of RV filling and pericardial disease.
**d.** He has mild ischemia and can be treated medically.

**10.** A 58-year-old man, with cardiac risk factors of tobacco use, hypertension, and hypercholesterolemia, presented to the emergency department a few days ago with an acute onset of left-sided chest pain. His evaluation revealed a diaphoretic man in moderate discomfort. An ECG was performed and showed a pattern consistent with an inferior wall acute MI. The patient was treated with thrombolytics. Forty-five minutes after the initial dose of the thrombolytics, he felt better and had complete resolution of his symptoms and normalization of the ECG. On the third day after the event, he reports midsternal chest pain, vague in nature, with mild diaphoresis and shortness of breath. An ECG is performed, as shown in Figure 12–6. Which of the following should you tell the patient is the next step in managing his condition?

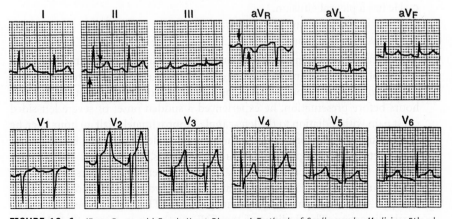

**FIGURE 12–6** (From Braunwald E, ed. *Heart Disease: A Textbook of Cardiovascular Medicine*, 5th ed. Philadelphia: WB Saunders; 1997, with permission.)

**NOTES**

a. There is evidence of reocclusion of the infarct-related artery, and a percutaneous intervention is needed.

b. There is evidence of reocclusion of the infarct-related artery, and re-bolus with thrombolytics and heparin is indicated.

c. He is showing signs of early postinfarction pericarditis, and a nonsteroidal anti-inflammatory medication should be started.

d. An LV aneurysm has developed, and a TTE is needed to evaluate the extent of the aneurysm.

11. A 19-year-old male college student presents to his local physician for evaluation of a dry cough. His symptoms started 3 days ago but now appear to be resolving. He had planned a trip overseas but was concerned and is now seeking advice. His physical examination is unremarkable. A CXR is performed and is read as showing an enlarged right cardiac silhouette. A TTE is ordered, which is shown in Figure 12–7. The patient most likely has which of the following conditions?

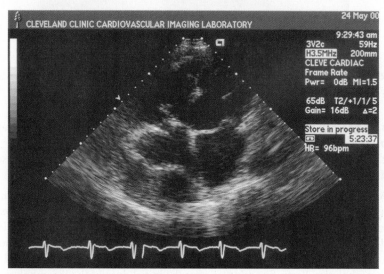

**FIGURE 12–7**

a. He has a pericardial cyst that is benign; no further treatment should be offered.

b. He has cardiac tamponade requiring a pericardial tap.

c. He has a pleural effusion.

d. There is no pathology. The CXR was misread.

e. He has mesothelioma.

12. You are called to the emergency department to see a 74-year-old man. He has a history of heavy smoking and hypertension. The patient cannot remember his medications, but he reports not taking them on a routine basis. In the past few hours before presentation, he experienced a sudden onset of severe left-sided chest pain with radiation to the left scapula. Approximately half an hour later, he noted some difficulty breathing. In the emergency department, he is noted to be diaphoretic and in significant respiratory distress. His physical examination reveals a BP of 160/90 mm Hg, elevated jugular venous pressures, and a quiet precordium. His ECG is reported as sinus tachycardia with no acute ST-T changes. After initial pain and BP management, a TEE is performed to rule out aortic dissection. The findings of the TTE are shown in Figure 12–8. What is your recommendation?

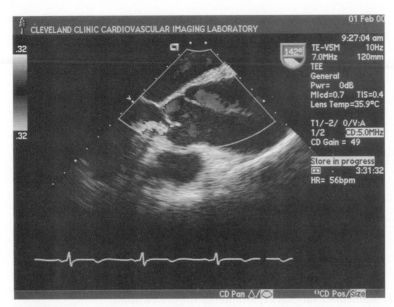

**FIGURE 12–8**

a. The patient should have immediate surgical intervention.

b. The patient needs BP control and surgical evaluation once he is medically stabilized.

c. The patient should have percutaneous pericardial drainage to manage the cardiac tamponade and then a surgical evaluation.

d. The diagnosis is unclear; a CT scan or an aortic angiogram is needed.

13. A 42-year-old man was referred for evaluation of symptomatic MR. He was diagnosed with mitral valve prolapse that was not suitable for repair. Given his family history of CAD and tobacco use, he underwent a coronary angiogram, which revealed no evidence of obstructive coronary disease. He underwent an uneventful mitral valve replacement. He was extubated and transferred from the ICU 48 hours after the operation. On postoperation day 3, you note the patient to be pale and lethargic and in mild respiratory distress. His BP is 100/60 mm Hg. His cardiac and lung examination is compromised by the presence of rapid breathing and chest tubes. His ECG reveals NSR at 97 bpm with no acute ST-T changes. A TTE is performed. Selected views are shown in Figure 12–9A. As the patient continues to deteriorate and becomes hypotensive, a TEE is performed next, as shown in Figure 12–9B. What should you recommend?

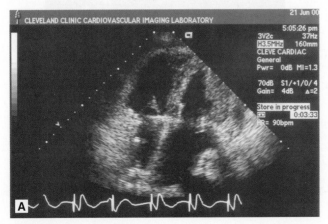

**FIGURE 12–9**    (*Continued*)

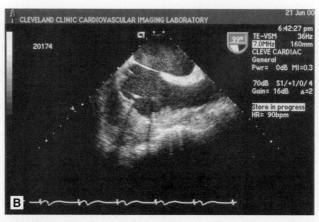

**FIGURE 12–9**

**a.** Immediate surgical exploration of the pericardium.
**b.** Percutaneous aspiration of the fluid present in the pericardium.
**c.** Immediate surgical intervention for malfunction of the prosthetic mitral valve.
**d.** A 500-cc bolus of IV normal saline solution should be started because the patient is dehydrated, and no further intervention is needed.

**14.** A 49-year-old black man with hypertension and chronic renal insufficiency presents with dyspnea and fluid overload with decreased urine output. He is treated in the hospital with diuretics, and his symptoms improve. However, his renal function continues to deteriorate with an increasing BUN of 90 and a creatinine of 5.4. In addition, the patient is noted to have several bruises on his arms from needlestick blood draws and IV lines. On hospital day 4, the patient is noted to be hypotensive and tachycardic: BP, 80/40 mm Hg; heart rate, 110 bpm. No jugular venous distention is noted, but heart sounds are diminished, and a loud pericardial rub is heard. His TTE is shown in Figure 12–10. What is the next step in management?

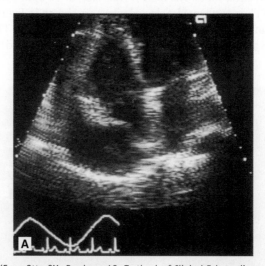

**FIGURE 12–10**   (From Otto CM, Pearlman AS. *Textbook of Clinical Echocardiography*. Philadelphia: WB Saunders; 1995, with permission.) (*Continued*)

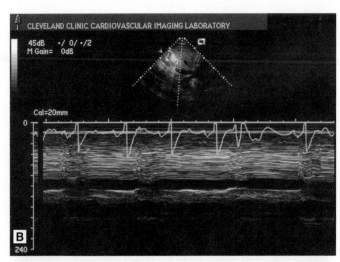

**FIGURE 12–10** (*Continued*)

**a.** urgent pericardiocentesis

**b.** IV hydration

**c.** immediate dialysis

**d.** the continuation of diuretics with serial TTE

15. A 42-year-old white male chef is brought into the emergency department after a motor vehicle accident in which he fell asleep at the wheel and ran into a tree. He is reporting anterior chest discomfort and shortness of breath. He relates no prior medical conditions and takes no medications. Vitals are stable with a BP of 120/60 mm Hg and a heart rate of 90 bpm. His ECG is shown in Figure 12–11A. A TTE is performed. Diastolic images are shown in Figure 12–11B. Laboratory tests show modest elevation of creatinine phosphokinase at 240. Which of the following is the most reasonable next step in managing this patient?

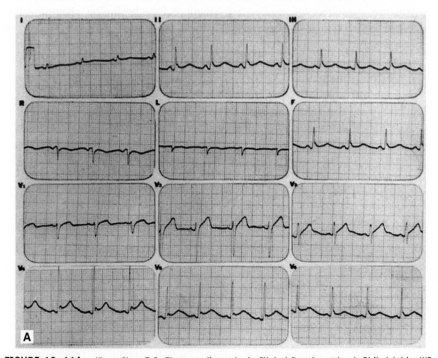

**FIGURE 12–11A** (From Chou T-C. *Electrocardiography in Clinical Practice*, 4th ed. Philadelphia: WB Saunders; 1996, with permission.)

**NOTES**

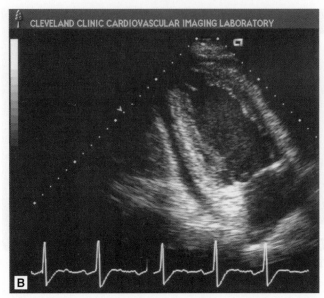

**FIGURE 12–11B**   (From Chou T-C. *Electrocardiography in Clinical Practice*, 4th ed. Philadelphia: WB Saunders; 1996, with permission.)

**a.** Start the patient on a nonsteroidal anti-inflammatory agent with follow-up as an outpatient in 1 week.

**b.** Admit the patient for observation on telemetry with a follow-up TTE.

**c.** The patient needs immediate percutaneous revascularization.

**d.** Send the patient for surgical treatment of pericardial rupture.

**16.** A 22-year-old white man is newly diagnosed with non-Hodgkin's lymphoma. He undergoes a metastatic workup that includes an MRI of the chest and abdomen, which is shown in Figure 12–12. The plan is for chemotherapy, but you are consulted for cardiac assessment before beginning chemotherapy. Radionuclide ventriculography shows a normal LV EF of 65%. What should you recommend?

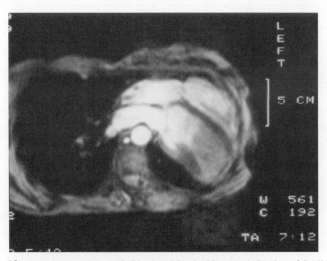

**FIGURE 12–12**   (MRI image was provided by Dr. Richard White, Head, Section of Cardiovascular Imaging, Departments of Radiology and Cardiovascular Medicine, The Cleveland Clinic Foundation.)

a. ordering a TTE to delineate the abnormality
b. cardiothoracic surgical consultation before starting chemotherapy
c. exercise stress testing
d. proceeding with chemotherapy without further cardiac evaluation

17. A 56-year-old Asian man, who recently emigrated from Thailand, presents to the emergency department with cough, fever, and chills. He is noted to have a BP of 80/50 mm Hg and a regular pulse at a rate of 135 bpm. CXR shows cardiomegaly. A two-dimensional echocardiography is shown in Figure 12–13A, and Doppler interrogation of the mitral inflow is shown in Figure 12–13B. All of the following are expected on physical examination *except*

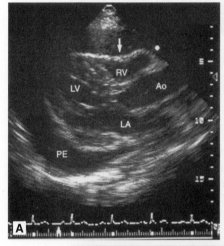
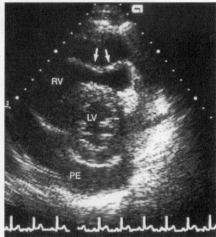
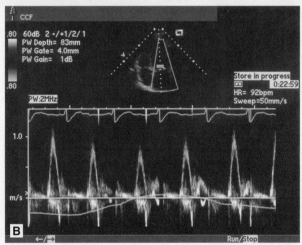

**FIGURE 12–13**

a. Kussmaul's sign
b. Ewart's sign
c. pulsus paradoxus
d. absent Y descent on jugular venous waveforms

18. A 64-year-old white woman, with a history of breast carcinoma in her 20s treated with mastectomy and radiation, is undergoing preoperative evaluation for knee surgery. She has not had a recurrence of breast cancer since her initial treatment, and she has no other medical problems. Her preoperative CXR demonstrates cardiomegaly. TTE is performed and is shown in Figure 12–14. Which of the following is the least likely cause of this patient's effusion?

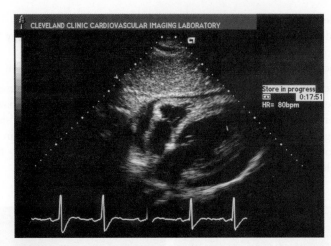

**FIGURE 12–14**

**a.** radiation pericarditis
**b.** hypothyroidism
**c.** viral pericarditis
**d.** recurrent malignant pericarditis

**19.** A 63-year-old white woman with a history of left-sided breast cancer, which was treated with lumpectomy and radiation therapy 30 years ago, presents with new-onset lower extremity edema, hepatomegaly, and ascites. The CT scan of the chest is shown in Figure 12–15. All of the following features may be present on TTE *except*

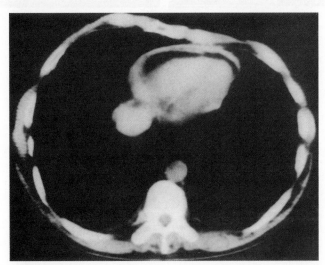

**FIGURE 12–15**

**a.** septal bounce
**b.** diastolic septal shudder
**c.** no respiratory variation of mitral inflow
**d.** myocardial tethering

**20.** For constrictive pericarditis, factors associated with a worse prognosis after peri-cardiectomy include all of the following *except*

**a.** older age
**b.** arrhythmia
**c.** history of irradiation
**d.** presence of pericardial effusion on preoperative TTE

**21.** A 44-year-old white man with rheumatoid arthritis is referred to your office for evaluation after his rheumatologist heard a loud heart sound. On questioning, the patient mainly reports joint pains in his fingers. He denies any chest discomfort or shortness of breath. He has been on methotrexate and prednisone for the past year. His examination is significant for mild erythema and swelling of his distal interphalangeal joints, rheumatoid nodules on his right forearm, clear lungs, distant heart sounds with a loud friction rub, and moderate peripheral edema. You order a TTE to further assess his heart. Selective images are shown in Figure 12–16. What is your recommendation?

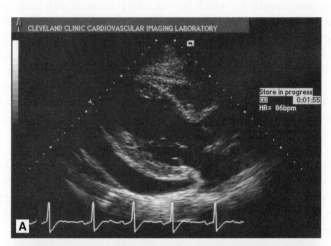

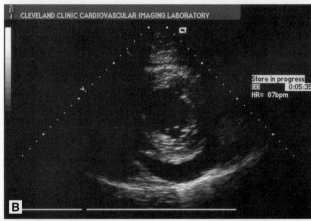

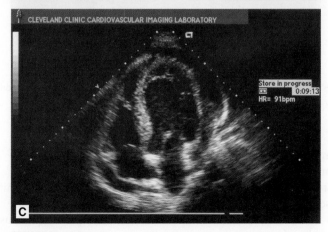

**FIGURE 12–16**

a. Because he currently has no cardiac symptoms, no further treatment is needed except to continue methotrexate and prednisone.

b. You want the patient to start indomethacin, continue methotrexate and prednisone, and follow-up in 4 weeks.

c. The best treatment at this time for his pericardial effusion is drainage with the instillation of steroids to prevent recurrence.

d. A surgical evaluation for pericardiectomy is necessary because the findings on his TTE indicate that he will develop problems in the future if this is not taken care of soon.

22. A 55-year-old white man presents for evaluation of chest pain. He has no prior medical problems, but he has noted burning epigastric and chest discomfort for the past few months for which he was taking antacids with some relief of his symptoms. However, because the symptoms persisted, he sought medical attention and was referred for an esophagogastroduodenoscopy, which was performed earlier today. He was found to have a fundal hiatal hernia with a gastric ulcer that was cauterized, and he was started on omeprazole. On returning home, he noted a new sharp anterior chest pain, somewhat positional related, that was not relieved with antacids or omeprazole. This pain progressively worsened over the next few hours, and he came to the emergency department. Examination in the emergency department revealed a temperature of 38.1°C, a heart rate of 110 bpm, and a BP of 120/70 mm Hg. Lung sounds were clear. Heart sounds appeared normal with the patient sitting upright, but they were diminished with the patient lying in the supine position. An ECG did not show any acute ST-T wave abnormalities to suggest infarction. A CXR was performed, as shown in Figure 12–17. You are called to further assess the patient. After reviewing the available data, which of the following is your next step?

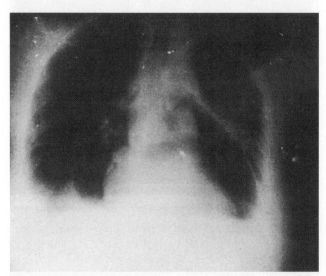

**FIGURE 12–17** (From Spodick DS. *The Pericardium: A Comprehensive Textbook*. New York: Marcel Dekker; 1997, with permission.)

a. Immediate surgical consultation.

b. Immediate pericardiocentesis.

c. Start a nonsteroidal anti-inflammatory medication and admit him for observation.

d. No further treatment is needed because his symptoms are caused by the hiatal hernia.

**23.** In patients who have congenital absence of the pericardium, which of the following is a common finding?

**a.** cardiac displacement to the left on CXR
**b.** sinus bradycardia on ECG
**c.** cardiac hypermobility with postural changes on TTE
**d.** absence of preaortic pericardial recess on CT
**e.** all of the above

**24.** A 71-year-old man presents to the hospital with palpitations of 2 to 3 days' duration. He has no known medical history, and he is not on any medications. Initial evaluation is unremarkable except for a BP of 160/90 mm Hg and an ECG showing AFib with a ventricular rate of 120 to 130 bpm. Given the duration of his symptoms, he is treated with beta-blockers for rate control and heparin for anticoagulation. On hospital day 2, he is referred for early transesophageal-guided cardioversion. The TEE reveals normal LV and RV function. There are no echocardiographic contraindications for cardioversion. An uneventful cardioversion is performed, and the patient converts to NSR. On hospital day 3, the patient is found in marked respiratory distress. On physical examination, he has a regular heart rate with a loud audible click over the precordium. A CXR is performed, as shown in Figure 12–18. What does this patient have?

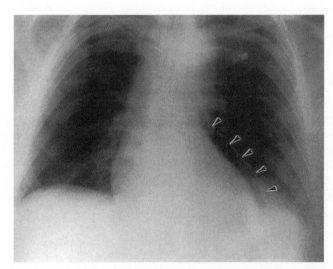

**FIGURE 12–18** (From Spodick DS. *The Pericardium: A Comprehensive Textbook*. New York: Marcel Dekker; 1997, with permission.)

**a.** He has a pulmonary embolism and should be treated with thrombolytics.
**b.** He has a hiatal/diaphragmatic hernia with compression of the heart by the fundus of stomach.
**c.** He has an iatrogenic pneumohydropericardium; immediate drainage and surgical attention are needed.
**d.** He has a recurrence of AFib.

**25.** Among the causes of pulsus paradoxus are all of the following *except*

**a.** large pericardial effusion
**b.** chronic obstructive lung disease
**c.** morbid obesity
**d.** constrictive pericardial disease

**26.** The etiologies of granulomatous pericarditis (Fig. 12–19) include which of the following?

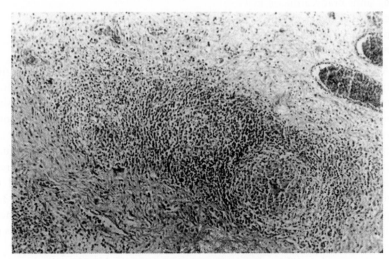

**FIGURE 12–19** (From Spodick DS. *The Pericardium: A Comprehensive Textbook*. New York: Marcel Dekker; 1997, with permission.)

    **a.** infections: tuberculosis, histoplasmosis
    **b.** connective tissue diseases and rheumatoid arthritis
    **c.** environmental exposures: silicosis, asbestosis
    **d.** idiopathic pericarditis
    **e.** all of the above

**27.** A 59-year-old woman with a history of chronic renal insufficiency presents to the emergency department with anterior left-sided chest pain. She reports that the chest pain started after her last dialysis 7 days ago. She appears lethargic and in mild respiratory distress. The physical examination demonstrates a BP of 160/90 mm Hg and a heart rate of 100 bpm. On cardiac auscultation, a loud friction rub is heard. An ECG is obtained (Fig. 12–20). What is the most important next step in this case?

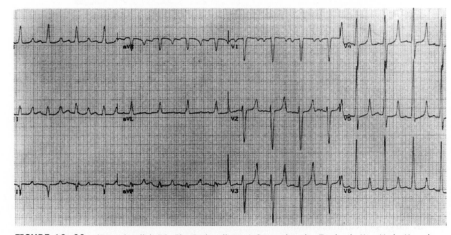

**FIGURE 12–20** (From Spodick DS. *The Pericardium: A Comprehensive Textbook*. New York: Marcel Dekker; 1997, with permission.)

**NOTES**

**a.** Perform emergency dialysis.
**b.** Obtain an echocardiogram.
**c.** Prepare for pericardiocentesis.
**d.** Admit the patient to the cardiac care unit to rule out MI.

**28.** An 82-year-old woman with no history of cardiac disease or malignancy is seen at your office for weakness, fatigue, constipation, and lower extremities swelling. Her daughter reports that she was in very good health until 6 months ago when she was admitted to the hospital with pneumonia. Her daughter noticed that she was discharged from the hospital on no medications. Her concern was that her mother had been on a pill for a long time for her "glands." On physical examination, the patient is an elderly woman who appears her age. She is pale, lethargic, and somewhat confused. Her skin is dry, and she has a BP of 100/60 mm Hg and a heart rate of 52 bpm. The chest examination reveals marked reduction in air entry in the lower third of her lung fields. She has normal heart sounds. Marked edema of the lower extremities is also noted. An ECG is obtained and is shown in Figure 12–21. The initial concern and management of this patient involves all of the following *except*

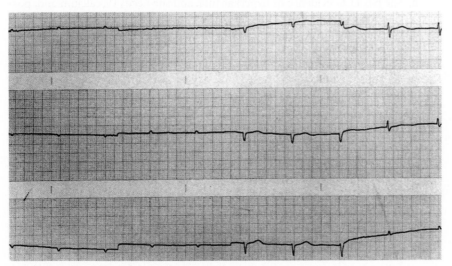

**FIGURE 12–21**   (From Spodick DS. *The Pericardium: A Comprehensive Textbook*. New York: Marcel Dekker; 1997, with permission.)

**a.** She is in cardiac tamponade and needs an immediate pericardial tap.
**b.** She is in a hypothyroid state and needs her medications restarted.
**c.** She is in CHB, and a pacemaker should be inserted.
**d.** She is in cardiogenic shock, and an IABP should be inserted.

**29.** A 29-year-old woman with known insulin-dependent diabetes mellitus was found unconscious 1 hour after an office party. Initial assessment by the emergency medical service team showed a BP of 90/60 mm Hg. Her pulse was 120, and her blood sugar was 870 mg/dL. She was given SC insulin and rushed to the emergency department. You are called to see her because of her abnormal ECG (Fig. 12–22). She is noted to be semiconscious. The emergency physician has already started her on IV insulin drip and hydration. What is your recommendation at this juncture?

**NOTES**

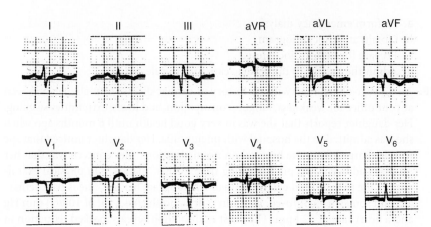

**FIGURE 12–22** (From Spodick DS. *The Pericardium: A Comprehensive Textbook*. New York: Marcel Dekker; 1997, with permission.)

**a.** She is having an acute MI, and immediate restoration of coronary flow is essential.

**b.** She has ECG evidence of hyperkalemia, and she needs IV calcium and, possibly, dialysis.

**c.** Continue the current management; the ECG will improve with the resolution of ketoacidosis.

**d.** Her ECG predicts high-degree AV block; a standby external pacemaker should be available.

**30.** Which of the following is the most common neoplastic pericardial tumor in adults?

**a.** neuroma

**b.** hemangioma

**c.** mesothelioma

**d.** teratoma

# ANSWERS

1. **c.** Respiratory difference >20 cm/second in superior vena cava flow velocities does not support constrictive physiology. The limitation on ventricular expansion imposed by the constricting pericardial sac will lead to ventricular "competition" for volume during the filling phase. The respiratory variations in the superior vena cava are typically <20 cm/second in constriction.

2. **c.** Reassure the patient and observe him over the next 3 months for worsening of symptoms. The natural history of acute viral or idiopathic pericarditis is usually short and self-limited. Occasionally, mild forms of constriction may develop weeks after the initial event, but they usually resolve without any specific treatment. No further treatment is indicated unless he becomes more symptomatic or develops signs of cardiac tamponade.

3. **b.** All of the answers except for B are true. Pericarditis after acute MI is usually associated with larger infarcts, as indicated by their more common presentation with anterior Q-wave infarctions.

4. **c.** Give a nonsteroidal anti-inflammatory medication. The clinical presentation of a few days of severe chest pain does not favor an acute MI. Furthermore, the ECG tracing supports the diagnosis of pericarditis. Therefore, cardiac catheterization or thrombolytics are not appropriate. The only reasonable answer is to start the patient on anti-inflammatory medications and obtain a TTE to rule out pericardial effusion.

5. **c.** Blood samples for liver function testing and hepatitis are not appropriate diagnostic tests. The patient is a young adult immigrant. Her chronic symptoms mainly suggest RV and LV failure. The CXR shows typical changes of calcific pericardial disease. All of the listed tests except those in choice C would be appropriate to help confirm the diagnosis. A right and left heart catheterization could probably confirm the diagnosis, although assessing the coronary arteries is not indicated. TEE could have been used before obtaining the CXR to evaluate the etiology of the biventricular failure. Passive congestion of the liver is common in patients with constrictive pericarditis.

6. **a.** Constrictive pericardial disease. This patient did not have evidence of ischemia on a recent stress test. Furthermore, there is no evidence of obstructive disease in his coronaries or grafts. His tracings mostly support the diagnosis of constriction, given the diastolic equalization of pressures in the cardiac chambers and the typical square root sign. Amyloidosis would typically show signs of restrictive hemodynamics with no respiratory variation. Echocardiography typically shows increased LV wall thickness. Additionally, a diagnosis of tamponade should have been evident by echocardiography, which the patient had before heart catheterization. Otherwise, hemodynamic tracings of cardiac tamponade would look exactly the same as for constriction.

7. **b.** This patient has significant diastolic dysfunction, and his prognosis is guarded. He has evidence of restrictive LV filling (advanced diastolic dysfunction) in the absence of CAD. The differential diagnosis in his age group includes amyloidosis (especially considering concomitant renal dysfunction), hemochromatosis, and other infiltrative processes.

8. **a.** Hypertrophic obstructive cardiomyopathy should not be included on the differential. The physical findings described in this case are seen in superior vena cava syndrome, obstructive lung disease, and tamponade. The presence of pulsus paradoxus is not observed in hypertrophic obstructive cardiomyopathy because the less compliant LV resists the phasically changing pericardial pressure.

9. **c.** His symptoms are related to impairment of RV filling and pericardial disease. This patient with the main presentation of dyspnea has an increased cardiac

silhouette. The nuclear image provided shows a circumferential echolucency surrounding the heart. This is consistent with a large pericardial effusion, and he most likely has right atrial and RV diastolic compromise. There is no evidence of a perfusion defect to suggest ischemia.

10. **c.** He is showing signs of early postinfarction pericarditis, and a nonsteroidal anti-inflammatory medication should be started. This patient had an MI 72 hours ago that was successfully treated with thrombolytics. The ECG shows diffuse ST elevation with PR depression. These findings support the diagnosis of post-MI pericarditis. The ECG changes are new and nonlocalizing. Most patients improve with nonsteroidal anti-inflammatory medications.

11. **a.** He has a pericardial cyst that is benign; no further treatment should be offered. The TTE and CXR show a pericardial cyst. Pericardial cysts are usually smooth structures containing transudative fluid. They are frequently only 2 or 3 cm in diameter, often located at the right cardiodiaphragmatic angle, and clinically silent. However, cysts can be associated with chest pain, dyspnea, cough, and arrhythmias likely caused by compression of adjacent tissues. They can also become secondarily infected. In this patient, whose nonspecific symptoms appear to be resolving, no further treatment is needed.

12. **a.** The patient should have immediate surgical intervention. This patient has evidence of acute type A aortic dissection with extension to the pericardium, as evidenced by the pericardial effusion on the TEE. He should be immediately referred for surgical repair. If the diagnosis were not certain based on the TEE, then CT, MRI, or aortic angiography would be needed to better define the anatomy. The safest and most efficient management of patients with aortic dissection is to carry out all diagnostic procedures in the operating room. Pericardial drainage often gives only temporary relief or no relief of the tamponade, and the subsequent increase in BP disrupts sealing clots, accelerating intrapericardial leakage.

13. **a.** Immediate surgical exploration of the pericardium. The TTE and TEE demonstrate a pericardial hematoma compromising right atrial and RV filling. This is an indication for surgical exploration and evacuation of the hematoma.

14. **b.** Intravenous (IV) hydration. This patient has evidence of pericarditis likely related to uremia, as he is close to requiring dialysis. Although his TTE shows signs of tamponade (right atrial collapse, moderate-sized effusion, and respiratory variation across the mitral inflow), there is no jugular venous distention, and the inferior vena cava is small sized, indicating that this patient has been overdiuresed. His hypotension and tachycardia are related to dehydration. He should, therefore, be treated with IV hydration.

15. **b.** Admit the patient for observation on telemetry with a follow-up TTE. The ECG shows findings consistent with an anterior wall injury, and the TTE shows a small pericardial effusion. Given this patient's history, he most likely has a cardiac contusion. Although the prognosis for recovery is generally excellent, these patients require careful monitoring and follow-up for late complications, which range from ventricular arrhythmias to cardiac rupture. Hence, the most logical answer to this question is to admit the patient to a telemetry bed with follow-up TTE.

16. **d.** Proceeding with chemotherapy without further cardiac evaluation. This patient's MRI shows congenital absence of the pericardium. This is a benign condition usually found incidentally. No specific cardiac treatment is needed unless there is entrapment of one of the cardiac chambers.

17. **a.** Kussmaul's sign is not expected on physical examination. This patient has findings of cardiac tamponade on his TTE with large pericardial effusion and respiratory variation of mitral inflow pattern. In constrictive pericarditis or restrictive cardiomyopathy, the jugular venous pressure may not fall appropriately or may

even increase with inspiration, a finding known as Kussmaul's sign. This finding may also be seen with RV infarction, but it is very uncommon and seldom noted in cardiac tamponade in which intrathoracic pressures are transmitted through the pericardial sac. Ewart's sign—dullness to percussion of the left lung base—can be seen in any syndrome with a large pericardial effusion resulting in compression of the left lower lobe. Pulsus paradoxus, which is an exaggeration of the normal inspiratory drop in systolic arterial pressure exceeding 12 to 15 mm Hg, commonly occurs in cardiac tamponade. In addition, there is often a lack of a sharp *x* and *y* descent with sometimes absent *y* descent reflecting poor RV filling during diastole because of high intrapericardial pressures causing RV collapse.

18. **d.** Recurrent malignant pericarditis. It would be extremely unusual for a patient to develop recurrence of breast carcinoma 20 years after successful treatment, especially without other signs of recurrence. More often, these patients have pericardial effusions related to cardiac disease, hypothyroidism, radiation pericarditis, or idiopathic pericarditis.

19. **c.** This patient has evidence of pericardial calcifications and symptoms consistent with constrictive pericarditis. All of the above findings except for choice C are seen with constrictive pericarditis. The heart and pulmonary vessels are intrathoracic, and, normally, both are simultaneously affected by respiratory pressure changes. In constrictive pericarditis, transthoracic pressures are not transmitted to the cardiac chambers. Hence, when inspiration decreases intrathoracic and pulmonary pressures, cardiac pressures remain high. Consequently, total pulmonary venous flow is decreased during inspiration, decreasing LV filling. Thus, respiratory variation is observed on Doppler interrogation of mitral inflow.

20. **d.** Presence of pericardial effusion on preoperative TTE is not included. Poorer results after surgical pericardiectomy are seen (a) with inadequate resection; (b) in uncorrected coronary disease; (c) with higher New York Heart Association classifications for "congestive failure"; (d) in older age; (e) after radiation pericarditis; (f) with chronicity—including peripheral organ failure (especially renal and hepatic) and ascites or edema, or both, which are ominous; (g) with severe myocardial atrophy and fibrosis (detectable by CT and MRI); and (h) with significant arrhythmias reflecting myocardial impairment.

21. **d.** A surgical evaluation for pericardiectomy is necessary because the findings on his TTE indicate that he will develop problems in the future if this is not taken care of soon. The patient is currently symptomatic with edema of the lower extremities. Furthermore, he has a pericardial friction rub suggestive of an active pericardial process likely related to his rheumatologic disease process. He is already on methotrexate and prednisone as anti-inflammatory medications. Pericardial effusions related to rheumatoid arthritis often progress to constriction despite anti-inflammatory therapy, and early management consisting of pericardial stripping is recommended.

22. **b.** The next step is an immediate pericardiocentesis. This patient has signs of early sepsis. Furthermore, the CXR shows pneumopericardium that likely developed secondary to gastric perforation from the esophagogastroduodenoscopy and cauterization of the ulcer. This patient needs immediate referral to surgery for repair.

23. **e.** All of the above. All are common findings in congenital absence of the pericardium.

24. **c.** He has an iatrogenic pneumohydropericardium; immediate drainage and surgical attention are needed. This patient had a TEE that most likely resulted in an esophageal tear with communication to the pericardial sac. On the CXR, there is a lucent triangle outlining the pericardium with pericardial passage over the aortic arch.

**25. d.** Constrictive pericardial disease is not a cause of pulsus paradoxus. Pulsus paradoxus depends on increased RV filling volume with inspiration. In constriction, although the RV filling velocity increases with inspiration, there is minimal change in the RV volume.

**26. e.** All of the above. Granulomas are focal nodules or masses made of granulation tissue and fibrous tissue with a variable degree of leukocytic infiltration. All the above entities have been linked to formation of granulomas.

**27. a.** Perform emergency dialysis. This patient has missed her dialysis session and is now presenting with hyperkalemia (note peaked T waves on ECG) and uremic pericarditis. The most essential step is to start dialysis to treat the hyperkalemia.

**28. b.** This patient has myxedema caused by untreated hypothyroidism. The ECG shows sinus bradycardia, low QRS voltage, and nonspecific T-wave changes. The treatment is thyroid hormone replacement, which is almost always followed by steady regression of the effusion. Drainage is rarely needed in these situations, and if medical treatment is initiated early, one can avoid the precipitation of cholesterol in the pericardium and cholesterol pericarditis.

**29. c.** Continue the current management; the ECG will improve with the resolution of ketoacidosis. Patients presenting with diabetic ketoacidosis can have ECG features that are typical of stage I pericarditis and hypokalemia. The treatment is usually that of ketoacidosis. The ECG returns to normal after resolution of the acidosis.

**30. c.** Mesothelioma. Teratoma is the most common pericardial tumor in infancy and childhood. Neuroma and hemangioma are uncommon enough to be considered curiosities.

## Suggested Reading

Buck M, Ingle JN, Giuliani ER, et al. Pericardial effusion in women with breast cancer. *Cancer.* 1987;60(2):263–269.

Hoit BD. Management of effusive and constrictive pericardial heart disease. *Circulation.* 2002;105(25):2939–2942.

Klein AL, Asher CR. Diseases of the pericardium, restrictive cardiomyopathy, and diastolic dysfunction. In: Topol EJ, ed. *Textbook of Cardiovascular Medicine*, 2nd ed. Philadelphia: Lippincott Williams & Wilkins; 2002.

Spodick DS. *The Pericardium: A Comprehensive Textbook.* New York: Marcel Dekker; 1997.

# chapter 13

# Cardiac Imaging

ELLEN MAYER SABIK · BRIAN P. GRIFFIN

## QUESTIONS

1. Patient is a 70-year-old woman with a history of hypertension, but no prior cardiac history, who comes in with sudden onset of chest pain, which later migrates to her back. She is diagnosed with a CT of her chest to have a type I aortic dissection. Her blood pressure is 100/70 mm Hg and her heart rate is 115 bpm. Images from her transthoracic echocardiogram are in Figures 13–1A–C. The next step in her care would be

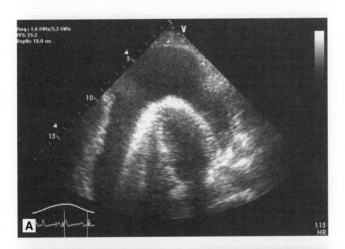

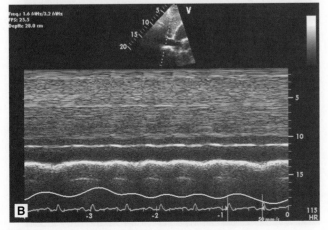

**FIGURE 13–1** (*Continued*)

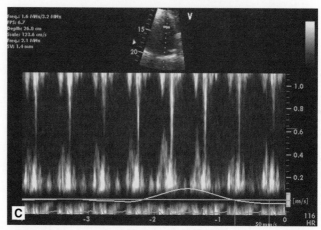

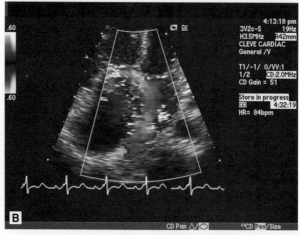

**FIGURE 13–1** **A.** Apical four-chamber view (TTE). **B.** M-mode through the IVC in the subcostal view (TTE). **C.** Continuous-wave Doppler through the mitral valve showing MV inflow pattern.

   **a.** aortic stent graft
   **b.** coronary angiography
   **c.** IABP placement
   **d.** pericardiocentesis
   **e.** emergent cardiac surgery

2. The finding in the transthoracic images in Figures 13–2A and B is commonly associated with which of the following lesions?

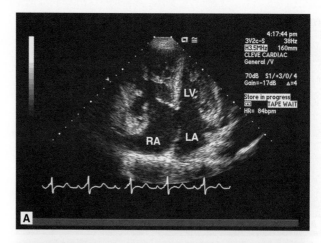

**FIGURE 13–2** **A.** Apical four-chamber view (TTE). **B.** (See color plate) Apical four-chamber view with color Doppler.

a. congenitally corrected transposition
b. cleft mitral valve
c. coarctation of the aorta
d. RV infarction
e. bicuspid aortic valve

3. A 36-year-old man with a history of hypertension on medications for 5 years presents to your office with complaints of dyspnea on exertion and is found by his internist to have a heart murmur. Below are some representative views from his transthoracic echocardiogram (Figs. 13–3A–E). What is the diagnosis?

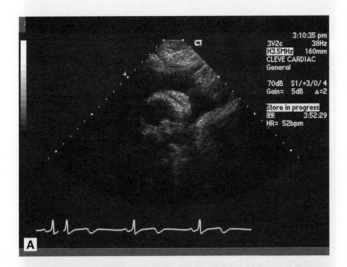

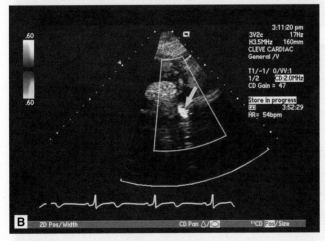

**FIGURE 13–3**   (See color plate) (*Continued*)

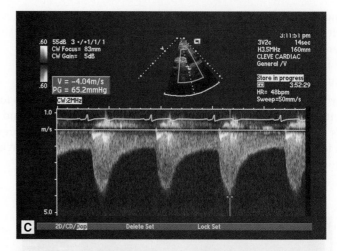

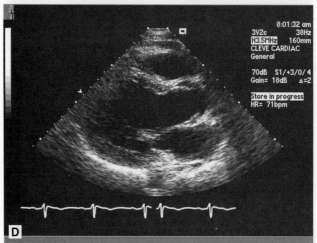

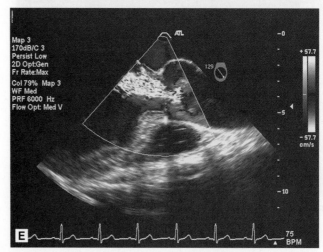

**FIGURE 13–3** **A.** Suprasternal notch view in 2D (TTE). **B.** Suprasternal notch with color Doppler. **C.** Continuous wave Doppler in the descending aorta from the suprasternal notch. **D.** Parasternal long axis view in systole. **E.** (See color plate) Parasternal long axis view with color Doppler.

**a.** PDA

**b.** rheumatic aortic valve (AV) with aortic insufficiency (AI)

**c.** rheumatic AS

**d.** coarctation of the aorta with bicuspid AV with AI

**e.** Marfan's with aortic dissection

**4.** A 37-year-old patient presents with fever, weight loss, and blood cultures that are positive for pseudomonas and the transthoracic echo finding in Figure 13–4. The patient's most likely demographic for this clinical scenario is

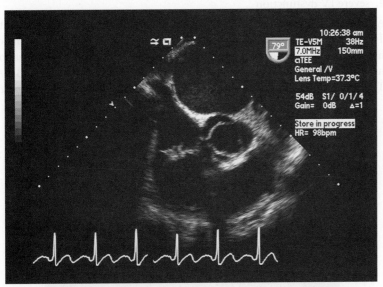

**FIGURE 13–4** Mid-esophageal short axis view of the aortic valve (TEE).

**a.** patient with HOCM who had a dental procedure 3 weeks ago
**b.** patient with myxomatous MV disease with MVP
**c.** patient with subaortic stenosis after dental procedure 3 weeks ago
**d.** patient with a patent ductus
**e.** IV drug abuser

**5.** This M mode tracing (Fig. 13–5) demonstrates a patient with

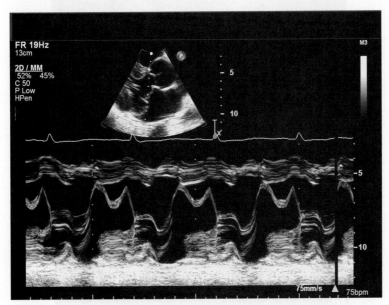

**FIGURE 13–5** M-mode through the mitral valve.

a. HOCM with systolic anterior motion (SAM) of the MV leaflets
b. MVP
c. AS
d. rheumatic MS
e. severe LV dysfunction

6. A 60-year-old man presents with 2 weeks of fever, night sweats, and weight loss. The patient had positive blood cultures for fungus. Upon further evaluation he has a small neurologic deficit with corresponding findings of embolization on head CT. Below are some representative images from his TEE (Figs. 13–6A–E). This patient's appropriate indications for surgery include the following *except*

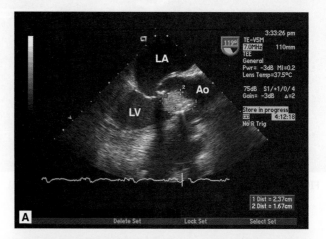

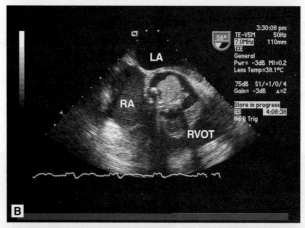

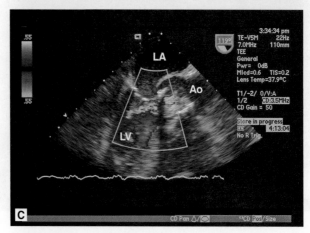

**FIGURE 13–6** *(Continued)*

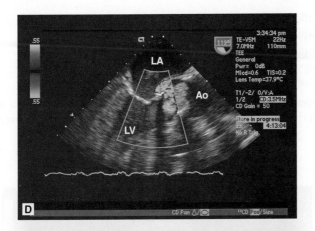

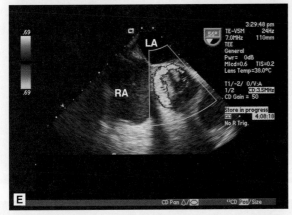

**FIGURE 13–6** **A.** Mid-esophageal long axis view of the aortic valve (TEE). **B.** Mid-esophageal short axis view of the aortic valve (TEE). **C.** (See color plate) Mid-esophageal long axis view of the aortic valve with color Doppler (diastole). **D.** (See color plate) Mid-esophageal long axis view of the aortic valve with color Doppler (systole). **E.** (See color plate) Mid-esophageal short axis view of the aortic valve with color Doppler (systole).

   **a.** fungal endocarditis
   **b.** degree of AI
   **c.** embolization with mobile vegetation >10 mm
   **d.** mobile vegetation >15 mm
   **e.** aortic stenosis caused by obstruction by vegetation

**7.** The following TEE image (Fig. 13–7) demonstrates a patient with

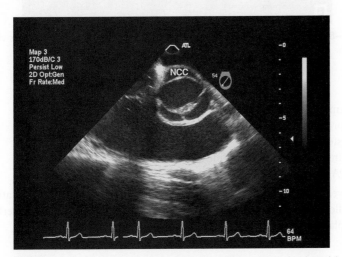

**FIGURE 13–7** Mid-esophageal short axis view of the aortic valve (systole).

a. trileaflet aortic valve
b. bicuspid aortic valve with fusion of RCC and NCC
c. bicuspid aortic valve with fusion of RCC and LCC
d. bicuspid aortic valve with fusion of LCC and NCC
e. unicuspid aortic valve

8. The patient is a 22 year old with a systolic and diastolic murmur with the following echo images (Figs. 13–8A and B). These images demonstrate

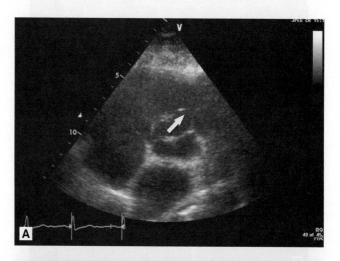

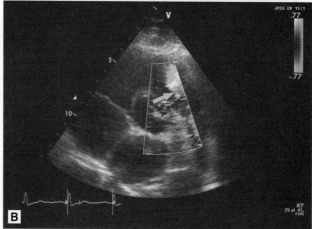

**FIGURE 13–8   A.** Parasternal short axis view. **B.** (See color plate) Parasternal short axis view with color Doppler.

a. membranous VSD
b. supracristal VSD
c. Ebstein's anomaly
d. Pulmonic Stenosis (PS)/Pulmonic Insufficiency (PI)
e. PDA

9. A 46-year-old woman with dyspnea on exertion with occasional palpitations has the following surface echo images (Figs. 13–9A–D). Her dyspnea on exertion can be explained by

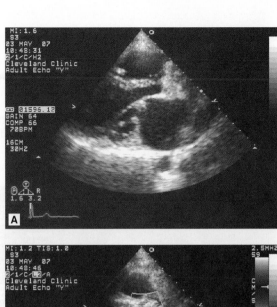

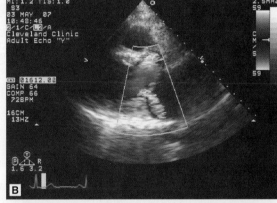

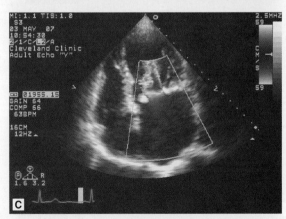

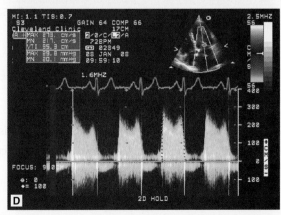

**FIGURE 13–9   A.** Parasternal long axis view. **B.** (See color plate) Parasternal long axis view with color Doppler. **C.** (See color plate) Apical four-chamber view with color Doppler of the mitral valve. **D.** Continuous-wave Doppler through the mitral valve.

    **a.** myxomatous MV disease with MR
    **b.** rheumatic MV disease with MS and MR
    **c.** endocarditis with vegetation causing MR
    **d.** severe mitral annular calcification
    **e.** cleft mitral leaflet

10. A 35-year-old patient had the following echocardiographic images (Figs. 13–10A and B). The pathology shown may be associated with any of the following complications *except*

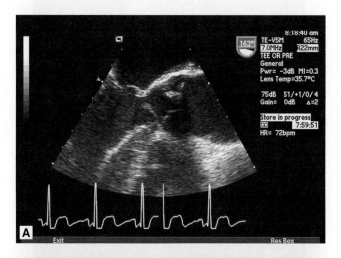

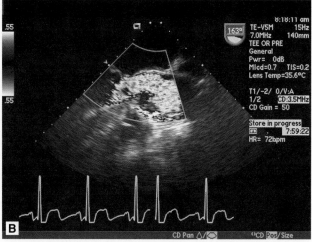

**FIGURE 13–10** **A.** Mid-esophageal long axis view of the aortic valve (TEE). **B.** (See color plate) Mid-esophageal long axis view of the aortic valve with color Doppler (systole).

    **a.** aortic insufficiency
    **b.** endocarditis
    **c.** left ventricular hypertrophy
    **d.** atrial arrhythmias
    **e.** may be difficult to assess aortic valve area by continuity in this situation

11. This parasternal short axis view (Fig. 13–11) would be most consistent with which of the following patients?

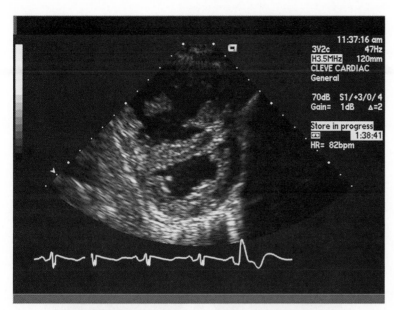

**FIGURE 13–11**  Parasternal short axis view (diastole).

**a.** patient with severe MR
**b.** patient with severe AI
**c.** patient with severe TR
**d.** patient with severe LV systolic dysfunction
**e.** patient with a subaortic membrane

12. The TEE images below are from a patient who has marked dyspnea on exertion and one episode of presyncope (Figs. 13–12A–C). The patient is now in the operating room for a procedure. The most appropriate operation for this patient would be

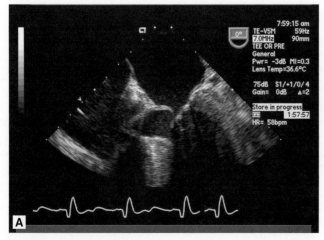

**FIGURE 13–12**  (*Continued*)

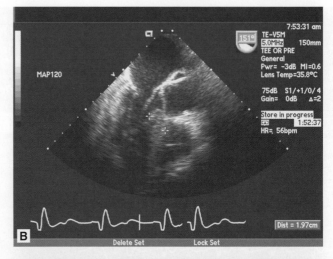

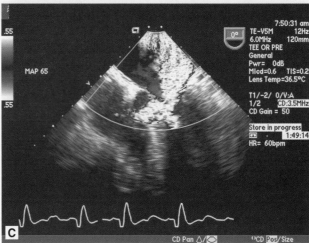

**FIGURE 13–12** **A.** Mid-esophageal four-chamber view (TEE). **B.** Mid-esophageal long axis view (TEE). **C.** (See color plate) Mid-esophageal four-chamber view with color Doppler.

    **a.** mitral valve repair
    **b.** septal myectomy
    **c.** mitral valve replacement
    **d.** CABG
    **e.** ascending aortic conduit

**13.** A 56-year-old man with a history of aortic stenosis underwent AVR with a bioprosthesis and now comes back 3 years later with shortness of breath, fatigue, weight loss, and night sweats. A transesophageal echocardiogram was performed and these are a few representative views (Figs. 13–13A–C). The important findings on this echo include all the following *except*

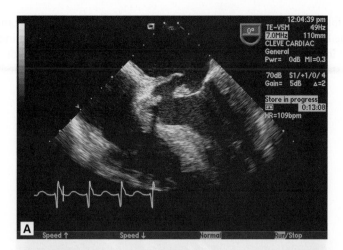

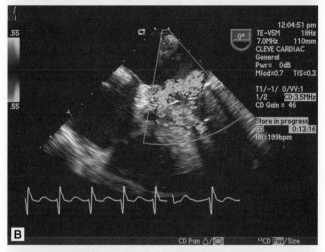

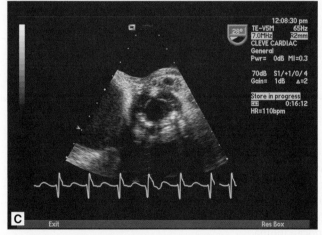

**FIGURE 13–13** **A.** Mid-esophageal four-chamber view (TEE). **B.** (See color plate) Mid-esophageal four-chamber view with color Doppler. **C.** Mid-esophageal short axis view of the aortic valve (TEE).

    **a.** large vegetation on the aortic prosthesis
    **b.** paravalvular abscess
    **c.** perforation at the base of the anterior mitral leaflet
    **d.** severe MR
    **e.** large vegetation on the TV

**14.** The following TEE images (Figs. 13–14A and B) demonstrate a large mass noted in the LV apex. This mass is located in a region of myocardial thinning and akinesis in a dilated LV. Although there is some mobility there does not appear to be a stalk. This mass is most likely which of the following possibilities?

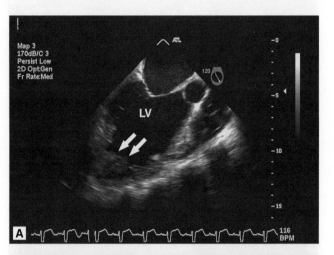

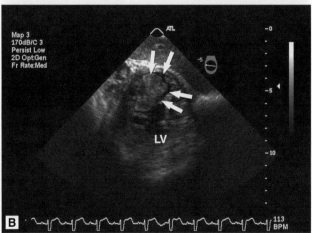

**FIGURE 13–14   A.** Mid-esophageal long axis view (TEE). **B.** Transgastric short axis view of the LV (TEE).

**a.** teratoma
**b.** myosarcoma
**c.** fibroelastoma
**d.** thrombus
**e.** adenocarcinoma

**15.** A patient with the shown anatomy (Fig. 13–15) is at increased risk or may have all of the following problems or complications *except*

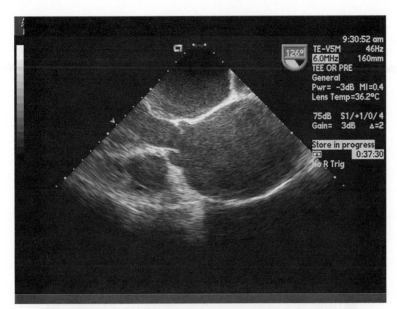

**FIGURE 13–15** Mid-esophageal long axis view of the ascending aorta (TEE).

**a.** aortic insufficiency
**b.** aortic dissection
**c.** aortic rupture
**d.** hoarseness
**e.** endocarditis

**16.** A 64-year-old woman with no known prior cardiac history comes in with an acute MI and received lytics at an outside hospital. She is transferred to your hospital pain free for further management. On cardiac catheterization the following day she has three-vessel disease; however, the infarct-related vessel has TIMI 3 flow. Four days later she develops chest pain and marked shortness of breath. Following intubation she had a TEE with representative images below (Figs. 13–16A–C). The appropriate therapy at this time is

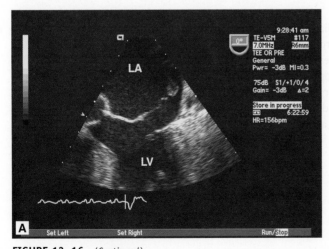

**FIGURE 13–16** (*Continued*)

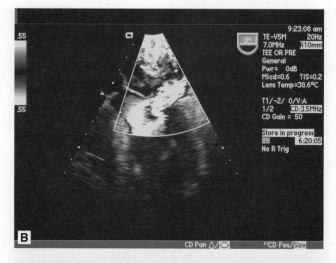

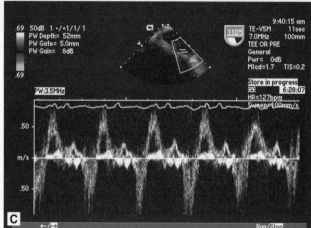

**FIGURE 13–16  A.** Mid-esophageal four-chamber view of the mitral valve. **B.** (See color plate) Mid-esophageal four-chamber view with color Doppler. **C.** Pulse-wave Doppler of the pulmonary veins.

**a.** cardiac catheterization with PTCA of the infarct-related artery for post-infarction angina
**b.** placement of IABP
**c.** nitroprusside (Nipride) as tolerated by BP
**d.** emergent cardiac surgery
**e.** a and b
**f.** b, c, and d

**17.** The patient is a 56-year-old man with HTN, diabetes, and obesity who was admitted 6 months ago to an outside hospital with a late presentation of an anterior MI. He presented approximately 3 days post MI and underwent cardiac catheterization at 1 week, which showed a total occlusion in the mid LAD, severe stenoses of the first and second diagonals, and no significant disease in either the RCA or LCx. The patient was then referred to your hospital for revascularization. The patient, however, failed to show for his appointment and finally presented 8 months later with chest pain and shortness of breath. Prior to revascularization you order a PET Rb/FDG using Rubidium$^{82}$/and F18$_A$ (Flourine-18)—labelled deoxyglucose). to determine the degree of inducible ischemia and viability. The images obtained are in Figure 13–17. The images from the PET scan demonstrate

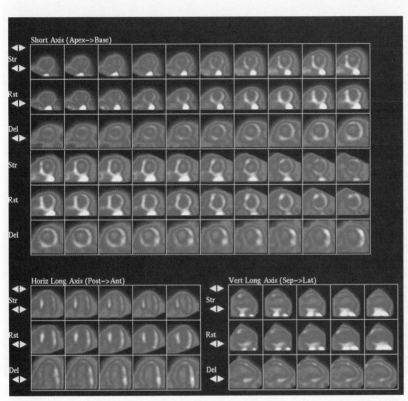

**FIGURE 13–17**  Rubidium/FDG PET scan with the stress images displayed on top, the rest images next, and the delayed metabolic FDG imaged displayed on the bottom.

**a.** scar in the LAD territory
**b.** inducible ischemia in the LAD territory
**c.** hibernating myocardium in the LAD territory
**d.** a combination of inducible ischemia and hibernation in the LAD territory
**e.** scar in the RCA territory

**18.** Patient is a 75-year-old man with hypertension, diabetes, hypercholesterolemia, and CAD who is 10 years s/p CABG: Lima to LAD, SVG to RCA, and SVG to OM1. He is asymptomatic on a good medical regimen, although he is relatively sedentary. TTE demonstrated normal LV systolic function with LVEF 60%, moderately severe LVH, and no significant valvular disease. The patient is now sent for cardiac evaluation prior to surgery on his dilated abdominal aorta (7.5 cm in diameter). An adenosine nuclear stress test is ordered for preoperative risk assessment. During the adenosine stress he remained asymptomatic although he developed 2-mm ST depressions in I, L V$_2$–V$_6$. There were no significant changes in blood pressure. Figure 13–18 shows the scan. The scan demonstrates

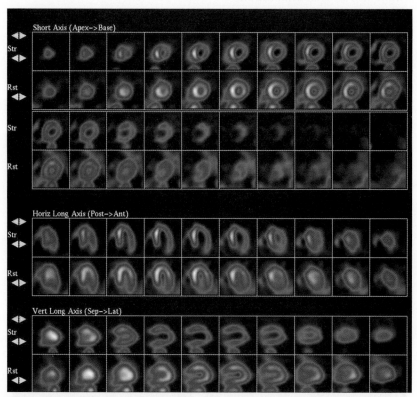

**FIGURE 13–18**  Adenosine technetium 99m nuclear stress test with the stress images on top and the resting images below.

**a.** marked attenuation
**b.** multivessel ischemia
**c.** infarct but no ischemia
**d.** mixture of infarct and ischemia
**e.** motion artifact

**19.** The patient is a 62-year-old man with CAD risk factors including diabetes (16 years), hypertension, family history of CAD, and obesity. The patient had a silent Inferior MI 2 years earlier by detected by ECG. The patient is now sent for preoperative evaluation for bilateral knee surgery. The patient has no chest pain with exertion; however, his exercise capacity is limited by knee pain. He does occasionally have mild post-prandial dyspnea. His medications include insulin, a statin, an ACE inhibitor, a beta-blocker, and an aspirin. A pharmacologic dual isotope (Thal/Tc) scan was performed and is shown in Figure 13–19. The gated images showed an LVEF of 42% with a wall motion abnormality in the infero-lateral wall. There were no ECG changes or symptoms during the adenosine infusion. The rest and post-stress images demonstrate

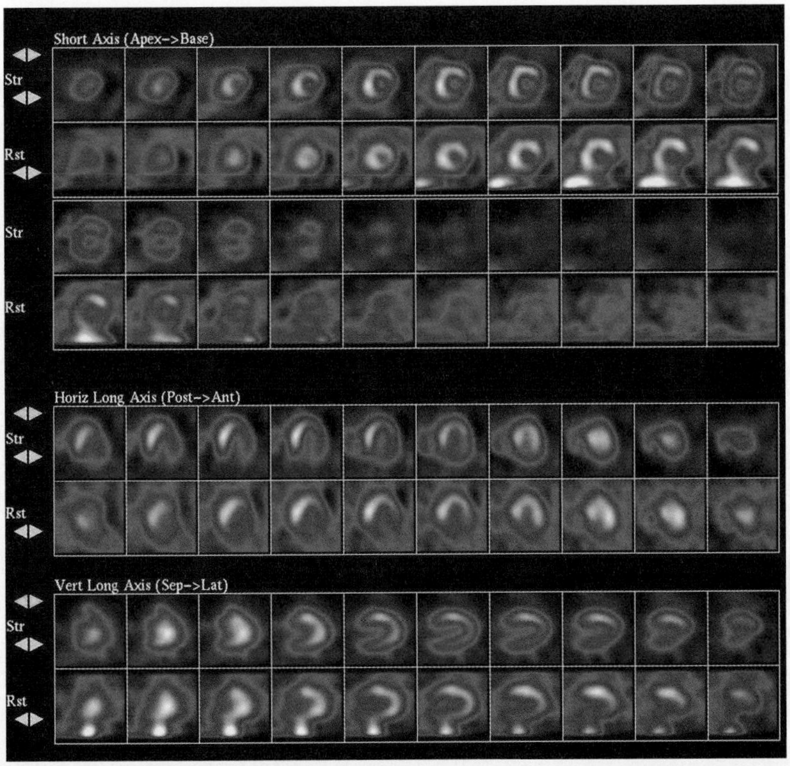

**FIGURE 13–19** A pharmacologic (adenosine) dual isotope (Thal/Tc) scan with the stress images displayed on top with the resting images below.

   **a.** scarred RCA/LCx territory
   **b.** scarred LAD territory
   **c.** normal test with artifacts
   **d.** scar and ischemia in the LCx/RCA territory
   **e.** scar and ischemia in the LAD territory

**NOTES**

20. The patient is a 60-year-old man with hypertension, diabetes (newly diagnosed), and CAD (s/p PCI with drug eluting stent [DES] in his mid LAD 5 years ago, and bare metal stent [BMS] to distal RCA and a posteroventricular branch 7 years ago). The patient is now sent for symptom evaluation. The patient notes the onset of chest pains with exertion while playing squash approximately 2 months ago. The pain occurs only with activity and resolves within a few minutes with rest. He denies other associated symptoms or discomfort at rest. A treadmill nuclear stress test was performed. The patient exercised using a standard Bruce protocol having completed eight METs and reached 98% MPHR. There was a normal ST-segment response to stress, and there was no chest pain with exercise. He did, however, develop new ST depressions in recovery and new atrial fibrillation in recovery, requiring treatment with beta-blockers. The scan images are shown in Figure 13–20. The appropriate interpretation of this scan is

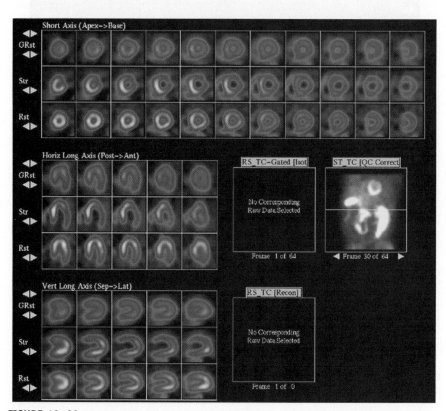

**FIGURE 13–20**  An exercise technetium 99m nuclear stress test with the stress images with the gated images (currently still) on top, the post-stress images next, and the resting images on the bottom.

    **a.** RCA territory infarct

    **b.** LAD territory infarct

    **c.** RCA territory ischemia

    **d.** LAD infarct with peri-infarct ischemia

    **e.** LAD and LCx versus left main ischemia

**21.** A 19-year-old female is referred to your office for evaluation of congestive heart failure and mitral regurgitation. She has a history of complete heart block and has previously undergone pacemaker implantation. On physical examination, her heart rate is 85 bpm, respiratory rate of 16, and blood pressure 108/65 mm Hg. Her jugular venous pulse is visible 6 cm above the sternal angle at 45°. The PMI is sustained but normal in location. She has a grade II/VI holosystolic murmur at the apex that radiates to the axilla. There is trivial bilateral pedal edema. A posterior-anterior and lateral chest x-ray demonstrates mild cardiomegaly. A transthoracic echocardiogram reveals moderately reduced left ventricular systolic function with an ejection fraction of 35%. There is 2+–3+ posteriorly directed mitral regurgitation. A cardiac CT with contrast is obtained to evaluate the coronary arteries (Fig. 13–21A and B). Which of the following is *true* regarding this patient's condition?

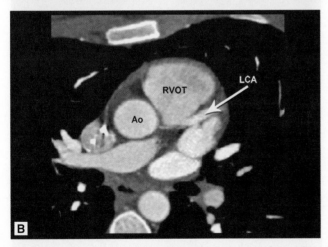

**FIGURE 13–21 A.** Double oblique image of the aortic root at the level of the right and left sinuses of Valsalva. Ao, aorta; LA, left atrium; RCA, right coronary artery; RVOT, right ventricular outflow tract. **B.** Oblique axial image at the level of the left coronary artery origin. LCA, left coronary artery.

**a.** This condition is a common cause of sudden cardiac death in athletes.
**b.** The anomaly shown represents origin of the left coronary artery from the right coronary ostium.
**c.** Surgical reimplantation of the anomalous coronary artery is indicated.
**d.** Patients with this condition who survive past childhood often present with varying degrees of heart failure, myocardial ischemia, and mitral regurgitation, depending on the development of collateral circulation.
**e.** This condition is usually inoperable and best left alone.

**22.** A 45-year-old female presents to your office for evaluation of atrial fibrillation. She had undergone prior open heart surgery for bypass grafting and has had atrial fibrillation intermittently since. Pulmonary vein isolation has been performed on one occasion since surgery because of atrial fibrillation refractory to medicines. She now complains of exertional intolerance and dyspnea, easy fatigue, and lower extremity edema. Her atrial fibrillation has returned. As part of her evaluation, a cardiac CT with contrast is ordered to evaluate her pulmonary venous anatomy prior to a possible second ablation procedure (Figs. 13–22A–D). Based on the CT scan images, which of the following is *true* regarding this patient's condition?

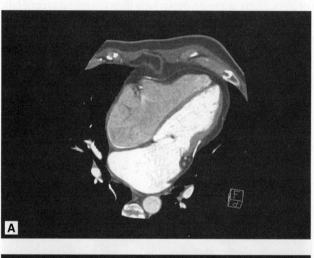

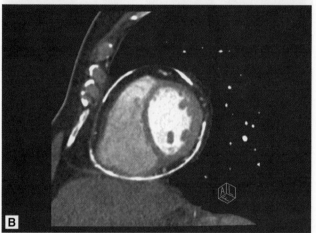

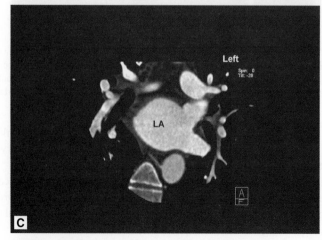

**FIGURE 13–22** (*Continued*)

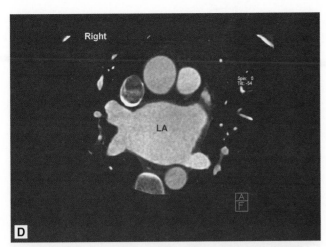

**FIGURE 13–22** **A.** Four-chamber view. **B.** Short axis mid-ventricular view. **C.** Oblique coronal view of the left-sided pulmonary veins. **D.** Oblique coronal view of the right-sided pulmonary veins.

a. An increase in tricuspid valve flow during inspiration would be seen on Doppler echocardiography.

b. Reduced perfusion in the lung segments affected by the stenosed pulmonary vein would be seen on quantitative V/Q scan of the lungs.

c. A pattern of diffuse delayed enhancement in a pattern consistent with a restrictive cardiomyopathy would be seen on cardiac MRI.

d. Right atrial pressure would be elevated, with a prominent $x$ descent and a diminished or absent $y$ descent on right heart catheterization.

e. None of the above.

23. A 72-year-old gentleman with a history of coronary artery disease, hypertension, peripheral vascular disease, and a chronic type B aortic dissection returns to your office for routine follow-up. On physical examination, his heart rate is 64 bpm, respiratory rate of 14, and blood pressure 148/85 mm Hg. His jugular venous pulse is unremarkable. The PMI is sustained but normal in location. $S_1$ and $S_2$ are normal. There is no pedal edema. Carotid and radial pulses are 2+ bilaterally; dorsalis pedis pulses are 1+ bilaterally. A cardiac MRI/MRA is ordered for follow-up of his aortic dissection (Figs. 13–23A and B). All of the following are true regarding this patient's condition *except*

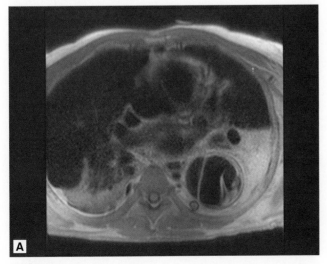

**FIGURE 13–23** *(Continued)*

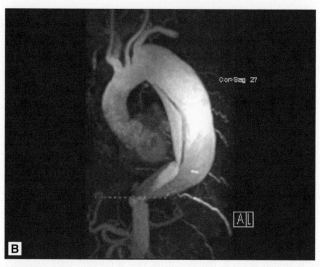

**FIGURE 13–23**    **A.** Axial spin echo MRI. **B.** Contrast enhanced MRA of the thoracic aorta.

a. Late deaths following dissection occur in 30% of cases and are caused by rupture of a second aneurysm or recurrence of the dissection.

b. The risk of late death from a type B dissection is highest in the first 2 years after diagnosis.

c. Severe chest and/or back pain, myocardial infarction, and/or acute aortic insufficiency are suggestive of proximal extension of the dissection.

d. Acute myocardial infarction caused by a type A dissection should be treated with primary PCI before surgery is considered.

e. Long-term management includes therapy with antihypertensive agents and referral for surgical or endovascular stent grafting for aneurysmal dilation of the dissected aorta.

# ANSWERS

1. **e.** The images demonstrate a patient with cardiac tamponade. Findings include significant respiratory variation of MV inflows (>25%) and RV diastolic collapse, RA inversion, and IVC plethora (dilated >2 cm and does not collapse normally with inspiration). A patient with a type I dissection and cardiac tamponade needs to go to emergent cardiac surgery as soon as possible for drainage of the pericardium and repair of the aorta. Pericardiocentesis could potentially cause complete rupture of the flap into the pericardium, causing cardiac arrest and death. An aortic stent graft is currently not the treatment of choice for a type I dissection and could certainly not address the problem of tamponade. Coronary angiography in this patient would only delay the definitive therapy (surgery) as well as possibly further propagate the dissection flap. Recall that delay of surgery in a patient with a type I dissection is associated with a 1% per hour increase in mortality in the first 48 hours of the process. (Note that this patient has not had prior cardiac surgery—if the person had prior cardiac surgery, that would likely change the need for cardiac catheterization prior to surgery, although in this patient emergent surgical drainage of the pericardium would be needed.)

2. **b.** The image displays an apical four-chamber view of a patient with a primum ASD. (Note Fig. 13–2B with color Doppler shows left-to-right shunting through the ASD.) This is part of either a partial or complete AV canal defect. A complete AV canal defect includes a primum ASD, a cleft anterior mitral leaflet, and a widened anteroseptal tricuspid commissure. A partial AV canal defect is as above but without the VSD. Note that because of the long-term, significant right-to-left shunt through the ASD in this patient the right side is dilated and there is RVH from pulmonary hypertension. The short axis view of the mitral valve (Fig. 13–24A) demonstrates the cleft anterior mitral leaflet, which "splits" in the center, as opposed to opening like a fish mouth as is seen with normal mitral valves. Figure 13–24B is a drawing showing normal short axis of mitral valve versus cleft mitral valve.

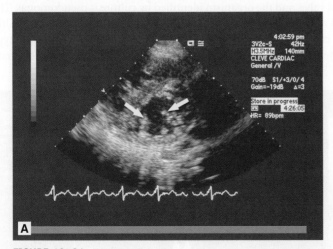

**FIGURE 13–24**  (*Continued*)

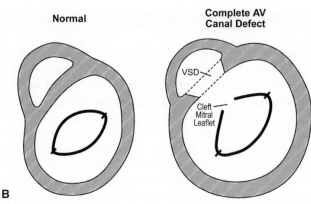

**FIGURE 13–24** **A.** Parasternal short axis view of the mitral valve (TTE). **B.** Drawing comparing the parasternal short axis view of a normal mitral valve to the opening of a cleft anterior mitral leaflet.

**3. d.** The patient is a young man with hypertension beginning in his late 20s or early 30s. Secondary hypertension must be considered and ruled out in this patient. When he was initially diagnosed he should have had his blood pressure checked in both arms and legs in consideration of a coarctation of the aorta. Note: Someone may also notice rib notching on a CXR. Other etiologies that should have been excluded include renal artery stenosis (more commonly seen in women if caused by fibromuscular dysplasia), pheochromocytoma, Cushing syndrome, or primary aldosteronism. This patient's heart murmur was a diastolic murmur from aortic insufficiency caused by prolapse of a bicuspid aortic valve. At least 50% of patients with a coarctation have a bicuspid aortic valve. Fewer patients with bicuspid aortic valve have a coarctation. Note that bicuspid aortic valves dome (doming aortic leaflets are seen in Fig. 13–3D) and could be mistaken on initial glance in long axis with a rheumatic AV. However, in addition to doming there is prolapse of the conjoined cusp (which would not be seen in a rheumatic valve) and the anatomic situation could be clarified with a good short axis view.

**4. e.** Right-sided endocarditis is less common than left-sided endocarditis. The TEE image (Fig. 13–25) shown demonstrates a patient with a vegetation on the tricuspid valve, and the organism identified by culture is pseudomonas. This is associated with IV drug use with contamination at the time of injection. Although the other clinical situations listed are at increased risk of endocarditis (typically left sided), pseudomonas would be a very unusual pathogen in those situations.

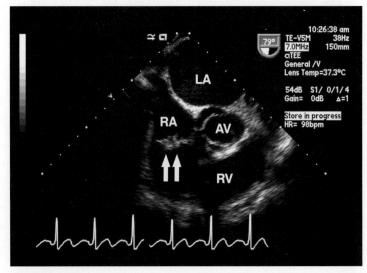

**FIGURE 13–25**

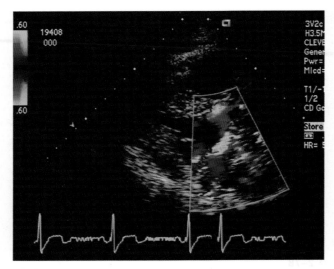

**FIGURE 2-1**

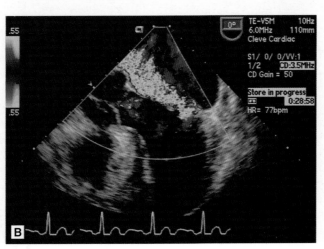

**FIGURE 2-5B**

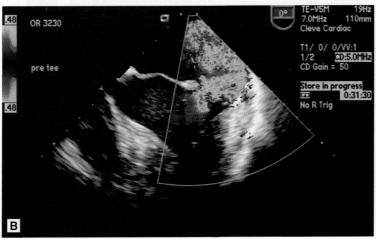

**FIGURE 2-6B**

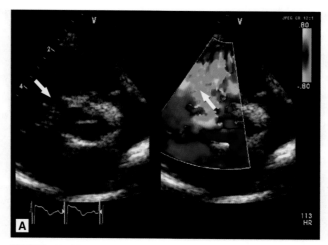

**FIGURE 13–28A**

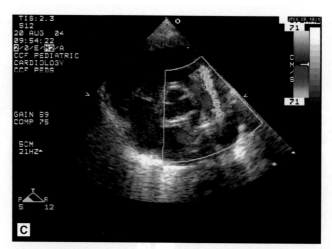

**FIGURE 13–28C**

**5. b.** The M-mode trace is performed through the mitral valve in a patient with myxomatous mitral valve disease with bileaflet prolapse. Note the marked dip backward of the MV leaflets after the closure point (Fig. 13–5). Note that there is full systolic range of motion creating the "M" trace of the anterior mitral leaflet and the normal "W" trace of the posterior leaflet. This is in contrast with a normal mitral valve M-mode, which would not have the systolic dip (Fig. 13–26A). Thus there is no rheumatic mitral stenosis, which would look like Figure 13–26B in which there are still pliable but tethered leaflets causing a loss of the normal "M" and "W" appearance of the mitral leaflets. More advanced mitral stenosis with thickened and calcified leaflets would have thicker and brighter appearance of the leaflets together with more restriction of the leaflet motion (Fig. 13–26C). M-mode for a patient with HOCM and SAM would appear like the images in Figures 13–26D and E. Note the systolic anterior motion of the mitral leaflets in Figure 13–26D and the early closure of the aortic valve in Figure 13–26E (compared to the M-mode of a normal aortic valve [Fig. 13–26F]).

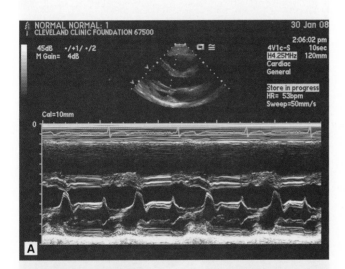

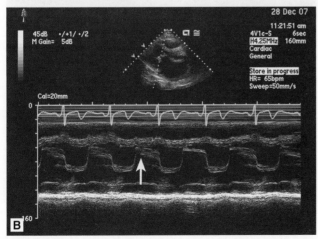

**FIGURE 13–26** *(Continued)*

**NOTES**

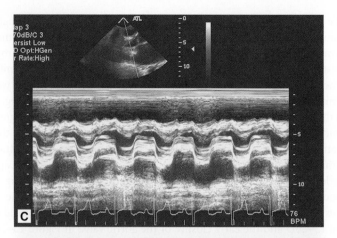

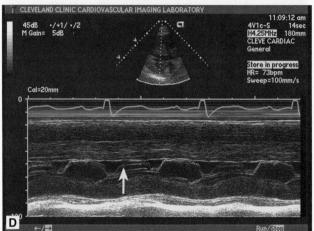

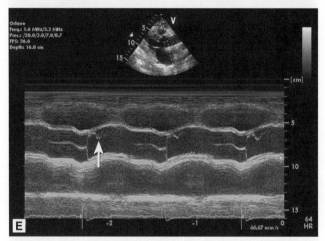

**FIGURE 13–26**   (*Continued*)

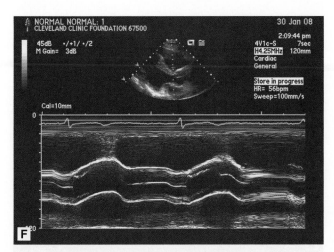

**FIGURE 13–26  A.** M-mode through the mitral valve. **B.** M-mode through the mitral valve. **C.** M-mode through the mitral valve. **D.** M-mode through the mitral valve. **E.** M-mode through the aortic valve. **F.** M-mode through the aortic valve.

6. **b.** The patient has fungal endocarditis involving his aortic valve with a very large vegetation. Although there is some AI, it is not severe, and the degree of AI in this patient would not be an indication for surgery. There is marked color acceleration antegrade across the AV, suggesting aortic stenosis caused by obstruction from the vegetation. This was confirmed by high gradients on continuous wave Doppler across the AV. Fungal endocarditis is an indication for AVR, as is the presence of a mobile vegetation. A mobile vegetation >15 mm on appropriate antibiotic therapy for greater than 7 to 10 days or an embolic event with mobile vegetation >10 mm is also an indication for surgery. Typically, vegetations associated with fungal endocarditis are large, "bulky" lesions. Valvular obstruction is also an indication for urgent surgery; the degree of AI alone in this patient (only moderate) would not be sufficient to warrant surgery. Note that in the setting of an active infection, a surgeon should consider placing an AV homograft to increase the likelihood of being able to clear the infection. Placing prosthetic material in an infected field increases the risk of the prosthesis to become infected, making the infection difficult to clear.

7. **c.** A bicuspid aortic valve with fusion of the right coronary cusp (RCC) and left coronary cusp (LCC). The 2D TEE mid-esophageal view (Fig. 13–7) demonstrates a bicuspid aortic valve in short axis. To determine cusp anatomy one must view the aortic valve in systole. If one looks for a "Mercedes Benz" image of the valve in short axis during diastole (Fig. 13–27A), one may mistake a bicuspid valve for a tricuspid valve, not realizing that one of the arms in the Mercedes Benz sign is actually a calcified raphe between two fixed cusps. Thus, it is important to look at the valve in systole to determine the true cusp anatomy. The most common form of bicuspid AV is fusion of the RCC and LCC. Bicuspid aortic valves are also associated with a dilated aorta with an aortopathy involving cystic medial necrosis. Another form of bicuspid AV is fusion of the RCC and NCC (Fig. 13–27B). There are other congenitally abnormal aortic valves, including unicuspid valves (Fig. 13–27C) and quadricuspid valves (Fig. 13–27D). The unicuspid and quadricuspid valves are much less common than bicuspid valves.

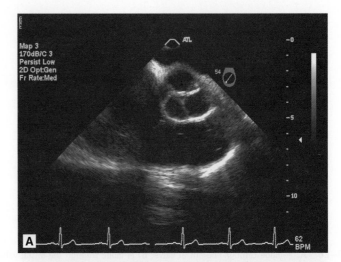

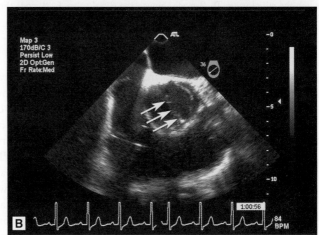

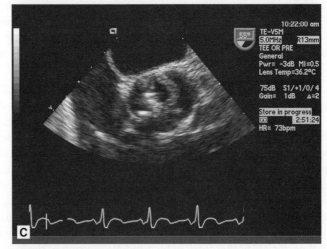

**FIGURE 13–27** *(Continued)*

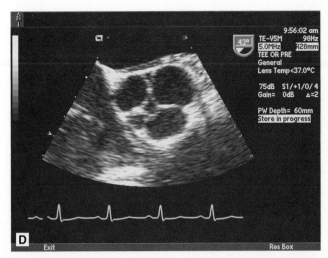

**FIGURE 13–27** **A.** Mid-esophageal short axis view of the aortic valve (diastole). **B.** Mid-esophageal short axis view of a bicuspid aortic valve with fusion of the RCC and NCC. **C.** Mid-esophageal short axis view of a unicuspid aortic valve. **D.** Mid-esophageal short axis view of a quadricuspid aortic valve.

**8. b.** This image demonstrates a supracristal VSD. The VSD is located just under the pulmonic valve—best seen in the parasternal short axis view (seen at at 1 o'clock). A membranous VSD would be seen at 10 or 11 o'clock in short axis view (Fig. 13–28A). Ebstein's anomaly involves apical displacement of the tricuspid valve with atrialization of some of the RV (Fig. 13–28B). Patent ductus can also be seen in the parasternal short axis view seen best by color Doppler showing a flow entering the PA (from the aorta) (Fig. 13–28C). Pulmonic stenosis is seen on 2D in the parasternal short axis view with doming pulmonic value leaflets with color acceleration across the valve. In diastole there may also be some PI as the leaflets may have restricted closing.

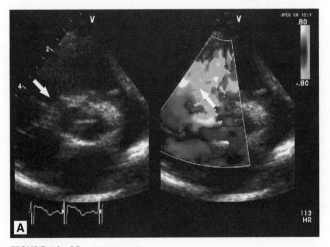

**FIGURE 13–28** *(Continued)*

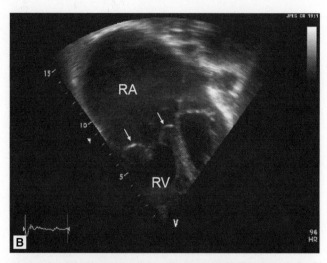

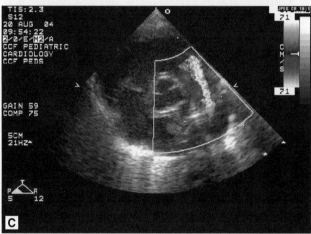

**FIGURE 13–28** **A.** (See color plate) Parasternal short axis view (both 2D and with color Doppler). **B.** Apical four-chamber view (pediatric display with atria at the top of the screen). **C.** (See color plate) Parasternal short axis view.

9. **b.** The images shown demonstrate a doming anterior mitral leaflet and a fixed posterior leaflet. There is color acceleration across the MV, suggestive of MS, which is supported by the high gradients found by continuous wave (CW) Doppler through the MV. There is also significant MR (posteriorly directed) seen in the systolic frame with color Doppler. The mechanism of MR in this case is restricted leaflet motion. Myxomatous MV disease (Fig. 13–29), in contrast, is characterized by markedly redundant, prolapsing leaflets, which prolapse back into the left atrium, occasionally with a torn chord causing a flail leaflet. Typically, the jet of MR is very eccentric if only one leaflet is involved (the jet is in the opposite direction from the most involved leaflet). If there is balanced bileaflet prolapse, the jet is usually centrally directed.

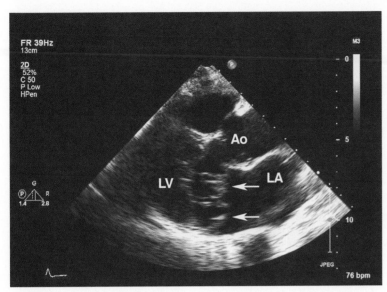

**FIGURE 13–29**  Parasternal long axis view of a patient with mitral valve prolapse.

**10. d.** The images shown are those of a patient with a subaortic membrane. This can best be seen as a linear structure across the LVOT in a long axis view (Fig. 13–30). Although sometimes seen on transthoracic echo, they are often better seen by TEE. Once the possible membrane is located by 2D images, color Doppler demonstrates the color acceleration that occurs prior to the aortic valve, showing that a hemodynamically significant obstruction is present below the valve, in the LVOT. The presence of a subaortic membrane puts a patient at an increased risk of endocarditis because of the turbulent flow caused by the subaortic membrane. Antibiotic prophylaxis was previously recommended; however, in 2007, the guidelines for antibiotic prophylaxis were narrowed, and antibiotic prophylaxis for a subaortic membrane is no longer recommended. In addition to the increased risk for endocarditis, the turbulent high velocity jets produced by the membrane damage the aortic valve over time and these patients often develop aortic insufficiency. A subaortic membrane is a fixed obstruction that the LV must overcome to eject blood into the aorta. The left ventricle responds to the increased load in a similar fashion as it responds to valvular aortic stenosis—it hypertrophies. Thus these patients commonly develop LVH in proportion to the degree of obstruction. Following resection these patients may have a recurrence of the subaortic membrane, although the exact frequency of this occurrence is unknown. Because there is a high velocity jet proximal to the valve and often some narrowing at the valve itself, it is often difficult to measure valve area by continuity or to assess the relative contribution of membrane and valve to the overall pressure gradient by Doppler.

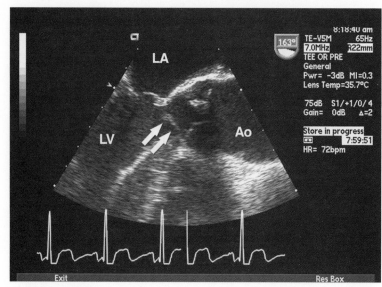

**FIGURE 13–30**

11. **c.** The parasternal short axis still frame in diastole demonstrates a patient with diastolic septal flattening. This is found in a patient with right-sided *volume* overload. You can also see patients with systolic septal flattening, which is consistent with right-sided pressure overload. The patient with severe TR has right-sided volume overload, and would have diastolic septal flattening as shown. Patients often have both diastolic and systolic septal flattening if they have both volume and pressure overload of the right side, for example, in a patient with chronic PEs who has developed pulmonary hypertension and also developed significant TR. The lesions of MR and AI are volume loads for the left ventricle, and the subaortic membrane is a pressure load on the LV.

12. **b.** The TEE images demonstrate a patient with HOCM. There is septal hypertrophy and the systolic frame demonstrates SAM, which is systolic anterior motion of the mitral leaflets (Fig. 13–31). The color Doppler images for this patient demonstrate severe mitral regurgitation that is posteriorly directed, which is classic for MR caused by SAM of the mitral leaflets. SAM can involve either the anterior or posterior leaflet alone, or a patient may have bileaflet SAM. Typically, if the mitral leaflet has not been too damaged by years of contact with the septum, performing a septal myectomy can fix the severe MR by eliminating the LVOT obstruction and eliminating the SAM. This type of MR is often hemodynamically labile depending on the loading conditions of the LV. The SAM can be brought out or accentuated by giving the patient amyl nitrite or isuprel. The SAM is decreased by volume loading the ventricle or increasing the systemic pressure. If the mitral leaflets, however, have been scarred by years of contact with the septum, a simultaneous MV repair or replacement may need to be performed. If the mitral valve has to be replaced, often the surgeon has to use a lower profile valve (typically a bileaflet mechanical valve) because of the narrowed LVOT. Neither a CABG nor an ascending aortic conduit would help this patient unless he had concomitant coronary artery disease or an ascending aortic aneurysm, in which case these procedures would have to be performed in addition to the myectomy.

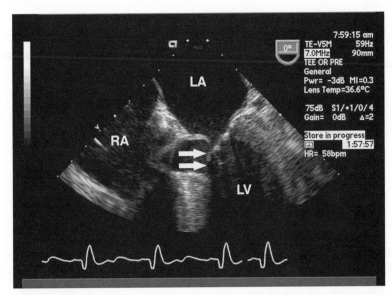

**FIGURE 13-31**

**13. e.** The four-chamber view in this patient demonstrates the perforation at the base of the anterior mitral leaflet (solid arrow in Fig. 13–32A). The color Doppler in this same view demonstrates the severe MR coming through the leaflet perforation. This view also shows a vegetation attached to the AVR seen extending into the LVOT (dotted arrow in Fig. 13–32A). The short axis view demonstrates an expansile cavity at 2 o'clock posterior and lateral to the sewing ring of the AVR (Fig. 13–32B). This is consistent with a paravalvular abscess. If the color Doppler images from the short axis view were included, you would have been able to see flow into this cavity. The short axis view also demonstrates the tricuspid valve (in a single limited view). This view, however, does not show a vegetation. When performing a TEE on a patient with endocarditis, it is important to perform a complete study examining all valves, even if pathology has already been found on one valve, to be sure to exclude any additional complications. In addition to vegetations, one needs to look for abscesses, perforations, or fistulae that can form as a result of widespread infection. This patient underwent extensive debridement of the paravalvular abscess with placement of an aortic homograft and debridement and closure of the perforation at the base of the mitral valve. Note that autologous pericardium was used to patch the perforation as opposed to prosthetic material to improve the likelihood of clearing the infection.

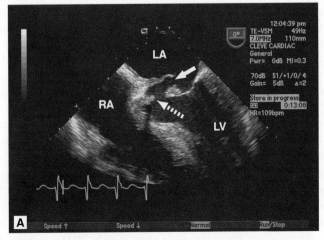

**FIGURE 13-32**   *(Continued)*

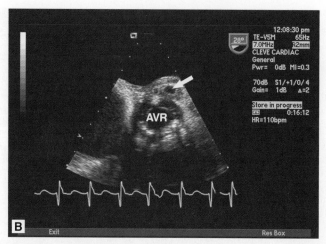

**FIGURE 13–32  A.** Mid-esophageal four-chamber view with the solid arrow demonstrating the perforation at the base of the anterior mitral leaflet and the dashed arrow showing the vegetation on the AVR. **B.** Mid-esophageal short axis view demonstrating a paravalvular abscess located at 1:00 or 2:00 around serving ring of AVR.

**14. d.** This patient had a very large anterior myocardial infarction and has significant thinning and akinesis of the anterior wall and LV apex. Because of this significant wall motion abnormality there is stasis of the blood and the patient is at risk of forming a thrombus, which this patient has done. The homogeneous nature of the mass with an echogenicity similar to that of the myocardium (or slightly less echogenic than the myocardium) suggests that the thrombus is relatively fresh. As this heals or organizes over time, calcium may be deposited, and old, organized thrombi in the heart are often quite echogenic. A sarcoma, on the other hand, would be an invasive mass and would not respect the boundaries of the myocardium, but rather would infiltrate the myocardium. Teratomas if found in the heart arise from the pericardium, not within the LV cavity. These are typically benign although may compress the heart. A teratoma would also have a more heterogeneous appearance on echo. Myxomas are the most common benign tumor of the heart and 80% of those are located in the LA, and most of the remaining ones are found in the RA. Papillary fibroelastomas are the second most common benign cardiac tumors, and are typically pedunculated (with a stalk) and mobile. Most (>80%) are located on heart valves.

**15. e.** The image demonstrates a patient with a large aortic aneurysm measuring approximately 7 cm in diameter. Patients with aortic aneurysms often have aortic insufficiency caused by distortion of the suspension of the aortic valve, even though the aortic leaflets themselves are structurally normal. This AI is typically centrally originating and centrally directed. As the ascending aorta becomes dilated there is an increasing risk of dissection as well as rupture as the vessel diameter increases. The surgical indications for aneurysms of the ascending aorta include aneurysms of 5.5 to 6.0 cm or greater for all comers, but 5 cm for patients with Marfan's disease or a bicuspid aortic valve (who also have an aortopathy), or aneurysms that have expanded more than 0.5 cm in 1 year, or patients with aneurysms that are causing symptoms or are of traumatic etiology. These patients are not typically at increased risk for endocarditis. Patients with ascending aortic aneurysms can present with hoarseness caused by stretching or pressure on the recurrent laryngeal nerve, or dysphagia caused by mass effect compressing the esophagus.

**16. f.** The images show a patient with a papillary muscle rupture causing severe MR. The typical time frame for a papillary muscle rupture to occur is 2 to 7 days post MI. Most commonly the patient with a papillary muscle rupture has not had a prior MI, and the posteromedial papillary muscle is involved much more often than the anterolateral due to the single blood supply (PDA) to the posteromedial muscle as opposed to the dual supply (LAD and LCx) to the anterolateral. Placement of a balloon pump and starting nitroprusside (Nipride) to improve forward flow and support the patient while the OR can be set up is only a temporizing treatment. Surgical repair of the mitral valve or replacement is the definitive treatment for this problem. PTCA of the infarct-related artery would not help correct the underlying problem in this patient. Luckily the patient had already had angiography so that the surgeon can perform bypass at the time he or she fixes the mitral valve problem. Note the appearance of the mitral valve on TEE. There is a flail of the mitral leaflet; however, at the end of the tissue prolapsing into the left atrium there is a mass, which represents the torn head of the papillary muscle. This appearance differs from a person with myxomatous mitral valve disease with a flail leaflet. In that situation there would only be torn leaflet and chordae seen within the LA, which would not have the bulk of the piece of muscle. The systolic flow reversal seen by the pulse wave Doppler in the pulmonary veins, as well as the large proximal isovelocity surface area (PISA) seen in the four-chamber view, confirms the severity of the MR.

**17. c.** There is a matched defect in the LAD territory seen on the resting and post-stress images involving the apex and four periapical segments as well as the mid-anterior and anteroapical segments. This is consistent with a large LAD territory infarct without any inducible ischemia. The metabolic FDG images show a perfusion/metabolism mismatch with FDG uptake seen in the previously mentioned LAD segments suggesting a large region of hibernation in the LAD territory without any significant scar. (Note that there is significant GI uptake near the inferior wall.) The degree of hibernation involved 40% of the myocardium (6% for each involved segment except for the apex, which represents 4% of the myocardium). A study by Hachamovitch et al.[1] in 2003 showed that revascularization was superior to medical therapy if the amount of myocardium at risk (ischemic and hibernating) exceeded 20%. Since the above patient demonstrated a large area of hibernating myocardium in the LAD territory, the patient would benefit from revascularization of the LAD territory as well as the diagonals. This patient underwent surgical revascularization of all three vessels.

**18. b.** The resting scan showed GI activity, but overall normal tracer uptake. There was increased septal uptake caused by the moderately severe LVH. Post stress there is severely reduced tracer uptake involving the mid and apical anterior, entire anteroseptal, and inferolateral walls and inferior wall and apex. There was also cavity dilation post stress. This is known as transient ischemic dilation (TID). The gated images that accompanied this study demonstrated hypokinesis of the above segments. Note that the post-stress gated images are acquired post stress, but at rest. That is to say that there is a delay between stress and imaging, which may allow for some recovery of function. This scan is high risk in that there is ischemia in all three vascular territories with TID and extensive wall motion abnormalities. Although the patient was asymptomatic under his baseline conditions, it was appropriate to order the adenosine nuclear stress test since the patient is diabetic with prior revascularization and with a questionable functional status who was going to undergo a high-risk surgical procedure (aortic aneurysm repair).

**19. d.** The full interpretation of the study was that there was marked GI activity in the rest images, but there was also a severe resting perfusion defect involving the basal and mid-inferolateral segments. Although GI activity can make the basal and mid-inferior segments difficult to interpret at rest, the post-stress images clearly show that the defect now involves the entire inferolateral and inferior walls, showing infarct with peri-infarct ischemia in the LCx/RCA territory. Cardiac catheterization demonstrated a total obstruction of the proximal LCx (a dominant LCx) with collaterals from the RCA and LAD. There were no obstructions in the RCA and LAD. Important points from this case include that diabetics are at high risk for CAD and clinical parameters do not predict ischemia (from the DIAD trial).

Myocardial perfusion imaging can be performed safely post MI to assess infarct size and the amount of myocardium at risk. It is also a good test to assess the adequacy of collateral blood flow.

20. **e.** The resting images demonstrate normal perfusion. Post stress, however, there are significant perfusion defects in the anterior, anterolateral, and inferolateral walls. There is also cavity dilatation, which is consistent with either left main disease or multivessel ischemia. The gated images showed new wall motion abnormalities in the LAD and LCx territories. The presence of stress-induced perfusion defects in multiple vascular territories, as well as transient ischemic dilatation and new wall motion abnormalities on the gated images, are all findings associated with high-risk scans. The cardiac catheterization in this patient demonstrated 70% stenosis in the proximal LAD, while the stent in the mid LAD was patent. There was a large obtuse marginal with a 90% proximal stenosis. There was mild disease in the proximal RCA, and the stents in posterior descending artery (PDA) and posteroventricular branch (PVB) were patent.

21. **d.** This CT demonstrates an anomalous origin of the left coronary artery from the pulmonary artery (ALCAPA). Also know as Bland-White-Garland syndrome, ALCAPA is a rare but serious congenital anomaly. It is caused by either (i) abnormal septation of the conotruncus into the aorta and pulmonary artery, or (ii) persistence of the pulmonary buds together with involution of the aortic buds that eventually form the coronary arteries. Occurrence is similar between males and females and is not considered an inheritable congenital cardiac defect. Because of the low pulmonary vascular resistance, left coronary artery flow reverses and enters the pulmonic trunk (coronary steal phenomena). As a result, the left ventricular myocardium remains underperfused, leading to infarction of the anterolateral left ventricular wall. This often causes anterolateral papillary muscle dysfunction and variable degrees of mitral insufficiency. Consequently, the combination of left ventricular dysfunction and significant mitral valve insufficiency leads to CHF symptoms (e.g., tachypnea, poor feeding, irritability, diaphoresis) in the young infant. Collateral circulation between the right and left coronary systems eventually develops. Approximately 85% of patients present with clinical symptoms of CHF within the first 1 to 2 months of life. Left untreated, the mortality rate in the first year of life is 90% secondary to myocardial ischemia or infarction and mitral valve insufficiency leading to CHF. In unusual cases, the clinical presentation with symptoms of myocardial ischemia may be delayed into early childhood. Rarely, a patient may stabilize following infarction and present with mitral valve regurgitation, periodic dyspnea, angina pectoris, syncope, or sudden death later in childhood or even adulthood, as in this patient. Treatment consists of surgical ligation of the anomalous coronary artery origin and bypass grafting to the left coronary artery. Reimplantation onto the native aortic root is typically not possible because of the friable quality of the anomalous left coronary artery ostium.

22. **a.** This CT demonstrates several classic features of constrictive pericarditis, including irregular thickening (>4 mm)/calcification of the pericardium, enlargement of one or both atria, and conical or tubular deformity of one or both ventricles. In this particular patient, indentations of both the right and left ventricles by the pericardium are also seen. Other classic morphologic characteristics include enlargement of the IVC, a shift of the interventricular septum toward the left ventricle during inspiration (most prominent during the first beat after inspiration on real-time imaging), and a diastolic bounce of the interventricular septum. The latter differs from abnormal motion of the interventricular septum caused by conduction abnormalities, pacemakers, or post-cardiac surgery, all of which occur during systole. Choice A describes the typical hemodynamic changes in constrictive pericarditis that are seen with echocardiography. There is no evidence of pulmonary vein stenosis to suggest an

alteration in pulmonary perfusion on quantitative V/Q scanning. There is no diffuse thickening of the ventricles or atria to suggest an infiltrative cardiomyopathy such as amyloidosis that would be better assessed by MRI or right heart catheterization, nor is there a pericardial effusion to such tamponade that would account for the changes in right atrial pressure waveforms of choice D.

23. **d.** This MRI demonstrates a typical type B dissection with aneurysmal degeneration of the dissected thoracic aorta. The dissection flap is clearly visible on both the axial spin echo and the MRA images. Acute myocardial infarction in the setting of a type A dissection is suggestive of extension of the dissection flap into a coronary artery and is an absolute contraindication to both thrombolysis as well as PCI. Immediate surgical treatment is indicated in this setting, although mortality is typically high in this setting. The other answer choices are correct.

## References

1. Hachamovitch R, Hayes SW, Friedman JD, et al. Comparison of the short-term survival benefit associated with revascularization compared with medical therapy in patients with no prior coronary artery disease undergoing stress myocardial perfusion single photon emission computed tomography. 2003 Jun 17. *Circulation,* 107(23):2900–2907.

# chapter 14

# Electrocardiographic Interpretation

DONALD A. UNDERWOOD

## CODING SHEET

### General Features

1. Normal ECG
2. Borderline ECG or normal variant (specify in other section)
3. Incorrect electrode placement

### P Wave Abnormalities

4. Right atrial abnormality
5. Left atrial abnormality
6. Nonspecific atrial abnormality
7. Sinoventricular condition with absent P wave

### Atrial Rhythms

8. Normal sinus rhythm (without other abnormalities of rhythm or AV conduction)
9. Sinus rhythm (in presence of abnormality of rhythm or AV conduction)
10. Sinus arrhythmia
11. Sinus bradycardia
12. Sinus tachycardia
13. Sinus pause or arrest
14. SA exit block
15. Ectopic atrial or junctional rhythm
16. Wandering atrial pacemaker
17. Atrial premature beats, normally conducted
18. Atrial premature beats, nonconducted
19. Atrial premature beats with aberrant intraventricular conduction
20. Atrial tachycardia (regular, sustained, 1:1 conduction)
21. Atrial tachycardia, repetitive (short paroxysms)
22. Atrial tachycardia, multifocal (chaotic atrial tachycardia)
23. Atrial tachycardia with AV block
24. Atrial flutter
25. Atrial fibrillation
26. Retrograde atrial activation
27. Supraventricular tachycardia, unspecified

## AV Junctional Rhythms

28. AV junctional premature beats
29. AV junctional escape beats or escape rhythm
30. AV junctional rhythm, accelerated rhythm (nonparoxysmal junctional tachycardia)
31. AV junctional tachycardia

## Ventricular Rhythms

32. Ventricular premature beat(s), uniform, fixed coupled
33. Ventricular premature beats, R on T phenomenon
34. Premature ventricular contractions, in pairs
35. Ventricular parasystole
36. Ventricular tachycardia
37. Accelerated idioventricular rhythm
38. Ventricular escape beats or rhythm
39. Ventricular fibrillation

## AV Conduction Abnormalities

(Also see items 48–53)

40. AV block, 1°
41. AV block, 2°—Mobitz type I (Wenkenbach)
42. AV block, 2°—Mobitz type II
43. AV block, 2:1, 3:1, 4:1
44. AV block, complete
45. AV block, varying
46. Short PR interval (with sinus rhythm and normal QRS duration)
47. Pre-excitation (Wolff-Parkinson-White) syndrome(s)

## Atrial Ventricular Interactions in Arrhythmias

(Also see items 40–47)

48. Fusion beats
49. Reciprocal (echo) beats
50. Ventricular capture beats
51. AV dissociation (without complete AV block)
52. Isorhythmic AV dissociation
53. Ventriculophasic sinus arrhythmia

## Abnormalities of QRS Voltage or Axis

54. Low voltage, limb leads only
55. Low voltage, limb and precordial leads
56. Left axis deviation ($>.30°$)
57. Right axis deviation ($>.+100°$)
58. Electrical alternans

## Ventricular Hypertrophy

59. Left ventricular hypertrophy by voltage only both voltage and ST-T segment
60. Left ventricular hypertrophy by changes
61. Right ventricular hypertrophy
62. Combined ventricular hypertrophy

## Intraventricular Conduction Disturbances

63. RBBB, incomplete
64. RBBB, complete
65. Left anterior fascicular block
66. Left posterior fascicular block
67. LBBB, complete with ST-T waves suggestive of acute myocardial injury or infarction
68. LBBB, complete
69. Intraventricular conduction disturbance, nonspecific type
70. Aberrant intraventricular conduction with supraventricular arrhythmia (specify rhythm)

## Transmural Myocardial Infarction

(Also see items 88–89)

|  | Age Recent or Probably Acute | Age Indeterminate or Probably Old |
|---|---|---|
| Anterolateral | 71. | 72. |
| Anterior | 73. | 74. |
| Anteroseptal | 75. | 76. |
| Lateral or high lateral | 77. | 78. |
| Inferior (diaphragmatic) | 79. | 80. |
| Posterior | 81. | 82. |

83. Probable ventricular aneurysm

## ST, T, U Wave Changes

84. Subendocardial or subepicardial nontransmural infarction
85. Normal variant, early repolarization
86. Normal variant, juvenile T wave
87. Nonspecific ST- and/or T-wave changes
88. ST- and/or T-wave changes suggesting myocardial ischemia
89. ST- and/or T-wave changes suggesting myocardial injury
90. ST- and/or T-wave changes suggesting acute pericarditis
91. ST-T segment changes secondary to intraventricular conduction distribution or hypertrophy
92. Post extrasystolic T waves
93. Isolated J-point depression
94. Peaked T waves
95. Prolonged QT interval
96. Prominent U waves

## Suggested Probable Clinical Disorder

97. Digitalis effect
98. Digitalis toxicity
99. Quinidine effect or toxicity
100. Hyperkalemia
101. Hypokalemia
102. Hypercalcemia
103. Hypocalcemia
104. Atrial septal defect, secundum

105. Atrial septal defect, primum
106. Dextrocardial, mirror image
107. Mitral valve disease
108. Chronic lung disease
109. Acute cor pulmonale including pulmonary embolus
110. Pericardial effusion
111. Acute pericarditis
112. Hypertrophic obstructive cardiomyopathy (IHSS)
113. Coronary artery disease
114. CNS disorder
115. Myxedema
116. Hypothermia
117. Sick sinus syndrome
118. Cardiac transplant

**ECG** INTERPRETATION AND CODING

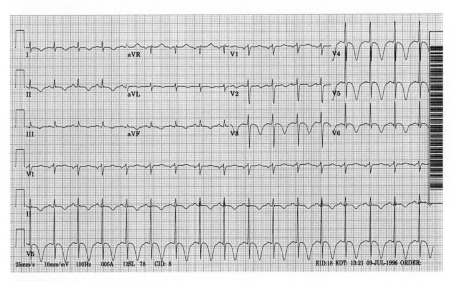

**FIGURE 14–1**

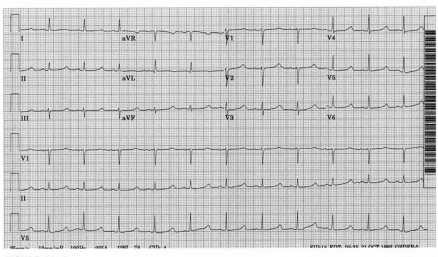

**FIGURE 14–2**

**FIGURE 14–3**

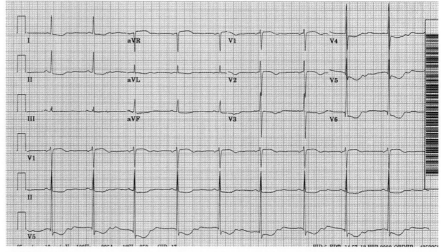

**FIGURE 14–4**

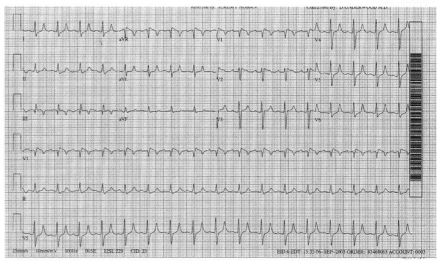

**FIGURE 14–5**

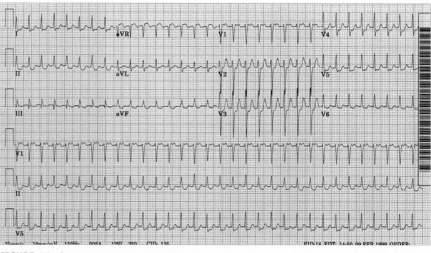

**FIGURE 14–6**

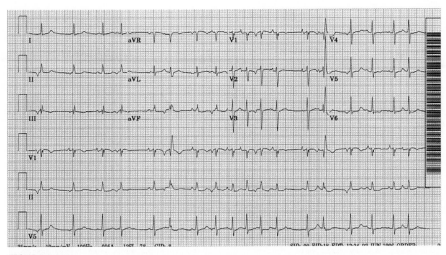

**FIGURE 14–7**

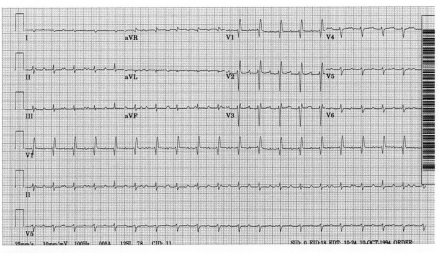

**FIGURE 14–8**

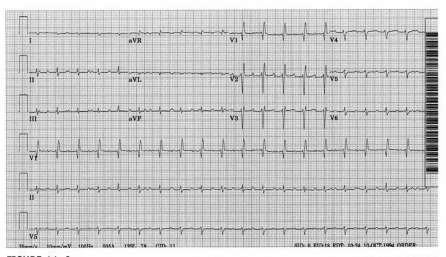

**FIGURE 14–9**

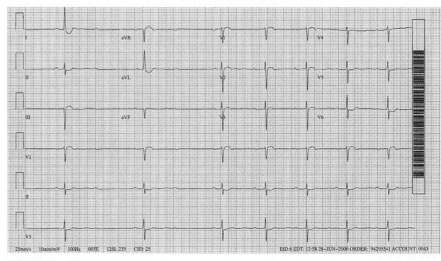

**FIGURE 14–10**

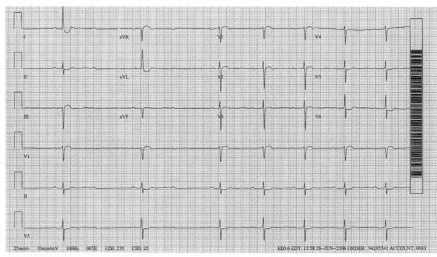

**FIGURE 14–11**

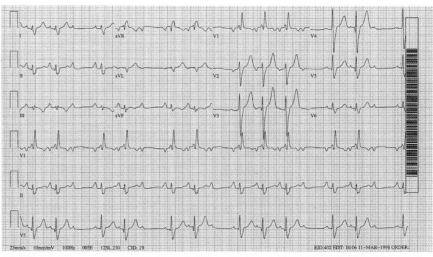

**FIGURE 14–12**

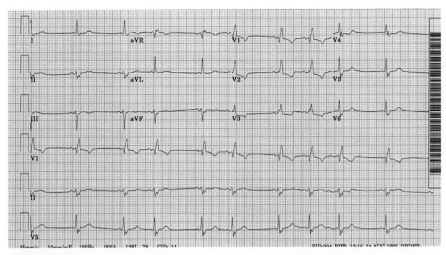

**FIGURE 14–13**

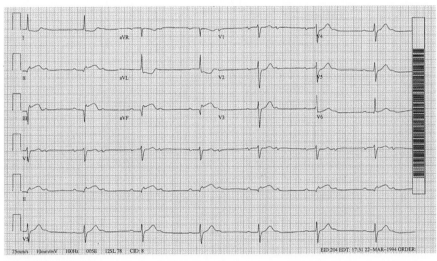

**FIGURE 14–14**

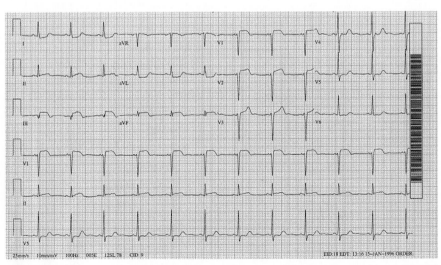

**FIGURE 14–15**

NOTES

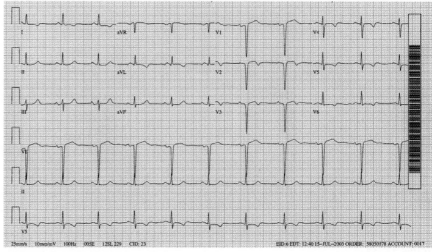

**FIGURE 14–16**

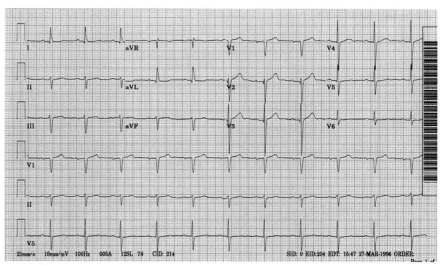

**FIGURE 14–17**

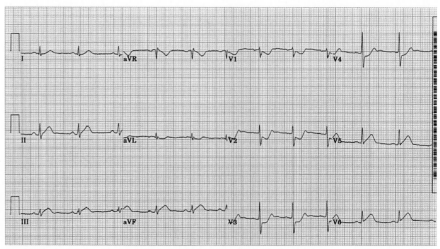

**FIGURE 14–18**

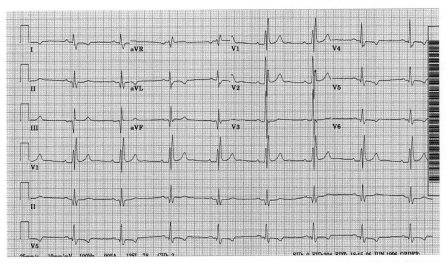

**FIGURE 14–19**

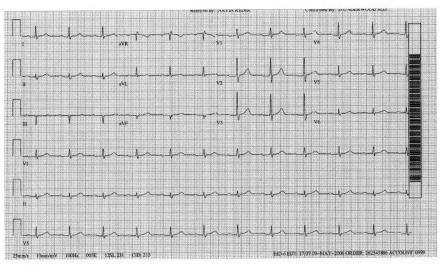

**FIGURE 14–20**

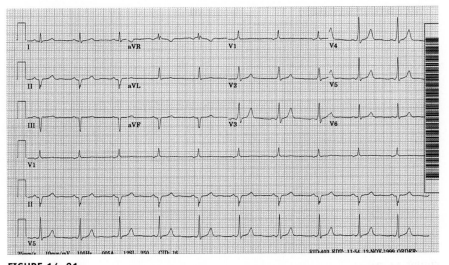

**FIGURE 14–21**

NOTES

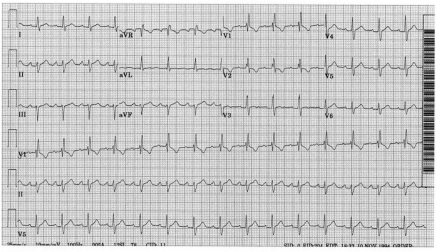

**FIGURE 14–22**

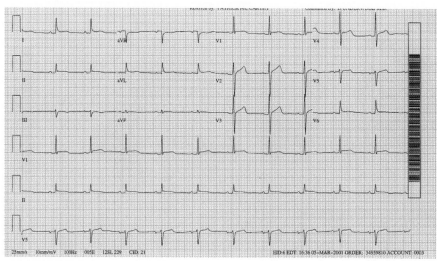

**FIGURE 14–23**

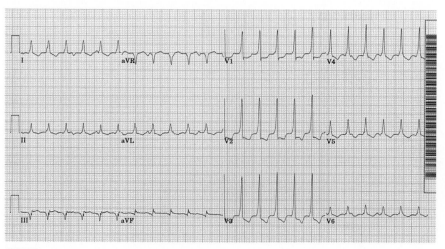

**FIGURE 14–24**

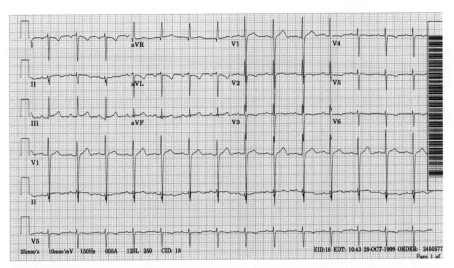

**FIGURE 14–25**

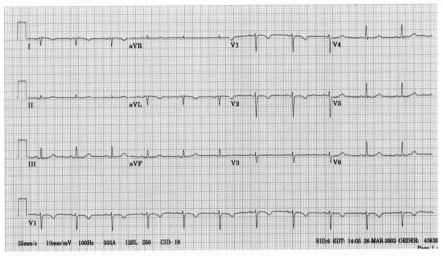

**FIGURE 14–26**

1. FIGURE 14–1: On this electrocardiogram, there is a sinus tachycardia. The voltage is low and in the $V_1$ and II rhythm strips, electrical alternans can be seen. This is an ECG from a patient with cardiac tamponade. Electrocardiographic coding is 12, 58, and 110.

2. FIGURE 14–2: This electrocardiogram shows a sinus tachycardia. There is generalized T-wave inversion. The T waves are symmetric, deep, and have a long QT interval. This is an electrocardiogram from a patient with a major CNS event such as a subarachnoid or intraventricular hemorrhage. Electrocardiographic coding would be 12, 95, and 114.

3. FIGURE 14–3: This electrocardiogram shows a sinus rhythm. There is prolongation of the QT interval. The T wave has a fairly normal duration and contour, however. This is an example of hypocalcemia. (Type III congenital long QT syndrome also has this appearance.) Electrocardiographic coding would be 8, 95, and 103.

4. FIGURE 14–4: On this electrocardiogram, there is a sinus rhythm. It is sinus bradycardia. There is a prolongation of the QT interval. In this case, there is ST-segment depression, T-wave flattening, and TU fusion with prominent U waves in the lateral precordial leads. This should suggest hypokalemia. Another possibility is digitalis plus an antiarrhythmic drug's effects (such as quinidine or procainamide). Electrocardiographic coding would be 11, 96, and 101.

5. FIGURE 14–5: This patient has a sinus tachycardia. There is symmetry of the T waves and there is a degree of QT prolongation. This is an example of a mixed electrolyte abnormality, hyperkalemia, and hypocalcemia. Values at the time were potassium of 7.2 and calcium of 8.0. This would be coded 12, 94, 95, 100, and 103.

6. FIGURE 14–6: On this electrocardiogram, there is a narrow complex tachycardia. The complexes are regular. In lead $V_1$, there is an atrial wave that has a short RP, long PR relationship. This is an example of supraventricular tachycardia or AV nodal reentrant tachycardia (AVNRT). If the atrial wave seen in $V_1$ extends 70 or 80 milliseconds out into the ST segment, then this type of tracing could be an example of AV reentrant tachycardia (AVRT), which usually involves a larger reentrant loop and a bypass tract. Electrocardiographic coding is 27.

7. FIGURE 14–7: Here there is a narrow complex tachycardia. It is chaotically irregular and there are multiple P-wave vectors. This is not atrial fibrillation, which also is chaotic, but instead is multifocal atrial tachycardia. This patient also shows aberrancy in the sixth and fourteenth beats. Electrocardiographic interpretation is 22, 87, 70, and 108.

8. FIGURE 14–8: This patient has a regular rhythm but the baseline as seen in lead $V_1$ is chaotic. It is an example of atrial fibrillation with a regular ventricular response. This is actually an accelerated junctional rhythm most likely caused by digitalis excess. In lead $V_6$ there is ST-segment sagging that is smooth and associated with QT interval shortening. This suggests digitalis "effect." Digitalis effect is seen in the repolarization changes with ST-segment scooping. Digitalis "excess" usually is suggested by arrhythmias and, in this case, the accelerated junctional rhythm. The coding would be 25, 30, 97, and 98.

9. FIGURE 14–9: This patient shows an rSR′ pattern in lead $V_1$ that might suggest a volume overload RVH. That is supported in part by the right axis deviation. However, in looking at the rhythm strip in lead II, there is a basic sinus rhythm with a first-degree AV block and, in addition, there is a second atrial rhythm that is dissociated from the basic PQRS sequence. This is accessory atrial activity related to cardiac transplantation. This would be coded 9, 40, 57, 63, and 118.

10. FIGURE 14–10: On this electrocardiogram, there is a regular atrial activity but the P waves are inverted in the inferior leads, suggesting an ectopic atrial tachycardia. This conducts with group beating and gradual PR prolongation. This is an example of atrial tachycardia with Mobitz type I AV block. This would be coded 23 and 41.

11. FIGURE 14–11: This electrocardiogram shows a sinus rhythm. There is a first-degree AV block and intermittent 2:1 block. In addition, there is ST-segment depression that is scooping in quality in the lateral leads. This is an example of digitalis excess with intermittent second-degree AV block and digitalis effect. It would be coded 11, 41 or 42, 97, and 98.

12. FIGURE 14–12: This patient has a right bundle branch block and left axis deviation. He also has pauses. In this case, the P waves are regular and the PR intervals do not change. This is an example of Mobitz type II second-degree AV block. The P-wave vectors are prominent in both leads II and $V_1$, suggesting left atrial enlargement. This would be coded 8, 42, 5, 56, and 64.

13. FIGURE 14–13: This patient has a right bundle branch block. There is also left axis deviation, which probably is enough to qualify as an anterior hemiblock. There are occasional pauses. In this case, the pauses are preceded by P waves, which are within the preceding T waves, and so this is an example of blocked PACs and not an example of more advanced AV block associated with bifascicular block. This would be coded 11, 18, 64, 56, and 65.

**14.** FIGURE 14–14: This patient shows a sinus rhythm with a 2:1 AV block. This can either be a Mobitz type I or Mobitz type II AV block. It is impossible to tell which. This also shows ST-segment elevation with Q waves in the inferior leads with reciprocal changes in leads I and aVL, and is an example of an acute inferior infarction with 2:1 AV block. This would be coded 8, 43, and 79.

**15.** FIGURE 14–15: This patient shows a sinus rhythm. There is ST elevation in the inferior leads, especially leads III and aVF. There are reciprocal depressions in leads I and aVL. In leads $V_1$ and $V_2$, there is also ST elevation. This is an acute inferior infarction plus acute right ventricular infarct. This would be coded 8 and 79. At least on this code sheet, the ability to call right ventricular infarction would not be available to you.

**16.** FIGURE 14–16: This electrocardiogram has a sinus rhythm. There are lateral T-wave changes that are not specific, and there are QS waves in leads $V_1$ through $V_3$. This is an anteroseptal infarction of uncertain age. It would be coded 8, 76, and 87.

**17.** FIGURE 14–17: Here, there is a normal sinus rhythm and marked left axis deviation. There are small Q waves in leads I and aVL with a slight activation delay in aVL. This is anterior hemiblock. Anterior hemiblock produces small Q waves in the right precordial leads. The QRS pattern seen in $V_2$ often is very suggestive of anteroseptal infarction, but the specificity is much less in the presence of anterior fasicular block. This would be coded 8 and 65.

**18.** FIGURE 14–18: In this patient, there are symmetric, prominent T waves that are upright. These are seen in the inferolateral leads and are associated with ST depression in leads $V_1$, $V_2$, and $V_3$. There are no Q waves so this is not an acute infarct, but it is an acute current of injury. The rhythm is sinus. Electrocardiographic coding would be 8 and 89.

**19.** FIGURE 14–19: On this electrocardiogram, there is a sinus rhythm. It is slow so sinus bradycardia. There are significant inferior Q waves and also Q waves in leads $V_5$ and $V_6$. There is also a prominent R-wave vector in lead $V_1$, and the T waves are upright despite the presence of a right bundle branch block. Usually with a right bundle branch block, ST-segment and T-wave inversion is expected. In this case, the upright T wave is an example of a "primary" T wave. A prominent initial vector and upright T wave in $V_1$, associated with inferior and lateral Q waves, are interpreted as an inferoposterior and lateral infarct. Electrocardiographic coding is 11, 80, 82, 78, and 64.

**20.** FIGURE 14–20: This electrocardiogram has a sinus rhythm. There is a prominent initial vector in lead $V_1$ that is greater than the S wave. T wave is upright. This is compatible with posterior infarct. That is supported by the presence of pathologic Q waves in leads III and aVF. Electrocardiographic coding would be 8, 80, and 82.

**21.** FIGURE 14–21: This electrocardiogram shows a sinus rhythm. There are inferior Q waves and a prominent R vector in leads $V_1$ and $V_2$. This might suggest inferoposterior infarction, but in leads $V_3$ and $V_4$, especially, there is a short PR interval and a delta wave suggesting that this is pre-excitation or Wolff-Parkinson-White syndrome. Electrocardiographic coding would be 8 and 47.

**22.** FIGURE 14–22: This patient has a sinus rhythm. Lead II does suggest left atrial enlargement with a P wave that is broad and notched. There is an rSR' pattern in lead $V_1$ with T-wave inversion and R' greater than S. This type of pattern is commonly seen in volume-overload-type right ventricular hypertrophy (RVH). Volume-overload RVH and left axis should suggest osteum primum ASD. Usually an ASD will not affect P waves greatly, at least in the early phases of the process. Osteum primum ASDs, however, very often have mitral valve abnormalities, which was the case in this patient, who had a cleft mitral valve and notable mitral insufficiency plus left atrial enlargement. Electrocardiographic coding would be 8, 5, 63, 61, 56, and 105.

NOTES

23. FIGURE 14–23: This electrocardiogram shows a sinus rhythm. There was a very prominent vector in lead $V_1$ associated with upright T waves. This drops down to a more typical appearance in lead $V_2$. This is not an example of posterior infarction but instead is an example of switched leads, $V_1$ and $V_5$ having been transposed. There also is ST-segment elevation throughout and perhaps some PR-segment elevation in aVR. This suggests acute pericarditis. Electrocardiographic coding would be 8, 3, and 90.

24. FIGURE 14–24: This patient has a wide complex tachycardia. There is AV dissociation and there is anterior, positive concordance in the chest leads. This is ventricular tachycardia. Electrocardiographic coding would be 9, 51, and 36.

25. FIGURE 14–25: This patient has marked right axis deviation and loss of voltage across the precordium. The P waves are inverted in leads I and aVL. Inverted P waves in I and aVL (if it is not an ectopic atrial rhythm) are caused by either dextrocardia or switched arm wires. Loss of voltage across the precordium suggests that this is dextrocardia. Electrocardiographic coding would be 8 and 106.

26. FIGURE 14–26: This patient has a sinus rhythm and right axis deviation. The vectors in leads I and aVL are incompatible with those seen in the other lateral leads, $V_5$ and $V_6$. The discrepancies are explained by the inverted P waves in leads I and aVL, which suggest switched arm wires. This is a normal ECG with a technical error. This would be coded 8 and 3.

# Index

Page numbers followed by f refer to figures; those followed by t refer to tables